MAKHUL

PEYRONIE'S DISEASE

CURRENT CLINICAL UROLOGY

Eric A. Klein, MD, SERIES EDITOR

PEYRONIE'S DISEASE

A GUIDE TO CLINICAL MANAGEMENT

Edited by

LAURENCE A. LEVINE, MD, FACS

Rush University Medical Center, Chicago, IL

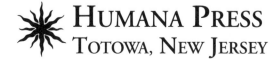

HUMANA PRESS
TOTOWA, NEW JERSEY

Due diligence has been taken by the publishers, editors, and authors of this book to assure the accuracy of the information published and to describe generally accepted practices. The contributors herein have carefully checked to ensure that the drug selections and dosages set forth in this text are accurate and in accord with the standards accepted at the time of publication. Notwithstanding, as new research, changes in government regulations, and knowledge from clinical experience relating to drug therapy and drug reactions constantly occurs, the reader is advised to check the product information provided by the manufacturer of each drug for any change in dosages or for additional warnings and contraindications. This is of utmost importance when the recommended drug herein is a new or infrequently used drug. It is the responsibility of the treating physician to determine dosages and treatment strategies for individual patients. Further it is the responsibility of the health care provider to ascertain the Food and Drug Administration status of each drug or device used in their clinical practice. The publisher, editors, and authors are not responsible for errors or omissions or for any consequences from the application of the information presented in this book and make no warranty, express or implied, with respect to the contents in this publication.

This publication is printed on acid-free paper. ∞
ANSI Z39.48-1984 (American Standards Institute) Permanence of Paper for Printed Library Materials.

Production Editor: Robin B. Weisberg

Cover design by Patricia F. Cleary

For additional copies, pricing for bulk purchases, and/or information about other Humana titles, contact Humana at the above address or at any of the following numbers: Tel.: 973-256-1699; Fax: 973-256-8341; E-mail: orders@humanapr.com; or visit our Website: www.humanapress.com

Photocopy Authorization Policy:

Photocopy Authorization Policy: Authorization to photocopy items for internal or personal use, or the internal or personal use of specific clients is granted by Humana Press, provided that the base fee of US $30.00 per copy is paid directly to the Copyright Clearance Center (CCC), 222 Rosewood Dr., Danvers MA 01923. For those organizations that have been granted a photocopy license from the CCC, a separate system of payment has been arranged and is acceptable to the Humana Press. The fee code for users of the Transactional Reporting Service is 1-58829-614-8/07 $30.00.

Printed in the United States of America. 10 9 8 7 6 5 4 3 2 1

eISBN 1-59745-161-4

Library of Congress Cataloging-in-Publication Data

Peyronie's disease : a guide to clinical management / edited by Laurence A. Levine.
    p. ; cm. -- (Current clinical urology)
  Includes index.
  ISBN 1-58829-614-8 (alk. paper)
  1. Penile induration. I. Levine, Laurence A. II. Series.
  [DNLM: 1. Penile Induration--therapy. WJ 790 P516 2007]
  RC896.P49 2007
  616.6'92206--dc22

                                        2006025987

Dedication

I dedicate this book to Linda, Jenna, Sasha, and Reilly Levine, whose love and support contributed to the success of this project.

Preface

I am delighted to present *Peyronie's Disease: A Guide to Clinical Management* as the first text dedicated to Peyronie's disease. As physicians, we are aware of the many frustrations associated with treating the man who presents with this difficult disorder. Much of the frustration is caused by the absence of a reliable and effective nonsurgical therapy and the fear that surgery may result in severe side effects, including impotence. In addition, the published literature has not been able to guide the treating physician clearly because most of the reported studies have been noncontrolled, have had a limited number of patients, and appear to be absent of objective measures of improvement. It is hoped that, as a result of attempts to establish a more internationally recognized and accepted evaluation protocol as well as a methodology for reporting on the outcomes from clinical trials, we will identify the most reasonable nonsurgical options. One thing that all treating physicians should remember in their consultations with men with Peyronie's disease is that it can be both physically and psychologically devastating.

Recent research in wound-healing disorders has provided models for study of Peyronie's disease; this has increased our understanding of its pathophysiology. A variety of techniques to perform this research has emerged, including tissue analysis, cell culture of fibroblasts derived from Peyronie's plaques, and animal models that attempt to mimic the in vivo process of tunica albuginea fibrosis while also providing an opportunity for manipulation with novel therapeutic options. All of these techniques have their limitations in terms of re-creating the true situation of the patient with Peyronie's disease, but they do provide an opportunity to study and gain further insights into this distressing disorder. The published research over the past decade has been exciting, elegant, and state of the art.

Peyronie's Disease: A Guide to Clinical Management places us precisely at the right time as major developments are occurring in the research of fibrotic disorders. I hope we will see the fruit of this research in the near future: effective and safe treatment. For those who suffer with Peyronie's disease in the meantime, this book reviews the current nonsurgical and surgical therapeutic options presented by recognized international authorities.

There are also many misconceptions about Peyronie's disease that need to be rectified so that the practicing physician will be able to diagnose, treat, or refer the patient with Peyronie's disease more appropriately. Too many men with Peyronie's disease are told that this is a rare disorder that simply will resolve with time. We now know from several recently conducted demographic studies that Peyronie's disease is not a rare disorder; in fact, its prevalence exceeds many cancers. In addition, spontaneous resolution is not the norm; recent studies of its natural history suggested that fewer than 10% of men can expect spontaneous resolution of penile deformity. Clearly, as a result of the sexual revolution that has occurred over the past several decades, as well as improved treatment options for erectile function, many more men with Peyronie's disease will likely present for evaluation and treatment.

Peyronie's disease is thought to be a disorder of middle-aged men and tends to occur most commonly in men in their 50s, but 10% of men with Peyronie's disease in two recent series were under the age of 40 years. Erectile dysfunction has been reported to occur in up to 90% of men with Peyronie's disease. It was previously thought that diminished rigidity was a result of the deformity. It is now recognized that men with Peyronie's disease often have erectile dysfunction because of the same factors occurring in men without Peyronie's disease, including vasculogenic and psychogenic components.

A wide variety of nonsurgical treatments has been used since the time of de la Peyronie (~1740), with limited benefit. As a result, many physicians do not offer nonsurgical therapy, assuming the disease will stabilize with time and can then be surgically corrected if necessary. The chapters reviewing nonsurgical therapies make it clear that it is reasonable to offer some nonsurgical treatments as early as possible after presentation. This is because the tissue changes within the tunica albuginea are likely to be most active and may be best manipulated at that time. Therefore, the misconception that intralesional therapy, in particular, should not be offered until the disease is stable is false, and in the appropriate patient, intralesional therapy may be offered in combination with other modalities (e.g., oral agents, topical drugs, or vacuum/stretching devices).

What should be clearly recognized by the treating physician is that, at this time, there is no nonsurgical cure for Peyronie's disease. We can tell our patients that we do not fully understand this disease, but we can also help them understand that it is a wound-healing disorder that results in a scar that causes penile deformity, pain, and frequently sexual dysfunction. Although there is no cure, there are treatments that may result in physical improvement or stabilize the scarring process. It is my opinion that there are medical treatments that make scientific sense and offer reasonable hope of making the patient more functional, which is better than offering no hope and no therapy. Unfortunately, a nihilistic, hands-off attitude prevails among many physicians, which leaves patients seeking answers elsewhere, like the Internet, which encourages them to use many empirical, completely untested, alternative remedies.

For those with more advanced disease, there are surgical options to correct the deformity in an effort to make the patients functional again. I strongly believe that a detailed discussion with the patient is needed before instituting any invasive therapy. The goal is to establish reasonable expectations for outcome as an informed patient is more apt to be satisfied with the treatment results once he understands the limits of the treatment. Specifically, no current therapy, including surgery, will reliably return the penis affected by Peyronie's disease back to its pre-Peyronie's state.

An exciting compliment to this textbook is the DVD surgical library. Many of the world's experts in surgery of Peyronie's disease have contributed written chapters that are further detailed in the DVD library. This will provide an opportunity to review how the expert performs an operation, with tips on patient selection and the surgical approach for the procedure.

The hope of the contributing authors is that *Peyronie's Disease: A Guide to Clinical Management* will provide an up-to-date summary of the etiology, natural history, and pathophysiology of this disease as well as present a review of the available medical and surgical treatment options.

Acknowledgments

I would like to congratulate all of the authors for an outstanding effort in making this not only the first, but also clearly a comprehensive and useful textbook on Peyronie's disease. I would also like to acknowledge Marah Hehemann for her extraordinary administrative skills and editorial assistance.

Laurence A. Levine, MD, FACS

Contents

Contributors

EMRE AKKUS, MD • *Department of Urology, Cerrahpasa School of Medicine, Istanbul University, Istanbul, Turkey*

FRANCESCO ATTISANI, MD • *Department of Surgery/Urology, TorVergata University, Rome, Italy*

ANTHONY J. BELLA, MD, FRCSC • *Department of Surgery, Division of Urology, St. Joseph's Health Center, The University of Western Ontario, London, Ontario, Canada*

GERALD B. BROCK, MD, FRCSC • *Division of Urology, Department of Surgery, St. Joseph's Health Center, The University of Western Ontario, London, Ontario, Canada*

CULLEY C. CARSON, III, MD • *Division of Urology, Department of Surgery, University of North Carolina, NC*

ROBERT C. DEAN, MD • *Department of Urology, University of California–San Francisco Medical Center, San Francisco, CA*

SAVINO M. DI STASI, MD, PhD • *Department of Urology, Tor Vergata University, Rome, Italy*

PAULO H. EGYDIO, MD, PhD • *Department of Urology–Hospital das Clinicas, University of São Paulo Medical School, São Paulo–Brazil*

PAUL F. ENGELHARDT, MD • *Department of Urology, Landesklinikum Thermenregion Baden, Austria*

MARTIN GELBARD, MD • *Department of Urology, UCLA School of Medicine, Los Angeles, CA*

ANTONELLA GIANNANTONI, MD, PhD • *Department of Urology, University of Perugia, Perugia, Italy*

NESTOR F. GONZALEZ-CADAVID, PhD • *Department of Urology, David Geffen School of Medicine at UCLA, and LABioMed at Harbor–UCLA Medical Center, Torrance, CA*

TULIO GRAZIOTTIN, MD • *Department of Urology, Santa Casa Hospital and Fundacao Faculdade Federal Ciencias Medicas, Porto Alegre, Brazil*

JASON M. GREENFIELD, MD • *Department of Urology, Rush University Medical Center, Chicago, IL*

DIMITRIOS G. HATZICHRISTOU, MD, PhD • *2nd Department of Urology, Papageorgiou' General Hospital, Center for Sexual and Reproductive Health, Aristotle University of Thessaloniki, Thessaloniki, Greece*

KONSTANTINOS HATZIMOURATIDIS, MD, PhD • *2nd Department of Urology, Papageorgiou' General Hospital, and Center for Sexual and Reproductive Health, Aristotle University of Thessaloniki, Thessaloniki, Greece*

EKKEHARD W. HAUCK, MD • *Department of Urology and Pediatric Urology, Justus Liebig University, Giessen, Germany*

WAYNE J.G. HELLSTROM, MD, FACS • *Department of Urology, Tulane University School of Medicine, New Orleans, LA*

EMMANUELE A. JANNINI, MD • *Department of Experimental Medicine, University of L'Aquila, L'Aquila, Italy*

ATES KADIOGLU, MD • *Departments of Andrology and Urology, Istanbul Faculty of Medicine, University of Istanbul, Turkey*

MUAMMER KENDIRCI, MD • *Department of Urology, Tulane University School of Medicine, New Orleans, LA*

L. DEAN KNOLL, MD • *Center for Urological Treatment and Research, Nashville, TN*

LAURENCE A. LEVINE, MD, FACS • *Department of Urology, Rush University Medical Center, Chicago, IL*

TOM F. LUE, MD • *Department of Urology, University of California–San Francisco Medical Center, San Francisco, CA*

VINCENZO MIRONE, MD • *Urology Department, University "Federico II," Naples, Italy*

JOHN P. MULHALL, MD • *Departments of Urology, Weill Medical College of Cornell University, New York Presbyterian Hospital, and Memorial Sloan Kettering Cancer Center, New York, NY*

JACOB RAJFER, MD • *Department of Urology, David Geffen School of Medicine at UCLA, Los Angeles, CA*

DAVID J. RALPH, MS, FRCS(Urol) • *Institute of Urology, London, UK*

CLAUS R. RIEDL, MD • *Department of Urology, Landesklinikum Thermenregion Baden, Austria*

ONER SANLI, MD • *Departments of Andrology and Urology, Istanbul Faculty of Medicine, University of Istanbul, Istanbul, Turkey*

ROBERT L. STEPHEN, MD • *(Deceased) Physion Laboratory, Medolla, Italy*

LUIGI STORTI, MD • *Department of Surgery/Urology, TorVergata University, Rome, Italy*

CLAUDIO TELOKEN, MD, PhD • *Department of Urology, Fundacao Faculdade Federal Ciencias Medicas and Santa Casa Hospital, Porto Alegre, Brazil*

PATRICK E. TELOKEN, MS • *Department of Urology, Fundacao Faculdade Federal Ciencias Medicas and Santa Casa Hospital, Porto Alegre, Brazil*

LANDON TROST, MD • *Department of Urology, Tulane University School of Medicine, New Orleans, LA*

GIUSEPPE VESPASIANI, MD • *Department of Surgery and Urology, Tor Vergata University, Rome, Italy*

WOLFGANG WEIDNER, MD • *Department of Urology and Pediatric Urology, Justus Liebig University, Giessen, Germany*

STEVEN K. WILSON, MD • *Department of Urology, University of Arkansas, Little Rock, AK*

DANIEL YACHIA, MD • *Department of Urology, Hillel Yaffe Medical Centre, Hadera, Israel*

Companion DVD

The companion DVD to this volume contains video segments in support of the book, organized in sections corresponding to the book. The DVD can be played in any DVD player attached to an NTSC television set. The DVD may also be viewed using any computer with a DVD drive and DVD-compatible playback software such as Apple DVD Player, Windows Media Player 8 or higher (Win XP), PowerDVD, or WinDVD.

1

Historical Review of Peyronie's Disease

de la Peyronie to Devine

Emre Akkus, MD

SUMMARY

François Gigot de la Peyronie, the famous French general surgeon, is very well known among urologists regarding the disease called by his name: Peyronie's disease. Because his father was also a surgeon, he followed his family tradition and became a doctor. He had gained most of his surgical skills during the civil wars in the 16th century. His academic career in France was outstanding. He was one of the two founders of the Royal Academy of Surgery. He was also the First Surgeon to King Louis XV. Even though he was a great surgeon and university professor, his legacy consists only of numerous case reports and not even one comprehensive textbook. However, his paper on induratio penis plastica attached his name and credit to the disease, and since then it has been called Peyronie's disease. This chapter consists of the history of the disease, starting with early assumptions of its pathophysiology and treatment up to the current knowledge, which still has dilemmas.

Key Words: History; penile curvature; Peyronie's disease.

The famous French surgeon François Gigot de la Peyronie is known as the man whose name has been credited with the discovery of Peyronie's disease (Fig. 1). Despite the fact that he was not the first to describe the condition, his name has become synonymous with this rather enigmatic, although not uncommon, disease. According to the French language, his name (actually last name) should be written as la Peyronie; hence, he signed his name as la Peyronie. But in Anglo-Saxon literature, by mistake or corruption, the name of the disease is called and remains Peyronie's disease. Today, Peyronie's disease is known as the accumulation of collagens at and onto the tunica albuginea of the penis, resulting in induration, nodule (plaque), penile curvature, painful erections, and erectile dysfunction.

LIFE OF DE LA PEYRONIE

La Peyronie was born in Montpellier in 1678 *(1)*. His father, Raymond, was a local barber surgeon. His mother, Elizabeth, was deeply religious; therefore, he received a

From: *Current Clinical Urology:*
Peyronie's Disease: A Guide to Clinical Management
Edited by: L. A. Levine © Humana Press Inc., Totowa, NJ

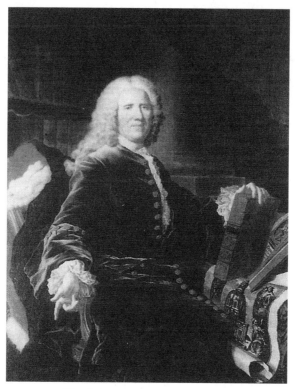

Fig. 1. François de la Peyronie.

strict Jesuit education. La Peyronie, which literally means "little stone" had followed his father's tradition of surgery and obtained his license at the city hospital in 1693. Then, he moved to Paris to advance his training with Georges Mareschal, who was the head surgeon of Charite Hospital and the "sun king." He developed and improved his surgical skills significantly under Georges Mareschal's mentorship and friendship. During that time, there was great animosity in Europe, particularly in France, among the barber surgeons, the surgeons, and the university-trained physicians.

When he returned to his hometown of Montpellier in 1700, he became the head surgeon at St. Eloi Hospital. He had continued to develop his surgical skills and engaged in teaching, which brought him the chair of the anatomy and surgery clinics at the university. In 1702, he was the commander of the medical corps in the military of Louis XIV. He had participated in the war against the peasants and guerrillas north of Montpellier; during the war, he had extended his talent and skills at abdominal-bowel surgery. He had evolved and developed the end-to-end anastomosis of enterostomy from the war and battlefield conditions *(2)*.

His reputation and good relationship with physicians and nonmedical academic departments helped him to build bridges among them, which resulted in the foundation of the Academy of the Sciences of Montpellier in 1706. In 1715, he returned to Paris for a more lucrative career. He became very famous, and he treated the kings of Poland and Prussia. He founded the Royal Academy of Surgery in 1731 with his former teacher Georges Marechal. He became the First Surgeon to Louis XV after the death of Georges Marechal. He had persuaded the king to acknowledge the tuition given by Ecole de Chirurgie *(3)*.

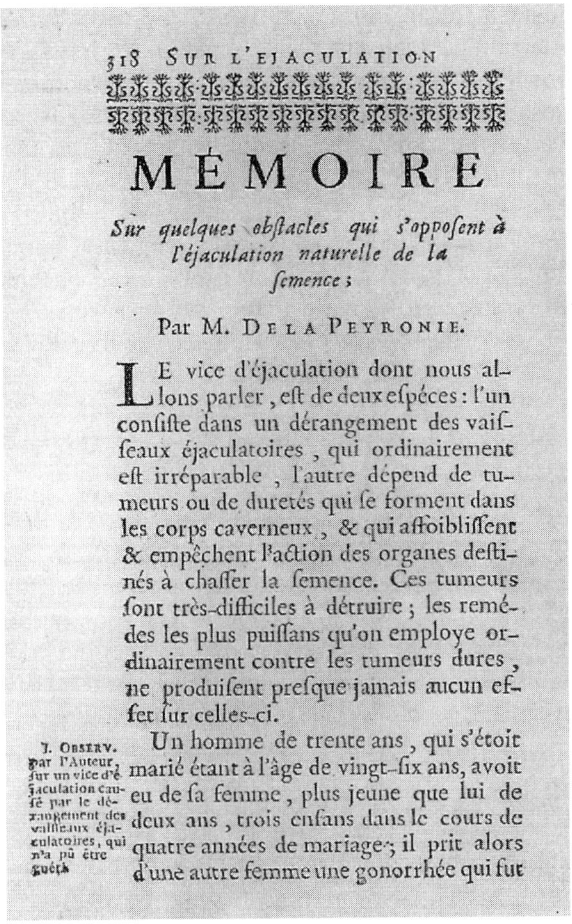

318 SUR L'EJACULATION

MÉMOIRE

Sur quelques obstacles qui s'opposent à l'éjaculation naturelle de la semence;

Par M. DE LA PEYRONIE.

LE vice d'éjaculation dont nous allons parler, est de deux espéces: l'un consiste dans un dérangement des vaisseaux éjaculatoires, qui ordinairement est irréparable, l'autre dépend de tumeurs ou de duretés qui se forment dans les corps caverneux, & qui affoiblissent & empêchent l'action des organes destinés à chasser la semence. Ces tumeurs sont très-difficiles à détruire; les remédes les plus puissans qu'on employe ordinairement contre les tumeurs dures, ne produisent presque jamais aucun effet sur celles-ci.

I. OBSERV. par l'Auteur, sur un vice d'éjaculation causé par le dérangement des vaisseaux éjaculatoires, qui n'a pû être guéri.

Un homme de trente ans, qui s'étoit marié étant à l'âge de vingt-six ans, avoit eu de sa femme, plus jeune que lui de deux ans, trois enfans dans le cours de quatre années de mariage; il prit alors d'une autre femme une gonorrhée qui fut

Fig. 2. Original paper of de la Peyronie.

This led to the liberation of the medical school of the university, and in 1743 surgeons in France finally were acknowledged as doctors.

François de la Peyronie died childless in Versailles in 1747, leaving behind a great library and immense estate to be used as scholarship. Even though he was a great surgeon and university professor, his legacy consists only of numerous case reports and not even one comprehensive textbook. However, his paper on induratio penis plastica (IPP) in the proceedings of the Royal Academy of Surgery *(4)* made his name labeled and credited with the disease and since then it is called as Peyronie's Disease.

LA PEYRONIE'S DISEASE

"Sur quelques obstacles qui s'opposent a l'ejaculation naturelle de la semence" is the original paper published in *Memoire de Academic Royale de Chir* in 1743 (Fig. 2). The English translation of the topic of his paper is "On Impaired Ejaculation. Dissertation on Some Obstacles to the Natural Ejaculation of the Semen." The description of IPP and his findings on those cases were as follows:

> The flexibility and elasticity of the ducts, the cells, and the fibers that form a part of the cavernous bodies, are another requirement for the ejaculation. The description of all

these muscles, and the mechanisms of their movements and action, belong to the animal economy, and are not the subject of this dissertation. We must only notice that these singular organs are subject to hard tumours which look like knots or ganglions, spreading sometimes in rosary beads from one end to another of these cavernous bodies. When it happens, the penis is not straight under erection, but it is full of knobs, which are bending and disfiguring it; if the erection is very hard, it is sometimes painful...I thought that this indurations could be venereal, or even, if they were not, could be well treated by mercury, a strong medicine in which I had more confidence than it deserved...His health which was somewhat impaired by the remedy was totally restored within 2 months; but the indurations of the penis remained as before, and even worse. I saw a great number of people who had some of these indurations in different parts of the cavernous bodies... If one of the indurations of the cavernous bodies is situated close to the middle of the right cavernous body, the penis instead of being straight will make a curvature to the right; if the induration is situated to the left, the curvature will be on the same side of the induration.

The bend is always on the side where the illness is; and this is probably the reason: the erection depends on the dilatation or on the swelling of the cavernous body cells. If they swell equally one of the two cavernous bodies does not dominate the other, they compete equally in the same action and the erection will be straight. But if an induration or a drying in one portion of the cavernous bodies prevent the dilatation of the cells of this portion, the cavernous body will be constricted, hard and dry in this portion; a ingression will take place, becoming the center of the curvature. This illness which is not rare among elderly men, particularly among those sexually very active, is sometimes also the result of the venereal disease. I saw a great number of persons, who in conjunction with syphilitic symptoms, had as well this kind of indurations.

La Peyronie had used mercurial rubs to treat the venereal disease, but these did not work for the penile indurations. Then, he suggested bathing in the holy waters of Barèges (spa therapy), which consequently worked and healed the indurations:

While the patient healed from his old injury, thanks to the waters, he took the shower over the induration, and observed that during a season of water treatment the induration decreased considerably. The first sign of success induced the patient to continue the same treatment. Repeated showers for one more season, completed the softening of this induration, the erections regained their old shape, and the semen its normal ejaculation.

However, the description of this unpleasant disease goes back to Theoderic of Bologna in the 13th century (5). Wilhelm from Salieto in 1476 (6), Gabriele Fallopio in 1561 (7), Andreas Vesal in 1543 (8), Arantius in 1579 (9), and Nicolaas Tulpius in 1641 (10) described similar symptoms. The first illustration of the penile curvature caused by to IPP on a cadaver was demonstrated by Dutch anatomist Fredrik Ruysch in 1691 (11). His article was actually on tubercules of the penis. These tubercules were hard, heavy, and stable during penile distension. In the United States, the disease was named Van Buren's disease in 1874 in the honor of one of its two investigators (12).

The etiology of la Peyronie's disease is still debatable and controversial. Assumptions or hypotheses go back to Emperor Heraclius, who had penile deformity and had been accused of having incestuous relations (13). In the 19th century French investigators' opinions and in 1942 Wesson's opinion were that the etiology of the disease was in a patient's sexual history (14). The theory of middle-aged people's prolonged ungratified sexual desires or violation of natural relations was thought to be the causative factor. This theory was concomitant to the partners' frigidity after the 40s because of menopause, which overlapped with the onset of la Peyronie's disease *(15)*. Forceful or vigorous penetration caused by annoying resistance of the partner was another theoretical opinion about the etiology *(12)*. Dorsal localization of the disease was related to the fact that this area was mostly subjected to mechanical strain during sexual intercourse *(16)*.

Like la Peyronie, other authors have also associated the disease with infections like gonorrhea and syphilis *(17,18)*. Relevance of Dupuytren's contracture was first reported in 1828 by Abernethy *(18)*. Dupuytren's contracture is a familial and genetic disorder known to be transmitted in an autosomal dominant pattern. That is why the theory of genetics was based in the etiology of Peyronie's disease. Vascular access in severe wartime wounds and injuries necessitated transfusion through the penis. Many of those men later developed Peyronie's disease *(19)*. Infections of corpora cavernosa and inflammation were also considered the cause of the disease, especially in young men *(20)*. Diabetes and gout were also considered to be involved in the etiology. There were also reports against this idea *(21)*. Vasculogenic effect and etiology were first reported by Weidoff in 1921 and were supportive of others that it happened to be the consequence of the atherosclerosis *(22)*.

However, since its first description little progress has been made in discovering the cause of this well-recognized disease, and the cause still remains obscure. Today, several hypotheses have been proposed to explain the etiology and pathophysiology of the fibrosis and plaque formation in la Peyronie's disease. These theories include vitamin E deficiency, microvascular traumas, genetics, autoimmune factors, excess production of fibrogenic cytokines, and cytogenetic aberrations. Devine et al. proposed trauma as the cause of the Peyronie's lesions *(23,24)*. Changes at the microscopic anatomy of the tunica albuginea caused by aging or trauma have also been shown to be relevant for the etiology of the disease *(25,26)*. Currently, the pathogenesis of la Peyronie's disease appears to be multifactorial, with the interplay of genetic predisposition, trauma, and tissue ischemia, and yet has not been fully elucidated.

The history of epidemiological data on la Peyronie's disease is also inconsistent. The first reported data were published by Polkey in 1928 and consisted of 550 cases *(27)*. In 1966, an Italian publication reported 3600 cases *(28)*. Ludvik and Wasserburger in 1968 reported a prevalence rate of 0.3–0.7% in a private clinic *(29)*. Lindsday et al.'s study in Minnesota revealed a 0.38% prevalence rate in 1991 *(30)*. Devine's result was 1% for those between 30 and 65 years of age *(31)*. The prevalence rate has been accepted to reach 7% in recent years.

The historical perspective of the treatment of la Peyronie's disease goes back to the treatment suggested by la Peyronie. Bathing in the holy waters of Barèges was the first suggested treatment *(4)*. Since then, substances such as mercury and mineral water, potassium iodide, bromides and hyperthermia, sulfur, copper sulfate, salicylates, estrogens, thiosinamin, acidification with disodium phosphate, arsenic, fibrinolysin, and milk have been suggested as oral or topical agents for la Peyronie's disease *(27)*. Of particular historical note is the early success of procarbazine (Natulan), a cytotoxic alkylating agent used in the treatment of Hodgkin's disease, which resulted with significant improvement of the accompanying Dupuytren's contracture *(32)*. However, later reports of azoospermia caused by the therapy led investigators to quit such therapy for la Peyronie's disease *(33)*. Vitamin E has been used as an antioxidant as a treatment modality since 1946 *(34)*. Response rates to vitamin E therapy were between 0 and 70% between 1952 and 1982. Devine and Horton reported resolution of plaques (20%) and penile curvate (33%) with vitamine E therapy (35). However, with additional follow-up subsequently they reported that, although 99% of the cases experienced a decrease in pain, 70% noted no objective improvement.

Potaba® (potassium paraaminobenzoate) was introduced in 1959 by Zarafonetis and Horax (36). Intralesional injections to the plaques had been tried since 1901, when Walsham and Spencer injected mercury and iodide (37). Intralesional steroids were first administered in 1954 by Teasley (38). Further reports were published by Bodner et al. in 1954 (39) concerning the use of intralesional cortisone and hydrocortisone. Winter and Khanna published their results on the use of mechanically aided injection of dexamethasone in 1975 (40). In 1980, Williams and Gren described the use of intralesional triamcinolone, a long-acting glucocorticoid with low solubility (41), which later was also shown to benefit Dupuytren's contracture and hypertrophic scars (42). Intralesional collagenase, parathyroid hormone, orgotein were also studied in the treatment of the disease (43). Recent intralesional treatments consist of verapamil and interferon as potential therapeutic alternatives.

The insertion of radium seeds into the Peyronie's plaques was reported to be successful by Kumer in 1922 (44). Later results demonstrated that it was useless and might have detrimental effects on the penis, and radium treatment was withdrawn.

Diathermy was used as local heat in 1926 by Corbus to treat the plaques. In 1960, the histamine iontophoresis technique was introduced with limited success (45). Ultraviolet light therapy was another trial in the treatment of the plaques in 1957. However, such therapy never gained popularity and had very limited success (46). In contrast, ultrasonographic treatment has gained some popularity with the addition of extracorporeal shock wave lithotripsy. This is probably with the encouragement of the first introduction by Heslop et al. in 1967 (47).

The history of surgical treatment goes back to the 19th century. The technique was simple excision of the plaques (48). In 1926, Young and Davis developed the procedure of freeing the plaque and suturing it to the undersurface of the penile skin (49). In 1950, Lowsley and Boyce added fat graft to the excised area of the plaque (50). Nesbit in 1965 described elliptical excisions of the tunica albuginea and a plication technique, which was then popularized and still is performed (51). This technique has been accepted as giving the best results and is the method of choice for most men (52). On the other hand, plaque excision was generally unsuccessful until a dermal graft replacement of the tunica albuginea was described by Bystrom et al. in 1972 (53). Finally, Devine and Horton reported that, despite satisfactory early results, longer term results were unsuccessful and disappointing (54). Therefore, after the 1990s Peyronie's plaque surgical excision currently has been replaced by incision and grafting methods (55).

CONCLUSION

Despite several theories for the etiology of la Peyronie's disease, it is still an enigma. We are probably getting closer to its real-life etiological factors with the advancement of diagnostic technology and understanding the basics of genetics and cell pathophysiology. Not only the etiology and pathophysiology but also the treatment modalities are still controversial and debatable. Today and the future are the reflection of history. Perhaps one or some of the theories and treatment alternatives may be modified and will be presented in the near future as the real etiology and treatment of the disease. Maybe someday in the near future we will again try the holy waters of Barèges in the treatment of the disease. What is real today is the real prevalence of the disease is higher than what we knew before, the treatment of the disease is still not specifically proven, and surgical treatment is not treatment of the disease but of the curvature or accompanying erectile dysfunction. With the warnings of the investigators and French colleagues, the name of the disease should be pronounced as la Peyronie's disease and not Peyronie's disease.

ACKNOWLEDGMENT

My special thanks to Dr. Ekkehard Hauck and Dr. Dirk Schultheiss for providing me the English translation of la Peyronie's original article.

REFERENCES

1. Hauck EW, Weidner W, Nöske HD. François de LaPeyronie: The first complete clinical description of Induratio penis plastica. In: Classical Writings on Erectile Dysfunction (Schultheiss D, Musitelli S, Stief C, Jonas U, eds.). ABW Wissenschaftsverlag GmbH, Berlin, Germany, 2005, pp. 105–110.
2. LaPeyronie FG. Observations avec des reflexions sur la cure des hernies avec gangrene. Mem Acad Royale Chir 1743; 1: 337–342.
3. Grasset D. Urologie a Montpellier des origines a nos jours. Prog Urol 1991; 1: 1091.
4. La Peyronie F. Sur quelques obstaclesqui sópposent à l'éjaculation naturelle de la semence. Mem Acad Royale Chir 1743; 1: 425–439.
5. Borgogni T. Cyrurgia Edita et Compilata. Venice, 1498 (written 1265–1275).
6. Saliceto W von. Chirurgia. Book 1, Chap. 49, Venice, 1476.
7. Fallopio G. Observationes Anatomicae. Venetiis, 1561.
8. Vesalius A. De Humani Corporis Fabrica Libi Dece. Basel, 1543.
9. Aranzi GJ. Observationes Anatomicae. Basel, 1579.
10. Murphy LJT. The urological case histories of Nicolas Tulp. Br J Urol 1975; 47: 232–233.
11. Ruysch F. Thesauri Anatomici Decem. Amsterdam, 1691.
12. Van Buren WH, Keyes E. On a novel disease of penis with cases and remarks. NY Med J 1874; 19: 390–397.
13. Murphy LJT. Miscellanea: Peyronie's disease (fibrous cavernositis). In: The History of Urology. Thomas, Springfield, IL, 1972, pp. 485–486.
14. Wesson MB. Peyronie's disease (plastic induration). Cause and treatment. J Urol 1943; 49: 350–356.
15. Osler JJW. Peyronie's disease—strabisme du Penis. Boston Med Surg J 1903; 148: 245–251.
16. Lowsley OS, Kirwin TJ. The penis and the prepuce. In: A Textbook of Urology. Lea and Febiger, Philadelphia, 1926, pp. 147–148.
17. Hunter J. Of the treatment of occasional symptoms of the gonorrhea. In: A Treatise on Venereal Disease. 2nd ed. Nicol and Johnson, London, 1788, pp. 88–89.
18. Abernethy J. The consequences of gonorrhea. In: Lecture on Anatomy, Surgery, and Pathology: Including Observations on the Nature and Treatment of Local Diseases, delivered at St. Bartholomew's and Christ's Hospitals. Balcock, London, 1828, p. 205.
19. Bidgood CY. Traumatic lesions of the genitourinary tract. In: Urology in War; Wounds and Other Emergencies of the Genitourinary Organs, Surgical and Medical. Williams and Watkins, Baltimore, MD, 1942, pp. 4–6.
20. Thompson-Walker J, Walker K. Fibrous cavernositis. In: Genito-Urinary Surgery. 3rd ed. Cassell, London, 1948, pp. 919–922.
21. Hertzier AE. Induration of penis. J Missouri Med Assoc 1917; 14: 1–18.
22. Weidhoff O. Zur Histologie der Induratio penis Plastia (Histology of plastic induration of the penis). Beitr Z Klin Chir 1921; 111: 712–719.
23. Hinman F. Etiological factors in Peyronie's disease. Urol Int 1980; 35: 407–413.
24. Devine CJ Jr, Somers KD, Jordan SG, Schloseggel SM. Proposal: trauma as the cause of the Peyronie's lesion. J Urol 1997; 157: 285–290.
25. Gentile V, Modesh A, LaPerla G, et al. Ultrastructural and immunohistochemical characterization of the tunica albuginea in Peyronie's disease and venoocclusive function. J Androl 1996; 17: 96–103.

26. Akkus E, Carrier S, Baba K, et al. Structural alterations in the tunica albuginea of the penis: impact of Peyronie's disease, aging and impotence. Br J Urol 1997; 79: 47–53.
27. Polkey HJ. ID induratio penile plastica. Urol Cut Rev 1928; 32: 287–308.
28. Urologia. International inquiry on the therapy of induratio penis plastica. Trevisco 1966; 33: Fasc.2.
29. Ludvik W, Wasserburger K. Die Radiumbehandlung der induratio penis plastica. Z Urol Nephrol 1968; 61: 319–325.
30. Lindsay MB, Schain DM, Grambsch P, et al. The incidence of Peyronie's disease in Rochester, Minnesota, 1950 through 1984. J Urol 1991; 146: 1007–1009.
31. Devine CJ Jr. Editorial. International Conference on Peyronie's Disease. J Urol 1997; 157: 272–275.
32. Blandy J. Penis and the scrotum. In: Urology (Blackwell J, ed.). Oxford, London, 1976, pp. 1083–1084.
33. Chesney J. Peyronie's disease. Br J Urol 1975; 47: 209–218.
34. Scott WW, Scardino PL. New concept in the treatment of Peyronie's disease. South Med J 1947; 41: 173–177.
35. Devine CJ Jr, Horton CE. Bent penis. Semin Urol 1987; 5: 251–261.
36. Zarafonetis CJD, Horax TM. Retrospective studies in scleroderma: skin response to potassium para-aminobenzoate therapy. Clin Exp Rheumatol 1988; 6: 261–268.
37. Walsham WJ, Spencer WG. Sores on the penis. In: Surgery: Its Theory and Practice. 8th ed. Churchill, London, 1903, p. 1037.
38. Teasley GH. Peyronie's disease: a new approach. J Urol 1954; 71: 611–613.
39. Bodner H, Howard AH, Kaplan JH. Peyronie's disease: cortisone-hyaluronidase-hydrocortisone therapy. J Urol 1954; 134: 400.
40. Winter C, Khanna R. Peyronie's disease: results with dermojet injection of dexamethasone. J Urol 1975; 14: 989–1000.
41. Williams G, Gren NA. The non-surgical treatment of Peyronie's disease. Br J Urol 1980; 52: 392–395.
42. Pentland A, Anderson T. Plantar fibromatosis respond to intralesional steroids. J Am Acad Dermatol 1985; 2: 212–214.
43. Lue TF, Gelbard MK, Gueglio GH, et al. Peyronie's disease. In: Erectile Dysfunction (Jardin E, Wagner G, Guiliano F, Khoury S, Padma-Nathan H, Rosen R, eds.). Plymouth Distributors Ltd., Plymouth, UK, 2000, pp. 439–475.
44. Kumer L. Uber die radum bechandlung der induratio penis plastica. Dermat Wcshner Leipzig v Hamburg 1922; 125: 673–677.
45. Corbus CB. Chronic cavernositis cured by diklothermy. J Urol 1926; 16: 313–314.
46. Burford EH, Burford CE. Combined (ultraviolet and vitamin E) therapy for Peyronie's disease. J Urol 1957; 78: 265.
47. Heslop RW, Oakland DJ, Maddox BT. Ultrasonic therapy in Peyronie's disease. Br J Urol 1967; 39: 415–419.
48. Dunsmuir WD, Kirby RS. François de LaPeyronie (1678–1747). The man and the disease he described. Br J Urol 1996; 78: 613–622.
49. Young HH, Davis DM. Operations on the penis. In: Young's Practice of Urology. Saunders, Philadelphia, 1926, pp. 647–648.
50. Lowsley OS, Boyce WH. Further experiences with an operation fort he cure of Peyronie's disease. J Urol 1950; 63: 888–898.
51. Nesbit RM. Congenital curvature of the phallus: report of three cases with description of corrective operation. J Urol 1965; 93: 230–232.
52. Pryor J, Akkus E, Alter G, et al. Priapism, Peyronie's disease, penile reconstructive surgery. In: Sexual Medicine Sexual Dysfunctions in Men and Women (Lue TF, Basson R, Rosen R, Guiliano F, Khoury S, Montorsi F, eds.). Health Publications, Paris, France, 2004, pp. 385–408.
53. Bystrom J, Johanson B, Edsmyr F, Korlof B, Nylen B. Induratio penis plastica (Peyronie's disease): the results of the various forms of treatment. Scand J Urol Nephrol 1972; 6: 1–5.
54. Devine CJ, Horton CE. Surgical treatment of Peyronie's disease with a dermal graft. J Urol 1974; 111: 44–49.
55. Lue TF, El-Sakka AI. Venous patch graft for Peyronie's disease. Part 1: technique. J Urol 1998; 160: 2047–2049.

2

Epidemiology of Peyronie's Disease

Ates Kadioglu, MD and Oner Sanli, MD

SUMMARY

Epidemiological studies of Peyronie's disease (PD) reported the prevalence of this
condition as much higher than once thought, highlighting the potential physical and psy-
chosocial impact of the disease on society. For this reason, knowledge of the epidemiology of PD is important for allocating and managing health care resources and assessing
intervention strategies. The true prevalence of PD is unknown; it is estimated as between
3.7% and 7.1%, but the actual prevalence of this disease may be higher because of patients'
reluctance to report this embarrassing condition to their physicians for cultural and
psychological reasons. Several risk factors, such as hypertension, diabetes, hyperlipidemia, and smoking, have been suggested. The estimated prevalence of PD at younger ages
is around 8% and shows a more acute onset and a lower incidence of associated erectile
dysfunction. This chapter reviews the contemporary state of knowledge of the epidemiology of PD.

Key Words: Epidemiology; penis; Peyronie's disease; prevalence; risk factors.

Peyronie's disease (PD) is an acquired disorder of the tunica albuginea characterized
by the formation of the plaque of fibrous tissue that may be associated with erectile dysfunction (ED) and pain on erection. There may be difficulty of penetration as a result of
the curvature, and the condition may be accompanied by some impairment of erectile
capacity *(1)*.

Although the "nodus penis" had been described centuries before, François de la Peyronie
described the disease that bears his name in 1743 *(2)*. He considered chronic irritation
through sexual abuse as well as sexually transmitted disease to be causative factors.
Despite the negative impact of PD on patient quality of life, neither the etiological factors
of the disease nor the exact pathophysiological mechanisms are clearly understood. One
of the causes of the poor understanding of the disease is the lack of definite epidemiological data.

Epidemiology deals with the distribution and determinants of health-related states
or events in specified populations, and the application of this study is to control health
problems *(3)*. Briefly, epidemiology deals with frequency and nature of diseases and

From: *Current Clinical Urology:*
Peyronie's Disease: A Guide to Clinical Management
Edited by: L. A. Levine © Humana Press Inc., Totowa, NJ

identification of risk factors. Epidemiology may be considered as minor to physical sciences because it does not investigate the biological mechanism leading from exposure to disease. But, without epidemiological data, the extent of a disease in a community cannot be determined, and the etiology or cause of a disease and the risk factors cannot be identified. Also, data obtained from epidemiological studies are vital for allocating and managing health care resources and assessing intervention strategies.

This work reviews the contemporary state of knowledge of the epidemiology of PD. Studies used in the context of the chapter were identified using a PubMed search on April 1, 2005, for "Peyronie's disease" for all available years in modern literature. The selected articles were all in peer-reviewed journals and in the English literature. Basically, the studies performed on the epidemiology of PD were divided into cross-sectional studies or case series. A study was considered cross sectional if all cases of PD in a defined population were reported (4). On the other hand, a study was considered as a case series when the size of the population from which cases were drawn was not known. This search revealed a number of cross-sectional studies undertaken to quantify the incidence and prevalence of PD. *Incidence* is defined as the number of new cases with a certain condition during a specific time period in relation to the size of the population studied (4). *Prevalence* characterizes the proportion of a given population that at a given time has the condition.

The negative impact of PD on patient quality of life is significant. A questionnaire based study done by Gelbard et al. demonstrated that 77% of patients with PD complained of "physiological effects" of this condition (5). For this reason, defining the prevalence of this disease is important. However, in the case of PD, the incidence and prevalence are usually measured using different instruments, such as the definition of PD (curvature vs plaque) or the means of detection (questionnaire vs examination) (1). Moreover, in the literature, epidemiological studies conducted in a multinational fashion using large pool data are still lacking.

CROSS-SECTIONAL STUDIES

Cross-sectional studies provide descriptive data on prevalence of diseases useful for health care planning. To our knowledge, there are only two population-based epidemiological cross-sectional studies that addressed the prevalence of PD; these studies were from the United States and Germany. The report by Lindsay et al. provided the first cross-sectional study giving the incidence and prevalence rates on PD (6). Their study was carried out in Rochester, Minnesota, using the Mayo Clinic's centralized medical records linkage system. A search of the indexing system for diagnoses of PD was assessed. They calculated the age-adjusted incidence rate of 25.7 per 100,000 population per year, and the prevalence rate was 388.8 per 100,000 (0.39%) population. They estimated that approx 423,000 men in the United States had PD at that time; thus, there should be 32,000 new cases annually. Moreover, the authors calculated that the diagnosis rates per 100,000 increased from 13.6 to 24.6 during a 35-yr period, for an average increase of 3.3% per year. Mean patient age at diagnosis was 53 yr (range 19–83 yr). The highest incidence (66%) was reported for the 50- to 59-yr age group. The prevalence of PD was 4.3, 4.6, 30.2, 46.3, 7.8, and 19.1% for men 20–29, 30–39, 40–49, 60–69, 70–79, and greater than 80 yr old, respectively (Table 1). Also, they noted that rheumatoid arthritis (7.9%) and hypertension (16.8%) were more common comorbid diseases among the patients with PD compared to the Rochester population.

Table 1
Incidence or Prevalence of Peyronie's Disease According to Age

Cross–sectional studies	Age (yr)					
	Overall	<40	40–49	50–59	60–69	>70
Lindsay et al. (6)	0.39	0.089[a]	30.2[a]	66.0[a]	46.3[a]	7.8[a]
Sommer et al. (7)	3.2	4.5	3.0	3.0	4.0	6.5
Case series						
Rhoden et al. (14)	3.67	NR	NR	3.19[b]	4.49[b]	3.81[b]
Mulhall et al. (15)	8.9	—	2.8	8.6	9.7	10.9
La Pera et al. (16)	7.1	NR	NR	5 (50–54 yr) 5.9 (55–59 yr)	7.6 (60–64 yr) 9.1 (65–69 yr)	NR
Kadioglu et al. (27,33)	1	9.4	20.5	44.2	23.4	2.28

NR, not reported.

[a]Incidence rates per 100,000 population for PD by age groups at diagnosis.

[b]Number of men examined stratified by age with Peyronie's plaques.

The German study performed by Sommer et al. provided the first prevalence rates for PD in a cross-sectional study in Europe (7). The study was a validated questionnaire survey of 8000 men 30–80 yr old in greater Cologne; and 142 (3.2%) of 4432 men who responded to questionnaire reported palpable plaque in the penis. The prevalence of the disease was 1.5, 3.0, 4.0, and 6.5% for men 30–39, 40–59, 60–69, and greater than 70 yr old, respectively. They found a statistically significant relationship between diabetes mellitus (DM) (18.3 vs 6.0%) and therapy with β-blockers (22.5 vs 14.2%). However, they found no association of PD with other comorbid diseases such as heart insufficiency and atherosclerosis, hernia, history of other drug therapies and any other operations, lower urinary tract symptoms, pelvic surgery, drinking alcohol, and smoking.

CASE SERIES

From the aspect of the case series, the epidemiological data on PD are variable. Polkey reported on 550 case reports up to 1928, and an Italian publication, published in 1966, described 3600 affected patients (7–9). In 1968, Ludvik and Wasserburger established a rate of 0.3–0.7% in all male patients seen in one urological practice (10). During the same time period, Smith reviewed 100 consecutive autopsies of patients who had no history of symptoms of PD. In 23, there was histological evidence of fibrosis in the subtunical sheath, but no involvement of the corpus spongiosum was reported (11). In 1989, Vorstman and Lockhart described a prevalence of 3 in 300 (1.0%) occurring within a given medical school faculty (12). In one of the first studies on the natural history of PD, Gelbard et al. noted that the prevalence of PD at the Wadsworth Veterans Administration Hospital in Los Angeles was greater than 10 times the prevalence of renal cell carcinoma in the same population (5). Meanwhile, Devine reported on two separate populations of male physicians, with 1% prevalence of a symptomatic PD, which was widely accepted as the prevalence of PD until recent data (13).

Since 1995, great effort has been made to understand the pathophysiology and treatment of PD by urologists. One of the consequences of this effort is the constitution of large series by the centers of excellence on PD. Like the historical case series, data based on case series published since 1995 contributed a number of advances and scientific understanding about its epidemiology and pathophysiology.

In one of these studies, Rhoden et al. aimed to ascertain the prevalence of PD in a male population over 50 yr old who originated from southern Brazil and attended a prostate cancer screening program *(14)*. In addition to the prostate digital examination, all patients were examined for the presence of a palpable plaque with extension of the penis. Of 954 men, 35 individuals were found to have palpable plaque that had not been previously diagnosed. The prevalence of PD in this group of patients was 3.67%. The mean age in this population was 60.7 yr. The distribution of patients in accordance to the age of men showed that 3.19% of these were between the ages of 50 and 59 yr, 4.49% were aged 60–69 yr, 3.81% were aged 70–79 yr, and 0% were over 80 yr.

With a similar study design to that of Rhoden et al., Mulhall et al. made an analysis of the prevalence of PD in a population of men presenting for prostate cancer screening *(15)*. Of 534 men, 48 patients were found to have a palpable penile plaque on physical examination, for a prevalence rate of 8.9%. The mean age of men with PD was 68.2 yr compared with a mean 61.8 yr in men without PD. The prevalence of PD based on age groups in decades was 2.8% for those 40–49 yr, 8.6% for patients 50–59 yr, 9.7% for those 60–69 yr, 10.9% for those 70–79 yr. In this series, specifically the prevalence of hypertension (43.8 vs 27.7%) and DM (25 vs 11.4%) was significantly increased in patients with PD. Coronary artery disease (10.4 vs 8.5%) and hyperlipidemia (33.3 vs 27.1%) were more common in PD cases but did not attain statistical significance. Dupuytren's contracture was also found more frequently in patients with PD (8.3 vs 0%). On the other hand, smoking was significantly less common in patients with PD.

In another study, La Pera et al., from Italy, evaluated the results of a questionnaire administered by an andrologist at each of 10 centers throughout the country in men aged 50–69 yr *(16)*. Their cohort of men revealed a prevalence of 7.1% for PD. The prevalence of the disease varied in different age groups, with a higher prevalence in older men. It was 5% at 50–54 yr compared to 9.1% at 65–69 yr. In addition, the prevalence of the disease at 55–59 yr and 60–64 yr was 5.9 and 7.8%, respectively. Further analysis of the study revealed that the probability for smokers developing PD was 4.6 times higher than for nonsmokers. The authors also detected a significant correlation in the subjects who had smoked 10,000 packs during their life, which is equal to a pack per day for 28 yr. However, statistical analysis did not reveal any significant correlation between PD and cardiovascular diseases, DM, drugs or alcohol.

RACIAL DIFFERENCES
IN THE EPIDEMIOLOGY OF PEYRONIE'S DISEASE

There are only a few studies giving data on the racial differences in PD. In one of these, Shaw et al. retrospectively reviewed data from three hospitals in New Orleans from 1994 to 2000 *(17)*. The racial distribution for PD was as follows: 77.6% Caucasian, 9.4% African American, and 2.9% Hispanic. In the Brazilian study conducted by Rhoden et al., 88.6% of patients diagnosed as having PD were Caucasian, and 11.4% were African American *(14)*.

NATURAL HISTORY OF PEYRONIE'S DISEASE

PD has been previously characterized as a process of gradual spontaneous resolution *(18)*. In one of the first studies on PD including patients with PD for a duration of 1–5 yr, Gelbard et al. reported that 13% of the patients with PD will gradually resolve, 47% will remain stable, and 40% will worsen *(5)*. Certain features that predispose against spontaneous resolution include PD greater than 2-yr duration at presentation, presence of Dupuytren's contractures, plaque calcification, and curvature greater than 45°.

We observed the natural course of PD in 63 (20.5%) of 307 patients presenting with acute disease for a duration of 5.8 mo and received no treatment *(19)*. In this series, 30.2% of the patients reported progression of the deformity, and 66.7% had stable disease after a mean follow-up of 8.4 mo without any treatment. Complete spontaneous resolution of the penile deformity was observed only in 2 cases in this group. In the chronic phase, which begins when disease duration is greater than 12 mo, the deformity does not change during this stable period.

Lania et al. investigated the natural history of PD in a total of 125 patients maintaining sexual activity and not requiring surgical treatment *(20)*. They were followed for at least 5 yr without any treatment. Regarding curvature and number and size of fibrotic nodules, the authors observed a consistent tendency to stabilize in the group of patients older than 50 yr compared with the patients younger than 50 yr. The percentage of patients who needed surgery for PD was 68 and 31.5% for the former and latter group of patients, respectively. The authors concluded that patients diagnosed before the age of 50 yr have a greater chance that the disease will worsen and require a surgical approach.

PEYRONIE'S DISEASE IN YOUNGER MALES

In the literature, patients with PD are represented by a wide age range, between 20 and 84 yr, with the youngest affected male reported at 19 yr *(6,13,21)*. On the other hand, it is generally observed that PD usually affects male individuals between 40 and 70 (87%) yr *(6)*. The classical image of the patient with PD is a man typically presenting in his 50s and 60s with compromised sexual function caused by penile deformity and, not infrequently, diminished rigidity. However, in studies that give the prevalence rate of PD, mostly men under 50 yr were not taken into consideration because of the much lower prevalence of PD.

In their large community-based study, Lindsay et al. calculated the prevalence rate of patients with PD between 20 and 29 yr and between 30 and 39 yr as 4.3 per 100,000 (0.043%) and 4.6 per 100,000 (0.046%) population, respectively *(6)*. In this study, the percentage of patients with PD who were under 40 yr among all patients was 9.9%. In the study by Sommers et al. that used a mailed questionnaire, only 1.5% of the group between 30 and 39 yr noticed induration on the penis *(7)*.

In our experience, it was reported that the prevalence of patients with PD who presented under age 40 yr is 8.2%, which is similar to the report by Lindsay et al. Of these younger patients, 78.9% presented during the acute phase of the disease, and pain on erection was a part of presenting symptom complex in 52.6% *(21)*. The majority (84%) had a degree of penile curvature less than 60°. Dorsal penile curvature was the most common type of deformity and was observed in 42% *(8)* of patients, whereas lateral curvature was observed in 36.8% *(7)* of the patients. ED was present in 21% of these patients. After a minimum 2-yr follow-up, improvement in penile deformity was observed in 36.8%, and 42.1% had stable disease; 21% experienced deterioration of penile curvature. The authors concluded that, despite the low prevalence of ED in patients with PD, the onset of PD is clinically more active and acute in patients presenting under age 40 yr, and this should encourage the clinician to treat these individuals more vigorously.

In another study, Levine et al. aimed to characterize disease presentation, symptomatology, natural history, and results of therapy in their institution *(22)*. The prevalence of

PD in men younger than 40 was calculated as 4.8% (30 of 626). The mean age at presentation in this group was 31 yr, and the most common complaints were penile pain and palpable nodule. There were 57% of the men who believed it was caused by a specific traumatic event, and 97% of the patients were able to achieve full erection with the deformity. On physical examination, all patients presented with a palpable penile plaque, and the mean curvature of the erect penis was 21°.

Overall, the characteristics of patients with PD who were mentioned in studies performed by our group and Levine et al. at younger ages are as follows: palpable plaque, significant pain, less-severe curvature, good quality of erections, and ability to have intercourse. Levine et al. *(22)* further discussed the main difference of patients with PD younger than 40 yr in comparison with a typical patient with PD by reviewing literature information for more than 1500 patients. They detected that there was a difference in the direction of the curvature; 41 and 81% of the younger men reported dorsal and lateral curvature, respectively, whereas the literature review of a patient classical PD yielded 77% dorsal and 20% lateral curvature. They mentioned that the clinical significance of this is not clearly understood. On the other hand, all the younger males presented with a palpable nodule, whereas in only 67% of typical patients was a plaque identified. Finally, a midshaft plaque was found in 20% of younger men, whereas this finding was reported in 42% of the reviewed patients. These may be because of a different mechanism of injury leading to a more accelerated or robust scar formation response in younger males *(22,23)*.

A third group investigated the clinical presentation of PD with 20 patients under 40 yr compared with 28 patients over 40 yr *(24)*. They reported that the difference between IIEF domain scores and subjective reduction of penile length was significant between the two groups. Also, they noted the only significant risk factor for PD was hypercholesterolemia. Overall, they confirmed the conclusions obtained from the studies by our group and Levine et al. that PD in younger patients shows a more acute onset and a lower incidence of associated ED.

COMORBID DISEASES IN RETROSPECTIVE COHORTS

The exact etiology of PD is still unknown, but current research suggests that PD represents a localized aberration of the wound-healing process *(25)*. The impact of systemic disorders such as DM, hypercholesterolemia, hyperlipidemia, and hypertension has been hypothesized to have a role in the pathogenesis of PD.

In one of the first studies for this issue, Carrieri et al. investigated the role of risk factors in a case-control study consisting of 134 men with PD and 134 age-related male controls *(26)*. Patients who underwent invasive procedures on the penis (i.e., urethral catheterization, cystoscopy transurethral prostatectomy) had 16.1-fold (13% of cases and 1% of controls) increased risk for PD; nearly a three-fold increase was observed among patients who had genital or perineal trauma. A history of urethritis (3.1-fold), uricacidemia (5.4-fold), and lipoma (5.2-fold) was also significantly associated with an increased risk of PD. Among cases, 20% were affected by Dupuytren's contracture, and 4% reported a family history of PD; none of the controls reported such conditions. Furthermore, a familial history of gout was more common among cases than among controls. Interestingly, no associations with risk of PD were noted with a history of diabetes and hypertension. In addition, this was the only study that interviewed both cases and controls on the past diseases of the genital tract of the female partner. The results of this survey revealed that inflammatory (3.7-fold) and fibromatous lesions (2.5-fold) or surgical intervention in the genital tract of the partner were more common by the cases.

Usta et al. evaluated the impact of risk factors on the severity of penile deformity in a total of 469 patients *(27)*. In their series, the most frequently documented comorbid conditions in association with PD were hypertension in 27.3% (128) of cases; smoking in 25.5% (120); hypercholesterolemia in 18.3% (86); DM in 17.2%, with 2.1% (10) of those with type 1 and 15.1% (71) of those with type 2; hyperlipidemia in 15.7% (74); history of penile trauma in 13.2% (62); previous pelvic surgery in 1% (5); and a urethral catheterization in 0.08% (4). Of these patients with PD, 68% had at least one of these comorbidities (Table 2). Also, 31.7, 16.4, and 19.6% of patients had one to three comorbidities, respectively. Statistical analysis of the study revealed no positive linear trend between individual comorbidities and the severity of the penile deformity.

In our experience, at least one risk factor for systemic vascular disease, with hypercholesterolemia the most common, was identified in 67.5% of 307 patients *(19)*. A positive family history was obtained in 3 (0.01%) of the cases. A detailed questionnaire revealed history of penile trauma during sexual intercourse in 26 (8.5%) men and a history of urethritis related to sexually transmitted diseases in 8 (2.6%). In this series, 13 (4.2%) patients had a history of pelvic surgery such as transurethral prostatectomy in 8 (2.6%), open prostatectomy in 3 (0.9%), and radical retropubic prostatectomy in 2 (0.6%); 5 (1.6%) patients had transurethral manipulation or catheterization.

In the update of this series, 484 patients were retrospectively evaluated in terms of risk factors for systemic vascular diseases and ischemic heart disease to assess the impact of these risk factors on the severity of penile deformity *(28)*. Of 484 patients, systemic vascular disease such as hypercholesterolemia (35.1%) was the most common, followed by DM (28.3%), hypertriglyceridemia (21.1%), and hypertension (16.7%); ischemic heart disease (9.1%). The comorbidities were identified in 62.4% (302) of the patients. Of the patients with severe deformity (>60°), 82.4% had at least one of these risk factors. In patients with deformity less than 30°, no risk factor was detected in 40.2% of the patients. The authors concluded the impact of risk factors on the severity of penile deformity is obscure, but the patients with at least one risk factor were more likely to have a deformity greater than 60°.

In another study, Perimenis et al. retrospectively evaluated 134 cases to investigate the clinical features of the disease *(29)*. They found that in 11 (8.2%) the onset of disease was noticed after autoinjections of vasoactive drugs, and 18 (13.4%) had a history of penile trauma (fracture) during sexual activity. Of patients with PD, 8 (6%) had DM, and 3 (2.2%) had Dupuytren's contracture.

In conclusion, there are contradictory results in the literature about the role of risk factors for systemic vascular diseases such as smoking, DM, hyperlipidemia, and hypertension and drugs. Further research with large epidemiological studies is needed to identify the definitive relationship between PD and these comorbidities. Further details on the etiology and pathophysiology of PD are discussed in other chapters.

EFFECT OF ORAL PHARMACOTHERAPY ON THE PREVALENCE OF PEYRONIE'S DISEASE

Most of the opinion leaders in this field note that the number of patients with PD has increased since the advent of oral pharmacotherapy for the treatment of ED *(30,31)* because up to 80% of patients with PD may have concurrent ED *(32)*. With more men successfully treated for ED, an increasing number of Peyronie's cases are becoming manifest and presenting for evaluation. PD may be diagnosed during a standard diagnostic evaluation for ED.

Table 2

Comorbid Factors Among Peyronie's Disease in Different Studies

Cross-sectional studies	Most common comorbid factors among patients with Peyronie's disease (%)									
	DM	Arthritis	β-Blockers	HT	DC	CAD	HL	HC	Smoking	PT
Lindsay et al. (6)	6.9	7.9	5.9	16.8	4	NR	NR	NR	NR	NR
Sommers et al. (7)	18.3	NR	22.5	NR	NR	NR	NR	NR	NR	NR
Case series										
Mulhall et al. (15)	25 OR 2.6	NR	NR OR 2.3	43.8	8.3	10.4	33.3 OR 0.32	NR	15	NR
La Pera et al. (16)	NR	NR	NR	OR 0.7	NR	OR 1.7	NR	NR	OR 4.6	NR
Kadioglu et al. (27)	33.2	—	—	14.7	NR	8.1	28.3	NR	NR	NR
Carrieri et al. (25)	16 OR 1.6	NR	NR OR 1.6	31	20	NR	NR	NR	76	13
Usta et al. (26)	17.2	—	—	27.2	0.08	2.3	15.7	18.3 OR 19.3	25.5	13.2
Kadioglu et al. (33)	25.2	NR	NR	16	NR	8.92	21.8	34.5	NR	NR
Perimenis et al. (29)	6	NR	NR	NR	2.2	NR	NR	NR	NR	21.6

CAD, coronary artery disease; DC, Dupuytren's contracture; DM, diabetes mellitus; HC, hypercholesterolemia; HL, hyperlipidemia; HT, hypertension; NR, not reported; OR, odds ratio compared to control; PT, penile trauma (including invasive procedures to the penis).

16

With colleagues, we analyzed the characteristics of these patients compared with patients presenting with classical complaints of PD during a 10-yr period in our institution *(33)*. Of 448 patients, 15.8% (71) were detected with PD during a diagnostic workup for ED, which consisted of a standard questionnaire for sexual function and combined injection and stimulation test. Of 7594 patients with ED who were seen at our outpatient clinic during this period, 1% (71) were found to have PD. The patients presenting with ED only were significantly older (57.4 yr) compared to the other patients with PD (52.2 yr). In this study, at least one comorbidity for systemic vascular diseases was observed in 73% of the cases, with DM (40.8%) and hypercholesterolemia (36.6%) the leading ones. The severity of deformity was significantly less in these patients compared to other patients with PD, which may be an important factor in their awareness of their disease. The mean degree of deformity was 31.5° in these patients; it was 41.1° in the other patients with PD.

On the other hand, pure notching deformity may be another factor for incidentally diagnosed PD during standard diagnostic workup. We compared the erectile status of patients with isolated notching deformity (57) with patients having any kind of penile curvature by history (534). We found that the leading presenting symptom was ED in 31.5% of patients with pure notching deformity; it was 14.2% in patients with any kind of curvature. There is no study regarding the prevalence of PD in patients receiving oral pharmacotherapy.

CONCLUSIONS

Epidemiological studies of PD revealed that the prevalence of PD in the population has continuously increased during the last 30 yr, and now its prevalence is estimated as between 3.7 and 7.1%. It is much higher than previously believed. The increase in prevalence of PD in case studies was also confirmed by Lindsay et al.'s cross-sectional study *(6)*. In this study, it was reported that the prevalence rates per 100,000 population increased from 13.6 to 34.6 during a 35-yr period, for an average increase of 3.3% per year. Although it was previously considered a rare condition, its prevalence seems to be equivalent to that of important public diseases like diabetes or urolithiasis, both estimated in 3–4% of the general population and greater than many cancers *(7)*.

The actual prevalence of this disease may be higher because of a patient's reluctance to report this embarrassing condition to the physician because of cultural and psychological reasons. On the other hand, because the symptoms may not be disabling, individuals do not seek medical help, and therefore they are not examined and registered in the medical system. Of concern is the belief by some authors that even the most recent data (7.1%) underestimate the true prevalence of PD, and there is no study addressing actual prevalence of PD diagnosed by physical examination as well as penile ultrasonography. PD at younger ages seems to have notably different characteristics, such as clinical hallmarks and outcome.

REFERENCES

1. Pryor J, Akkus E, Alter G, et al. Priapism, Peyronie's disease, penile reconstructive surgery. In:Sexual Medicine, Sexual Dysfunctions in Men and Women (Lue TF, Basson R, Rosen R, Giuliano F, Khoury S, Montorsi F, eds.). Health Publications, Paris, France, 2004, pp. 383–409.
2. Dunsmuir WD, Kirby RS. Francois de La Peyronie (1678–1747). The man, the disease he described. Br J Urol 1996; 78: 613–622.
3. Last JM (ed.). A Dictionary of Epidemiology. 4th ed. Oxford University Press, New York, 2001.

4. Lilienfield AM, Lilienfield DE. Foundations of Epidemiology. 2nd ed. Oxford University Press, New York, 1980.
5. Gelbard MK, Dorey F, James K. The natural history of Peyronie's disease. J Urol 1990; 144: 1376–1379.
6. Lindsay MB, Sehain DM, Grambsch P, Benson RC, Beard M, Kurkland T. The incidence of Peyronie's disease in Rochester, Minnesota, 1950 through 1984. J Urol 1991; 146: 1007–1008.
7. Sommer F, Schwarzer U, Wassmer G, et al. Epidemiology of Peyronie's disease. Int J Impot Res 2002; 14: 379–383.
8. Polkey HJ. Induratio penis plastica. Urol Cut Rev 1928; 32: 287–308.
9. Urologia. International Inquiry on the Therapy of Induratio Penis Plastica. Trevisco, 1966: 33: Fasc II.
10. Ludvik W, Wasserburger K. Die radiumbehadlung der induratio penis plastica. Z Urol Nephrol 1968; 61: 319–325.
11. Smith BH. Subclinical Peyronie's disease. Am J Pathol 1969; 52: 385–390.
12. Vorstman B, Lockhart J. Peyronie's disease. Probl Urol 1987; 1: 507–509.
13. Devine CJ. Introduction to Peyronie's disease. J Urol 1997; 157: 272–275.
14. Rhoden EL, Teloken C, Ting HY, Lucas ML, Teodosio da Ros C, Ary Vargas Souto C. Prevalence of Peyronie's disease in men over 50-yr-old from Southern Brasil. Int J Impot Res 2001; 13: 291–293.
15. Mulhall JP, Creech SD, Boorjian SA, et al. Subjective and objective analysis of the prevalence of Peyronie's disease in a population of men presenting for prostate cancer. J Urol 2004; 171: 2350–2353.
16. La Pera G, Pescatori ES, Calabrese M, et al. and the Simona Study Group. Peyronie's disease: prevalence and association with cigarette smoking. Eur Urol 2001; 40: 525–530.
17. Shaw K, Puri K, Ruiz-Deya G, Hellstrom WJG. Racial considerations in the evaluation of Peyronie's disease. J Urol 2001; 165(5), suppl: 170.
18. Williams JL, Thomas GG. The natural history of Peyronie's disease. J Urol 1970; 103: 75.
19. Kadioglu A, Tefekli A, Erol B, Oktar T, Tunc M, Tellaloglu S. A retrospective review of 307 men with Peyronie's disease. J Urol 2002; 168: 1075–1079.
20. Lania C, Grasso M, Franzoso F, Blanco S, Rigatti P. Peyronie's disease, natural history. J Urol 2004; 171(4), suppl: 331.
21. Tefekli A, Kandirali E, Erol H, Alp T, Koksal T, Kadioglu A. Peyronie's disease in men under 40: characteristics and outcome. Int J Impot Res 2001; 13: 18–23.
22. Levine LA, Estrada CR, Storm DW, Matkov TG. Peyronie's disease in younger men: characteristics and treatment results. J Androl 2002; 24: 27–32.
23. Seftel AD. Peyronie disease in younger men. J Androl 2003; 24: 33–34.
24. Briganti A, Barbieri L, Deho F, et al. Clinical presentation of Peyronie's disease in young patients. Int J Impot Res 2003; 15(suppl 6): S44–S47.
25. Gholami SS, Gonzales-Cadavis NF, Lin C, Rajfer J, Lue TF. Peyronie's disease: a review. J Urol 2003; 169: 1234–1241.
26. Carrieri MP, Serraino D, Palmiotto F, Nucci G, Sasso F. A case-control study on risk factors for Peyronie's disease. J Clin Epidemiol 1998; 51: 511–515.
27. Usta MF, Bivalacqua TJ, Jabren GW, et al. Relationship between the severity of penile curvature and the presence of comorbid diseases in men with Peyronie's disease. J Urol 2004; 171: 775–779.
28. Oktar T, Kendirci M, Sanli O, Kadioglu A. The impact of risk factors on the severity of penile deformity in 484 Peyronie's patients. J Urol 2003; 169(4), suppl: 274.
29. Perimenis P, Athanasopoulos A, Gyftopoulos K, Katsenis G, Barbalias G. Peyronie's disease: epidemiology and clinical presentation of 134 cases. Int J Urol Nephrol 2002; 32: 691–694.
30. Hellstrom WJG, Bivalacqua TJ. Peyronie's disease: etiology, medical, and surgical therapy. J Androl 2000; 21: 347–354.
31. Hellstrom WJG. History, epidemiology and clinical presentation of Peyronie's disease. Int J Impot Res 2003; 15(suppl 5): S91–S92.
32. Jarow JP, Burrnet AL, Geringer AM. Clinical efficacy of sildenafil citrate based on etiology and response to prior treatment. J Urol 1999; 162: 722–725.
33. Kadioglu A, Oktar T, Kandirali E, Kendirci M, Sanli O, Ozsoy C. Incidentally diagnosed Peyronie's disease in men presenting with erectile dysfunction. Int J Impot Res 2004; 16: 540–543.

3

Experimental Models for the Study of the Cellular and Molecular Pathophysiology of Peyronie's Disease

Nestor F. Gonzalez-Cadavid, PhD and Jacob Rajfer, MD

SUMMARY

Research on the molecular and cellular pathophysiology of Peyronie's disease (PD) and the potential implications for the discovery of novel therapeutic targets for this prevalent condition has lagged considerably behind the advances in surgical techniques. However, two animal models have been generated based on the injection in the tunica albuginea of the rat of either transforming growth factor-β_1 (TGF-β_1) or fibrin to induce PD-like plaques and on the extensive characterization of fibroblast cell cultures from the human tunica albuginea and the PD plaque. These in vivo and in vitro models of PD not only replicate key molecular pathways and cell differentiation processes operating in most other types of tissue fibrosis, but also are excellent tools to test and validate new antifibrotic approaches of wider applicability. The fibrogenic roles of TGF-β_1, oxidative stress, fibrin, plasminogen activator inhibitor 1, myofibroblast differentiation, and others have started to be elucidated in the context of the PD plaque, and stem cells have been found in the tunica albuginea that may be involved in plaque calcification and ectopic osteogenesis. In addition, endogenous antifibrotic pathways have been found in the PD plaque, mainly the inducible nitric oxide synthase/nitric oxide/cyclic guanosine monophosphate cascade, antioxidant enzymes, anti-TGF-β_1 factors, and others, that may maintain the plaque in cellular and molecular turnover, particularly in terms of collagen deposition/breakdown and myofibroblast differentiation/apoptosis. Both the modulation of these defense mechanisms and some antifibrotic agents utilized in other conditions are starting to be tested therapeutically in human PD or its models or are potential targets for experimental research.

Key Words: Collagen; fibrosis; inducible nitric oxide synthase; myofibroblast; nitric oxide; oxidative stress; PDE5; PDE5 inhibitors; penis; reactive oxygen species; TGF-β; tunica albuginea.

Peyronie's disease (PD) continues to be underdiagnosed and overlooked in terms of the research effort invested in clarifying its etiology, pathology, and molecular pharmacology *(1–5)*. Recent advances have been made that demonstrate that the mechanisms of

From: *Current Clinical Urology:*
Peyronie's Disease: A Guide to Clinical Management
Edited by: L. A. Levine © Humana Press Inc., Totowa, NJ

fibrosis that occur in PD are also operative in other fibrotic conditions, such as wound healing *(6)*; more than likely, these same processes are involved in other fibrotic conditions as diverse as erectile dysfunction *(7,8)*, Dupuytren's disease *(9)*, heart failure *(10, 11)*, hypertension *(12,13)*, renal tubulointerstitial fibrosis *(14,15)*, arteriosclerosis *(16, 17)*, liver cirrhosis and nonalcoholic fibrosis *(18)*, and idiopathic pulmonary fibrosis *(19)*.

Indeed, what makes PD an interesting process to be approached experimentally is the fact that two animal models *(20–30)* and cell cultures *(25,31–37)* of the PD plaque have been developed, and a number of molecular and cellular biology concepts have been derived from these experimental models of PD and seem to play a role in many of the aforementioned more diffuse fibrotic processes. Simply stated, fibrosis is fibrosis regardless of the affected tissue, the pathological consequences, or the etiology of the fibrosis; as such, there must be a multitude of common processes indigenous to all these fibroses. Therefore, elucidation of therapeutic regimens to prevent or reverse the fibrosis in any one of these fibrotic conditions may be applicable to a number of the other fibroses.

In this chapter, we discuss (1) the cellular and molecular pathophysiology of PD in the context of general pathways and therapeutic targets of fibrosis in other non-PD conditions, highlighting the main concepts that are supported by experimental evidence derived from the studies using human PD plaque tissue and plaque tissue experimentally induced in the animal models and (2) possible avenues of research that may develop into new therapeutic strategies for not only PD but also any of the disorders of fibrosis.

PROFIBROTIC FACTORS AND COLLAGEN METABOLISM

Relationship Between TGF-β₁ and Collagen in PD as Illustrated by the First Animal Model of PD

Fibrotic diseases are characterized by the excessive production, deposition, and contraction of extracellular matrix (ECM), mainly collagen and proteoglycans, in association with the disorganization of both the collagen and elastin fibers, together with the relative loss of certain cells that are essential for the normal function of the affected tissues (e.g., smooth muscle, cardiomyocytes, myofibers) *(6,38)*. The result is a pronounced reduction in the cellular/collagen balance that may occur by the increase in collagen synthesis, reduction in collagen breakdown, and a decrease in cellular replication or induction of apoptosis. One of the main features of fibrosis is the appearance of new cell types, such as myofibroblasts, stellate cells, and mastocytes, that are actively involved in excessive collagen synthesis, contraction, or other abnormal processes with a tendency to replace the normal cellular milieu *(30–41)*. Fibrosis is usually triggered by an injury or other types of (endogenous or exogenous) insults that lead initially to an acute and later to a chronic inflammatory process that is considered to be critical in the overproduction of profibrotic factors *(42)*.

Although a number of growth and differentiation factors have been identified in the literature in most fibrotic conditions, it is transforming growth factor-β_1 (TGF-β_1) that has emerged as one of the key agents responsible for triggering the initial stages of fibrosis and its progression *(43–45)*. This protein is a multifunctional regulator of cellular activity that is maintained as a large (210-kDa) latent complex composed of (1) the noncovalently bound mature 25-kDa protein homodimer of two 12.5-kDa chains, which are cleaved at the carboxy terminus from a 53-kDa monomeric precursor; (2) the 40-kDa N-terminal protein processed from the precursor, named latency-associated protein (LAP); and (3) a 125- to 160-kDa protein named TGF-β_1-binding protein. The cleavage of the mature protein 12.5-kDa monomeric chains from the precursor by proteolysis (furins) and the release from the noncovalent link to the large complex are necessary steps for TGF-β_1 activation and are therefore potential targets for antifibrotic strategies since only the mature protein is able to bind to the TGF-β receptor.

TGF-β_1 belongs to a large family of proteins, the TGF-β_1 "superfamily," that is critical in cellular proliferation, differentiation, apoptosis, epithelial-mesenchymal transition, and production of ECM and includes TGF-β_2 and -β_3, the bone morphogenic proteins (BMPs), and myostatin, among many others (46,47). However, with the possible exception of myostatin and of BMPs in ossification, only TGF-β_1 acts as a major profibrotic factor that exerts its biological functions mainly through its downstream signaling molecules human mothers against decapentaplegic (Smad)-2 and, in particular, Smad-3 (43, 45). TGF-β1 also plays a key role in mediating fibrotic tissue remodeling by increasing the production and decreasing the degradation of connective tissue via several mechanisms. TGF-β_1 is a strong activator of collagen I synthesis and inducer of myofibroblast transition and, paradoxically, has powerful anti-inflammatory actions (45). This is important to consider because as in the case of nitric oxide (NO) and many other pleiotropic agents, TGF-β_1 may be either beneficial or deleterious in the context of fibrosis development, depending on the level of its overproduction/activation and the tissue milieu.

The identification by Lue's group in 1997 (48) of the association of TGF-β_1 overexpression, as measured by quantitative Western blot, with the typical focal or diffused elastosis, fenestration, and disorganization of the collagen bundles in the human PD plaque, was the first demonstration that this critical profibrotic factor was overexpressed in PD. In this setting, TGF-β_2 and TGF-β_3 protein expression was not enhanced. Another report had previously shown in the aging rat penis increasing TGF-β_1 expression by enzyme-linked immunosorbent assay, although at low levels (49). It was subsequently shown that TGF-β_1 could actually induce a PD-like condition in the rat, by injecting, into the tunica albuginea, a synthetic heptopeptide with TGF-β-like activity (cytomodulin) (23), thus leading to the development of the first animal model for PD. Chronic and cellular infiltration, focal and diffuse elastosis, thickening, disorganization, and clumping of the collagen bundles were associated with TGF-β_1 protein expression by 6 wk in this cytomodulin-injected rat model. Like that of the human plaque tissue, no TGF-β_2 or TGF-β_3 protein was observed in this animal model.

As in any other animal model, the histology of the PD-like plaque may not be absolutely identical to the one in the human condition, but it does strikingly resemble the latter, as demonstrated by ultrastructural changes denoting densely packed collagen, fragmented and scarce elastic fibers, separation of neuronal fibers by interposing clumps of packed collagen, and perivascular collagen deposition (21). Interestingly, trauma per se to the rat tunica albuginea via a surgical incision initially produces increased TGF-β_1 expression, but as in a normal wound elsewhere in the body, TGF-β_1 expression ceases, and a PD-like lesion does not ensue. This suggests that only a high self-sustained and localized TGF-β_1 expression will induce a plaque (50), resembling the acute phase of human PD. Injection of TGF-β_1 per se into the tunica albuginea, rather than cytomodulin, can also induce a PD-like plaque after 6 wk. When colchicine was given either together or subsequent to the TGF-β_1 injection, both TGF-β_1 expression and plaque size were reduced, with the most reduction seen at the earliest treatment with the colchicine (22).

The TGF-β_1-induced rat model of PD has been extensively used by two other groups to study additional aspects of PD pathophysiology (23–27), as discussed below. The resulting fibrotic process has also been further characterized by showing that the levels of the

immature form of collagen, collagen III, as measured by quantitative histochemistry by
Sirius red, increased in comparison to the levels of collagen I *(27)*. This observation in
the rat is in agreement with the initial determinations found in human plaque by two
other groups *(51,52)* but differs from a reported decrease in the collagen III/I ratio *(53)*,
probably because of the different procedures utilized to detect both collagen forms.
Although the determination of total collagen as measured by hydroxyproline *(24)* and
of collagen I and III messenger RNAs (mRNAs) by reverse transcriptase polymerase
chain reaction and DNA microarrays *(35,54)* showed an increase in collagen levels in
the human PD plaque as compared to the normal tunica albuginea, this observation has
so far not been conducted in the PD-like plaque in animal models. This is because the
animal model produces a very small plaque size, and this imposed that most determinations had to be performed on tissue sections by quantitative image analysis of Masson
trichrome staining *(24–27)*. It is not known whether other forms of collagen, like collagen V, which is present in the human plaque *(53)*, accumulate in the PD-like plaque
of the rat model.

FIBRIN/PAI-1 SYSTEM AND THE DEVELOPMENT
OF A SECOND ANIMAL MODEL OF PD

Another series of profibrotic factors that have been extensively characterized, particularly in the context of lung, kidney, and vascular fibrosis, are the ones related to the
fibrin/plasminogen activator inhibitor 1 (PAI-1) system *(55,56)*. Plasmin, the enzyme
responsible for fibrinolysis, favors the degradation of the ECM, either directly by removing glycoproteins from ECM or by activating matrix metalloproteinases (MMPs) that
break down collagen *(57,58)*. PAI-1 may prevent ECM degradation by blocking MMPs
and by inhibiting fibrinolysis through the blockade of plasminogen activator (t-PA)
activity. This leads to fibrin accumulation and exacerbation of fibrosis *(56,57)*.

In pulmonary fibrosis, fibrinogen participates in the activation and migration of fibroblasts and provides a fibrin scaffold for cell migration following induction of an acute
lung injury. The subsequent fibrinous intrapleural matrix leads to pleural fibrosis, which
ultimately results from disordered fibrin turnover, by which fibrin formation is upregulated
and fibrin breakdown is downregulated *(55,57)*. TGF-β and tumor necrosis factor (TNF)-
α facilitate the fibrin matrix formation. Fibrinogen and fibrin upregulate PAI-1, which
as discussed for TGF-β_1 and NO, should not always be considered deleterious since it
may have a protective role during fibrin-dependent diseases, such as experimental glomerulonephritis and aortic atherosclerosis *(55)*. In this context, PAI-1 is required for the
regulation of plasminogen activator-dependent and plasmin-independent processes, and
its expression in vivo modulates inflammation, potentially by its capacity to occupy vitro-
nectin-binding sites *(55)*.

In the case of PD, fibrin has been suspected as one of the main factors triggering PD
ever since fibrin was detected in the majority of specimens of human PD even years after
the development of the plaque *(59–63)*. Indeed, histochemical staining and immunoblotting demonstrated that fibrin was present in 95% of human PD specimens. This led
to the hypothesis that trauma or microtrauma to the erect penis with extravasation of
fibrin into the tunica albuginea was the initial triggering factor of an abnormal wound
healing process that eventually causes plaque formation *(61–63)*. Fibrinogen and fibrin
would trigger the initial acute inflammation process and the subsequent release of profibrotic factors. Fibrin would persist by the inactivation or inaccessibility of the fibrin-

olytic system, and this would impair wound formation and cause fibrosis. In other words, the PD plaque was seen as a scar *(61–64)*.

Based on these observations and assumptions, a new animal model was developed in which the PD-like plaque was not induced by TGF-β_1 injection into the tunica albuginea, but by a fibrin-generating preparation that clots within the tissue *(28)*. The immediate fibrin formation was seen as essential, rather than the simple injection of soluble fibrinogen, to trap the fibrogenic deposit within the tunica for a sufficient length of time. In this model, the process of plaque formation, as denoted by Masson trichrome and when compared to the TGF-β_1 model, was considerably accelerated (3 wk) after an early stage of acute inflammation. This was accompanied by the persistence of fibrin within the tunica as detected by both histochemistry and immunohistochemistry. Interestingly, TGF-β_1 was considerably expressed in the fibrin-induced PD-like plaque, and from this it was postulated that the fibrin-induced plaque was most likely mediated by TGF-β_1 expression. This study also furnished an explanation for the fibrin persistence by showing by (1) immunocytochemistry that PAI-1 was considerably increased in the PD-like plaque and by (2) Northern and Western blots that there were high levels of PAI-1 mRNA and protein in the human PD plaque *(29)*. Although PAI-1 is likely to act as a profibrotic agent in PD, the possibility remains that in the initial stage of acute inflammation, as is postulated in the kidney *(55)*, it may be an anti-inflammatory factor.

Some clinical studies have put in doubt the trauma origin of PD by either indicating the absence of the patient's recollection of a traumatic episode during sexual activity *(4)* or conversely by showing that a very strenuous torsion of the erect penis practiced by some ethnic groups *(65)* was not associated with a higher incidence of PD. This serves as a warning that the cause–effect relationship is not easy to demonstrate in PD, on one side because microtrauma may occur and still not become obvious to the patient, and on the other hand because there may be an ethnic difference in the susceptibility to translate an injury to the tunica albuginea into an abnormal wound-healing process. The association of PD with Dupuytren's disease and other conditions suggests that a genetic or immune-related process may determine predisposition to localized fibrosis in certain anatomical locations, and this may modulate the reaction after trauma or microtrauma. In this context, it should be reminded that PD occurs in 11% of patients after radical prostatectomy, a traumatic process that may lead to distant clot formation in the penis and even affect paracrinely the tunica albuginea *(66)*.

Chronic Inflammation, Oxidative Stress, and Fibrosis in PD

One of the most significant concepts that has recently evolved in pathophysiology is the recognition that (1) vascular complications of type 2 diabetes and aging such as atherosclerosis, hypertension, and arteriosclerosis; (2) some nephropathies; as well as (3) fatty liver disease are chronic inflammatory conditions leading to localized or generalized fibrosis in the affected tissue, and that oxidative stress is a major factor in this process *(67–70)*. This occurs via the production of reactive oxygen species (ROS) through oxidative enzymes such as xanthine oxidoreductase (XOR) or nicotinamide adenine dinucleotide oxidase in a process counteracted by antioxidant enzymes such as superoxide dismutase (SOD), hemeoxygenase I, catalase, or glutathione peroxidase/reductase *(71)*. ROS comprise free radicals such as superoxide ($O_2^{\bullet-}$) anion, hydrogen peroxide (H_2O_2), and hydroxyl ($OH^{\bullet}$) and peroxyl ($ROO^{\bullet}$) and can be measured directly in blood or tissues by the quantitation of the reduced/oxidized glutathione ratio (GSH/GSSG) of malonaldialdehyde or in tissues by a series of fluorescent probes or luminol-induced chemoluminescence. The indirect determination of ROS in tissues is based on the immunohistochemical detection of oxidant or antioxidant enzyme expression coupled to quantitative image analysis or the Western blot estimation of the levels of the respective enzymes.

In the case of diabetes, hyperglycemia promotes ROS formation, and angiotensin II is also a powerful ROS generator via the angotensin 1 receptor *(70)*. ROS induces peroxidation of lipids and subsequent membrane damage. Products of lipid peroxidation, such as 4-hydroxynonenal, stimulate collagen synthesis and are also toxic to the mitochondria *(72)*. This aggravates oxidative stress that contributes to endothelial dysfunction and to vascular wall permeability, leukocyte infiltration, tissue hypertrophy/proliferation, and fibrosis by stimulating nuclear factor (NF)κB and by upregulating adhesion molecules, cytokines, and chemokines, specifically TGF-β1, which also stimulates collagen deposition *(73)*.

The influence of chronic inflammation in the generation of the human PD plaque has been well documented through numerous reports showing an acute inflammatory phase that persists for 6–18 months, involving perivascular infiltration of lymphocytes, monocytes, and neutrophils, followed by a chronic phase persisting for years *(2)*. The early acute inflammation is recapitulated in the rat models of PD, and it is a process in both species that is conceivably maintained by the constant release of cytokines and other proinflammatory agents. This inflammatory response is critical for the generation of ROS *(71)*, and this has been shown by the increase in hemeoxygenase I immunostaining in both human PD and in the TGF-β-induced PD-like plaque in the rat in parallel to the increase in the content and disorganization of collagen fibers *(24–27)*. A similar association of oxidative stress and fibrosis in the fibrin-induced PD-like plaque was demonstrated by measuring the increase of both XOR and SOD *(28–30)* and by the fact that therapies that reduced the plaque in any of the animal models were accompanied by a decrease in oxidative stress, whereas interventions that exacerbated collagen deposition led to a parallel increase in ROS-related enzymes *(24–27)*.

Obviously, many cytokines and ancillary factors other than TGF-β are produced during inflammation by ROS/NFκB activation of their gene transcription, and the control of the inflammatory response may retard the fibrotic plaque formation. The application of DNA microarrays to discern which of these inflammatory factors and the respective downstream fibrotic genes are elevated in the PD plaque in comparison to the normal tunica albuginea has started to provide some valuable information *(35,54)*. DNA microarrays allow the determination of the differential profiles of multiple gene expressions that are altered in a given specimen as compared to its control. In a study using the Clontech Atlas Array for 1200 genes as well as the Affymetrix GeneChip for more than 10,000 genes, some mRNAs for proinflammatory genes were detected as upregulated in the PD plaque, mainly monocyte chemotactic protein 1 (MCP-1), whereas TGF-β modulators were downregulated *(54)*.

The observation regarding MCP-1 was confirmed in two other studies *(74,75)*, but surprisingly MCP-1 was not found upregulated in a larger cohort where PD plaque changes over the normal tunica albuginea were compared with Dupuytren's tissue against normal ligament using DNA microarrays *(35)*. This suggests that inflammation is not necessarily present at all stages of PD, but it also supports the view that the identification by DNA microarrays and proteomics of profibrotic pathways other than the fibrin-ROS-TGF-β cascade should be conducted on animal models to try to find novel therapeutic targets that may be operative in PD. The problem in conducting such studies is that human PD tissue specimens are usually obtained surgically well beyond the early acute inflammatory phase. It may be possible to circumvent this issue by studying the PD-like plaque at different stages of development in the animal models of PD.

Collagen Breakdown and Matrix Metalloproteinases in Human PD

Most of the emphasis in the study of fibrotic processes has been placed on the factors that trigger collagen synthesis and generate, mostly in fibroblasts, myofibroblasts, and smooth muscle cells, the synthetic cellular phenotype producing collagen. However, a very important aspect in fibrosis is the fact that collagen breakdown may be inhibited, either by inadequate functioning of the enzyme system responsible for collagen degradation, the MMPs (58,73,76,77), or by crosslinking of collagen fibers that block the effect of the MMPs (16,78,79). There are about 20 MMPs, identified by numbers, and the ones most involved in the physiological degradation of collagen I are collagenase 1 (MMP-1) and collagenase 3 (MMP-13) and to a lesser degree MMP-2, -8, and -14. For collagen III, they are mainly MMP-1, -3, -10, and -13. MMPs are induced by TGF-β_1 and interleukin 1, which also stimulate their processing from larger precursors named latent MMPs or zymogens.

MMPs can be inhibited by specific inhibitors named TIMP-1 and -2 (tissue inhibitors of metalloproteinases 1 and 2), as well as by fibrinolytic inhibitors such as PAI-1, and therefore overexpression of MMPs may occur in fibrosis in the presence of defective collagen breakdown because of higher levels of the MMP inhibitors. For this reason, it is convenient to estimate MMP expression by Western blot or immunohistochemistry and MMP enzyme activity by different procedures such as zymography or special enzyme-linked immunosorbent assay and enzyme activity kits that detect specific MMPs. These procedures have allowed the identification of defective MMP activity or expression in a number of fibrotic conditions, such as liver fibrosis, hypertension, cardiac failure, arthritis, and others (7,76). However, in myocardial infarction, in atherosclerotic plaques, and in other vascular pathologies, the converse process of MMP induction (i.e., the activation of zymogens or the decrease of MMP inhibitors) leads at times to noxious excessive collagen degradation and inadequate tissue remodeling (11,80).

In conditions such as aging and diabetes, excessive amounts of advanced glycation end products (AGEs) are formed and react with proteins, particularly collagen, and in diabetes their formation is greatly enhanced with rising hyperglycemia (16,78,79). This leads to tighter collagen fibers because of AGE crosslinks that render collagen much more resistant to proteolysis by MMPs, and clinically this presents as tissue fibrosis and rigidity.

Despite the potential of initiating collagen breakdown as a therapeutic approach to fibrosis, very little research has been conducted on this topic in PD other than the early trials of collagenase for trying to "soften" the PD plaque. These trials did not bear fruition against the PD plaque (81,82). The studies utilizing DNA microarrays identified a paradoxical increase of mRNAs for two species, MMP-2 and MMP-9, and of the peptides named thymosins, which act as MMP activators, specifically thymosin-β_{10} and -β_4, in both the PD plaque and the Dupuytren's nodules (35).

These results can be interpreted in two different ways: (1) an actual intensification of MMP activity triggers tissue remodeling, like in the cardiovascular system (11,80), which in this case would not be noxious but part of a spontaneous defense process opposing fibrosis (see below); or (2) an MMP transcriptional gene activation reacts against higher levels of MMP inhibitors, like the observed PAI-1 increase, that may not overcome the MMP inhibitors and would eventually lead to considerable downregulation of MMP activity and the decrease in collagen breakdown. Further investigation should be carried out in the human PD specimens and in the animal PD tissues to determine whether MMP activity is actually reduced in the fibrotic tissue because of an increase in PAI-1 or TIMP and whether this imbalance varies according to the progression of fibrosis. A preliminary study (83) showed in the human PD plaque an elevation of all four TIMPs as compared to the perilesional tunica, which seems to support the hypothesis that the elevation of MMP activity is a compensatory mechanism against an increase of MMP inhibitors.

A question that so far is unexplored is whether the collagen fibers *per se* in the PD plaque are more resistant to proteolytic breakdown through the formation of AGE crosslinks. This is important for two main reasons: (1) AGEs are intensified by oxidative stress even under normal glycemia, so that this would lend more credence to the hypothesis of oxidative stress as a key factor in the fibrotic process; and (2) it may justify the trial of agents in PD that would reduce the formation of collagen crosslinks or directly break down the ones already formed (see below).

CELL MEDIATORS OF FIBROSIS

Myofibroblasts, Abnormal Repair, and the PD Cell Culture Model

One of the aspects that is essential in the study of fibrosis is the interplay and interrelation of fibroblasts in the connective tissue with myofibroblasts, a cell type that has been the focus of considerable attention in the context of normal and abnormal wound healing and various fibrotic processes in different organs (10,38–40). The myofibroblast shares the phenotype of fibroblasts and smooth muscle cells, and this can be detected by the expression of two immunochemical markers: vimentin, which is present in both fibroblasts and myofibroblasts, and α-smooth muscle actin (ASMA), present in myofibroblasts only. Myofibroblasts, under the light microscope, display actin fibers and have projections to contiguous cells; under the electron microscope, they have a distinctive morphology with nuclear indentation. Myofibroblasts accumulate during wound healing, exercising the contractile force that helps to bring together the edges of the wound, and actively synthesize the collagen required for extracellular formation during tissue repair after injury. They normally disappear by apoptosis, but when they persist and continue synthesizing collagen, an excessive scar is formed.

In most fibrotic conditions, the appearance and subsequent persistence of myofibroblasts are linked to the development of fibrosis, and although their origin is uncertain, they are thought to derive from fibroblasts, endothelial cells, or stem cells (10,38–40). In the case of the liver, myofibroblasts are postulated to originate from hepatic stellate cells, located between parenchymal cell plates and sinusoidal endothelial cells, in a differentiation or "activation" in which the stellate cells lose the lipid droplets and long processes (41), although this view has been challenged (84).

The presence of the myofibroblast in PD was initially established in 1978 (85), a few years after the discovery of this cell type by Gabbiani (38–40). Myofibroblasts were obtained in cell culture from the PD plaque in 1982, showing the typical actin cable formation, surface membrane blebs, nuclear indentation, and microvilli (86). Rather surprisingly, virtually no detailed studies of the myofibroblast in the context of PD were made for the next 15 yr, despite the abundant literature in an associated condition, Dupuytren's disease (87). One study in 1997 described the myofibroblasts in the PD plaque (88), and another one referred to "myofibroblast" cultures, although it is not clear whether they were different from corpora cavernosa smooth muscle cells *(89)*. In a series of subsequent reports, the role of the myofibroblast in PD was "rediscovered" by demonstrating that whereas myofibroblasts were virtually absent in the normal human tunica albuginea, their number, as determined by quantitative image analysis and Western blot for ASMA, was considerably increased in the PD plaque *(24,25)*, and that the same occurred in both the TGF-β_1-induced and the fibrin-induced PD-like plaque in the rat models, in comparison to saline-injected tunica *(24–30)*. Moreover, myofibroblasts were even more abundant when the size of the plaque and the level of oxidative stress were increased by experimental manipulation (*see* below) *(25–30)*.

Because the human tunica albuginea can be easily dissected, whereas the rat tunica is much more difficult to obtain, cell cultures have been developed from both the normal tissue and the PD plaque *(25,31–37)* and from the rat tunica albuginea and extensively characterized, showing that they contain a variable proportion of myofibroblasts within an essentially fibroblast population. These cells synthesize collagen I and III, fibroblast growth factor, and some of these processes are stimulated by incubation with TGF-β_1 *(25, 36)*. One of the laboratories studying these cultures has demonstrated: "(a) consistent morphologic transformation; (b) increased S-phase on flow cytometry; (c) decreased dependence on culture medium; (d) cytogenic instability; (e) excess production of fibrogenic cytokines; and (f) stabilization and dysfunctionalization of p53" *(31–34)*.

In addition, the human PD plaque, when compared with the tunica albuginea tissue by DNA microarrays, showed upregulation of early growth response protein, which is an activator of fibroblast proliferation, and of the myofibroblast markers α- and γ-smooth muscle actin, desmin, RhoGDP dissociation inhibitor, and others *(35)*.

Human Tunica Albuginea, Stem Cells, and Ossification in the PD Plaque

A stage in the progression of fibrosis that presents in certain tissues, such as the skeletal muscle or the arterial wall, is *ossification* or *calcification*, during which there are deposits of calcium that eventually evolve into the formation of a bonelike tissue, in which osteoblasts and markers of osteogenic differentiation are identified *(89,90)*. The mechanism of this ectopic ossification is unknown, although it is assumed that fibroblasts in the interstitial tissue of the skeletal muscle or in the adventitia of the arterial wall harbor stem cells that can differentiate into localized osteoblasts. In the arterial tree in particular, calcification is very prevalent in type 2 diabetes and aging, and this may be related to the persistent hyperglycemia and oxidative stress, respectively *(90)*. The presence of stem cells in adult tissues, also named *multipotent* cells (able to originate more than one cell lineage) to differentiate them from embryonic *totipotent* or *pluripotent* cells (able to originate all or most cell lineages), is well established *(91,92)*. The activation of resident "dormant" stem cells in the muscle may explain (1) fibrosis through their differentiation into myofibroblasts and other ancillary cell types, like keratinocytes in the skin, or (2) ectopic ossification through their differentiation into osteoblasts.

Ossification occurs in about a quarter of patients who have a palpable PD plaque *(93, 94)*, and there is some controversy whether the calcification can extend into the corpora cavernosa smooth muscle *(95)*. An in vitro study has shown the presence of stem cells in the human tunica albuginea and PD plaque *(36)* as identified in their respective cell cultures by (1) stem cell markers; (2) the ability to grow in soft agar, a clonogenic assay (only the PD cells); (3) their differentiation into myofibroblasts, smooth muscle cells, and osteoblasts; and (4) the secretion of paracrine factors that can modulate the differentiation of other multipotent cells in dual cultures. Specifically, the osteoblastlike cells were detected by immunocytochemistry, Western blot, and reverse transcriptase polymerase chain reaction using markers such as alkaline phosphatase, BMP-2 and osteopontin, and their formation was stimulated by TGF-β_1, implying that this cytokine triggers osteogenesis (as well as myofibroblast differentiation and fibrosis) and may be involved in in vivo ossification of PD plaques.

Formation of osteoblastlike cells in vitro occurs to about the same extent from fibroblasts derived from either normal tunica or PD plaques, and the normal tunical fibroblasts secrete differentiation factors similar to the ones produced by the PD plaque. This indicates that normal tissue is, *per se*, prone to fibrosis and ossification through transformation of endogenous cells, and this process is not dependent on migration of stem cells, myofibroblasts, or progenitor cells to the site of plaque development. This poses the interesting question of the relationship of the tunica albuginea with the corporal smooth muscle that hypothetically may be equated to the one between the adventitia and the media in the arterial wall as a source of stem cell differentiation and migration *(96)* since the penis and the corporal tissue specifically are in fact an extension of the vascular tree. If this is the case, then the tunical stem cells may be speculated to act as reservoirs for replenishing the corporal smooth muscle cells that are lost by apoptosis during aging, or alternatively on injury to the tunica, they would undergo conversion to myofibroblasts and fibrosis in the tunica (PD plaque) and at later stages conversion into osteoblasts (ossified plaque). This would resemble the putative adventitia/media interactions in arteriosclerosis and calcified atherosclerotic plaques.

In addition to the presence of stem cells, the PD cultures, but not the normal tunica albuginea cultures, harbor cells that appear to be malignant, as shown by the following lines of evidence: (1) PD cells can form colonies on soft agar *(36)*, a feature not only shared by stem cells but also may be suggestive of the presence of malignant cells; (2) the presence of aneusomies, recurrent deletions of the Y chromosome, and other chromosomal abnormalities that progress during culture, although these features are also present in tunical fibroblasts *(32)*; (3) prolonged S phase (DNA replication) and inactivation of the antitumor p53 gene, features that are consistent with uncontrolled replication *(34)*; and (4) the more direct demonstration that immunodeficient mice developed subcutaneous tumors when injected with PD cells but not with normal tunica cells *(33)*. This poses the question regarding why no penile tumors are associated with PD, even if myofibroblasts themselves can be responsible for the development of benign lesions (myofibroblastomas), locally aggressive fibromatosis (similar to PD), and even low-grade and high-grade sarcomas *(97)*.

ENDOGENOUS ANTIFIBROTIC MECHANISMS AND NEW THERAPEUTIC TARGETS FOR PEYRONIE'S DISEASE

Inducible Nitric Oxide Synthase/NO/ROS Balance in PD Plaque Development

The regression of fibrosis was considered until recently as a very rare event since fibrosis steadily progresses with time. However, more recently, regression of fibrosis has been claimed to occur occasionally in liver and kidney fibrosis *(98,99)*, and the mechanism may be assumed to involve the activation of a series of antifibrotic pathways that may overcome the effect of the profibrotic factors. Although these endogenous mechanisms of defense are not known, there is considerable evidence that NO may be one of the antifibrotic factors, at least in the case of heart and kidney fibrosis, based on the fact that (1) inhibition of nitric oxide synthases (NOSs) by isoform-unspecific inhibitors exacerbate fibrosis *(100,101)*, and (2) administration of L-arginine or gene transfer of NOS complementary DNAs (cDNAs) can ameliorate this process *(102–104)*.

The identity of the NOS isoforms involved in producing "antifibrotic" NO is not clear, but the inducible NOS (iNOS), which is not normally expressed in healthy tissues, is overexpressed in most inflammatory conditions and many fibrotic processes *(17,105,106)*. iNOS is regulable transcriptionally by the activation of its gene promoter by cytokines through a NFκB mechanism. This leads to a steady output of NO at supraphysiological levels, as opposed to the brief pulses released through the enzymatic activation of neuronal NOS during neurotransmission or the more prolonged synthesis of relatively low levels of NO by the enzymatic activation of endothelial NOS. It has been shown that the blockade of iNOS expression in the iNOS(–/–) mouse is associated with increased fibrosis of (1) the kidney after ureteral ligation *(107)*, (2) the liver following a high-fat diet *(108)*, and (3) the lung after ovalbumin instillation *(109)*.

In the case of PD, although in general the tunical plaques undergo progression in terms of their size and increasing curvature of the erect penis, it is assumed anecdotally that about 5–15% of PD plaques undergo spontaneous regression. As in other fibrotic processes, the mechanism is unknown, but evidence obtained by the application of DNA microarrays has suggested that, in both the PD plaques and the Dupuytren's nodules, an active tissue turnover occurs at both the cellular and the molecular levels; this summarized in the next section.

Within the context of beneficial fibrotic tissue remodeling, one of the plausible defense reactions is the production of NO through the cytokine-induced expression of iNOS. This process was shown to occur in the human PD plaque *(24)* and in the two animal models *(24–29)* by detecting iNOS in the fibrotic tunical tissue and showing a considerable increase in nitrotyrosine linked to proteins when compared to the normal tunica. Nitrotyrosine is an indicator of the generation of peroxynitrite, a product of the reaction of NO produced from iNOS with ROS. Therefore, the higher levels of nitrotyrosine in the tissue are a fingerprint of ROS quenching by NO, and this suggests that, by reducing oxidative stress, iNOS acts as an antifibrotic factor since peroxynitrite by itself does not seem to be profibrotic. In other words, the balance between the respective levels of NO and ROS, or between the downstream nitrosative and oxidative pathways, may modulate the development of the fibrotic plaque.

The support for the above-stated hypothesis comes from three other lines of evidence:

1. When iNOS was inhibited by *N*-iminoethyl-L-lysine (L-NIL), there was an increase in fibrosis as measured by the increase in the collagen/cellular area in the tunica, the stimulation of the collagen 1α promoter, the increase in profibrotic markers such as TGF-β$_1$ and PAI-1, higher oxidative stress as indicated by the increase in XOR and hemeoxygenase I, and the stimulation of fibroblast/myofibroblast differentiation measured by ASMA expression, when the activity of iNOS was specifically inhibited by long-term oral administration of L-NIL to the TGF-β$_1$ model of PD from the initiation of plaque development *(24,25)*.
2. Long-term oral L-NIL also intensifies fibrosis in both the penis (corpora cavernosa and penile artery) and the media of the vascular tree in aged rats *(17)*.

3. An increase in apoptosis in the PD-like tissue (presumably myofibroblasts) when either a cDNA for iNOS is injected into the tunica albuginea or long-term oral L-arginine (NOS substrate) was given to the fibrin-induced or the TGF-β_1-induced rat models (26,30).

The translation of these observations in the penis and vascular tree into a therapeutic clinical approach would require additional studies in animals utilizing long-term oral NO donors (110) and investigation of the antifibrotic mechanism in depth by demonstrating that (1) ROS is decreased in the tissue by NO through the formation of peroxynitrite, and this correlates with the inhibition of plaque development and specifically collagen synthesis; (2) NO may also favor collagen degradation by stimulating MMP activity; (3) there are no noxious effects of long-term NO release, such as stimulation of smooth muscle apoptosis or induction of priapism.

cGMP and Phosphodiesterase 5 Inhibitors in PD-Like Plaque in the Animal Models

The main downstream product of NO synthesis is cyclic guanosine monophosphate (cGMP) through the activation of guanylylcyclase by NO (7,105). This reaction in the smooth muscle of the penile corpora cavernosa and the media of the penile arteries is responsible for penile erection by the production of NO through activation of penile neuronal nitric oxide synthase (PnNOS) in the nerve terminals and endothelial NOS in the endothelial lining of the blood vessels and possibly the corporal cisternae of the penis. The currently available phosphodiesterase 5 (PDE-5) inhibitors (sildenafil, vardenafil, and tadalafil) increase the levels of cGMP by inhibiting its breakdown by PDE-5 (27).

Besides NO, cGMP also seems to act in certain conditions as an antifibrotic agent. This is evidenced by its inhibitory effect on collagen synthesis, myofibroblast differentiation, and AGE formation in cell cultures from tissues such as the heart and kidney (111,112) and by the demonstration that when sildenafil is given every other night for 6 mo following radical retropubic prostatectomy, it seems to prevent the fibrosis of the corpora cavernosa that may occur after this type of surgery (113). The cGMP-related effects may also result from activation of soluble guanylyl cyclase since a specific inhibitor reduced glomerulosclerosis in the rat (114). Higher cGMP levels from PDE-5 inhibition or guanylylguanylyl cyclase activation stimulate protein kinase G, an enzyme with antifibrotic effects since protein kinase G gene transfer also reduces collagen synthesis (115).

In the case of PD, it has been shown that cGMP inhibited collagen synthesis and myofibroblast differentiation and stimulated apoptosis in the cultures described above that were derived from human PD plaques and normal tunica albuginea (26). In addition, it was shown that long-term continuous administration of high doses of sildenafil prevented the development of the PD-like plaque in the TGF-β_1 rat model of PD, and that the target enzyme, PDE-5A, is expressed not only in the penile corpora cavernosa but also in the human and rat tunica albuginea and PD tissues and their respective fibroblast cultures (26). Oral long-term pentoxifylline, a nonspecific PDE inhibitor, exerted effects similar to sildenafil in this scenario.

A study has extended those findings by showing that long-term continuous or discontinuous oral administration of a moderate dose of vardenafil prevented the development of the PD-like fibrotic plaque in the TGF-β_1 rat model of PD and reduced the size of a preformed plaque (27). There was a marked decrease in the collagen/smooth muscle ratio and the collagen III/I ratio, accompanied by a similar reduction in the number of cells expressing TGF-β_1 and in the number of myofibroblasts, with a concomitant increase in the apoptotic index, presumably in myofibroblasts; this was restricted to this tissue since the corpora smooth muscle was not affected. It was proposed that these effects were mediated by the inhibition of PDE-5 present in the tunica albuginea, thus maintaining the high levels of cGMP produced by the spontaneous induction of iNOS. cGMP would reduce collagen synthesis by downregulating TGF-β_1 expression, thus reducing myofibroblast differentiation, and by inducing myofibroblast apoptosis, which would further reduce myofibroblast number. Both downregulatory effects would then decrease collagen synthesis in a process that would add to the direct reduction by NO of collagen synthesis and of the levels of the profibrotic ROS.

Antioxidants and Other Therapeutic Approaches Based on Endogenous Mechanisms of Defense

The induction of antioxidant enzymes, mainly SOD, appears to be an important mechanism in the reaction of tissues against oxidative stress induced by hyperglycemia, inflammatory processes, smoking, and many other conditions and its downstream consequences, particularly within the cardiovascular system *(67–69)*. This has led to a series of preventive clinical trial therapies to reduce the risk of atherosclerosis and vascular disease in general based on the administration of vitamin E and other antioxidants *(115,116)*. Failure to show an improvement is often assumed to derive from incorrect dosage, age at treatment, inadequate antioxidant agent, and other factors rather than disproving the oxidative stress theory.

Similarly, other endogenous mechanisms of fibrosis, or of defense mechanisms against this process, are under study as potential targets for the development of new therapeutic options, and some are focused on the fibroblasts and myofibroblasts *(10)* and TGF-β_1 *(117)*. Since it has been documented that decorin, a small leucine-rich proteoglycan that binds to the TGF-β_1 receptor, is produced during fibrosis *(117–119)*, several animal trials have been conducted with this product. Analogous therapeutic approaches are under testing with neutralizing antibodies against TGF-β_1 by giving compounds such as Smad-7 that block the Smad signaling pathway that is activated by TGF-β_1, by the inhibition of the proteolytic processing of its precursor, or by the release from its large complex *(44, 45,117,118)*. A member of the TGF-β family, BMP-7, is under study in the treatment of renal fibrosis *(120)*.

On the other hand, the activation of MMPs, or the counteraction of TIMPs and even PAI-1, are under exploration *(7,76)*. Perhaps one of the most promising interventions is to act either preventively to reduce the production of AGEs in the case of aging- and diabetes-related vascular fibrosis, which has already been shown to lead to collagen crosslinks and resistance to its breakdown by MMPs, or therapeutically by breaking those established crosslinks with compounds such as alagebrium chloride (ALT-711) *(16,78,79)*.

In the case of PD, the relative failure for advanced stages of the disease of previous antioxidant therapies such as vitamin E *(121)* has not deterred investigations with other approaches, and it should be considered in combination with pentoxifylline, as used for the treatment of radiation fibrosis *(122)*. Pentoxifylline, an isoform-unspecific PDE inhibitor, reduced considerably the TGF-β_1-induced plaque development in the animal model *(26)*. Considering also that this drug may be effective for the treatment of kidney and lung fibrosis *(123)*, it may be worth investigating whether the vitamin E/pentoxifylline combination may not only prevent but also regress the PD-like plaque in the animal models.

An interesting example of antioxidant therapy for PD is a study that was based on the application of recombinant human SOD in a liposome encapsulation as a topical gel that can reach the plaque in the treatment of the painful stage of PD in an attempt to combat inflammation rather than fibrosis *per se* *(124)*. Thirty-nine patients with PD and significant pain symptoms were treated with SOD or placebo for a 4-wk period, followed by a cross-over study design to ensure a total of 8 wk of SOD therapy. Pain, plaque, and curvature assessment was performed at study entry and every 4 wk until completion. Although the reduction of plaque size, consistency, and penile curvature, as compared to placebo, was not conclusive, the alleviation of pain and the statement of patient satisfaction were very significant. Since SOD cDNA has ameliorated erectile dysfunction in the aged rat model *(125)*, these clinical results should encourage the refinement of this approach in the animal models of PD to try to achieve plaque reduction.

On the other hand, decorin mRNA has been found consistently increased in human PD and Dupuytren's nodules *(35)*, suggesting that this is another mechanism of defense against the development of the plaque that may be investigated in the animal models. The use of PAI-1 small interference RNA, which breaks down the mRNA and "silences" gene expression *(126)*, is another avenue to explore based on the findings of a consistent elevation of PAI-1 in both the human PD and the animal PD-like plaque tissues *(28,29)*. Another potential agent is thymosin-β_4, which together with other thymosins has been found to be increased (as mRNA) in the PD and Dupuytren's plaques *(35)*. In fact, thymosin-β_4 is hydrolyzed by prolyl oligopeptidase into Ac-SDKP, a ubiquitous antifibrotic tetrapeptide that in long-term treatment decreases cardiac and renal fibrosis and inflammatory cell infiltration in hypertensive rats *(127)*. Therefore, thymosin-β_4 may act as an antifibrotic via the production of acetyl-*N*-ser-asp-lys-pro (AcSDKP) and may stimulate MMP activity.

FUTURE DIRECTIONS

The animal models, imperfect as they are in terms of mimicking the human disease, and cell culture to a more restricted extent, provide an invaluable tool for exploring what we believe are fundamental questions in the pathophysiology and medical therapy of PD: (1) to define the cellular and molecular markers of disease progression; (2) to demonstrate directly the role of the myofibroblast in the fibrotic development and the less-prevalent osteogenic phase of the disease and how to reduce their number by selectively stimulating their apoptosis; (3) to improve gel formulation in drug preparations to facilitate a noninvasive release of traditional and novel therapeutic agents; and (4) to utilize a combination of drugs and routes of administration, rather than a single agent, to reduce chronic inflammation and pain while stimulating the breakdown of the collagen fibers and the resolution of ectopic ossification if present. The last strategy could mean improving previous single-agent treatments that were not effective or only partially effective, such as collagenase or SOD, with novel strategies such as AGE crosslink breakers, NO donors, PDE inhibitors, and selected MMP formulations.

A more complex aspect that may not be addressed with experimental models of PD is the clarification on whether systemic factors, such as predisposing genes of autoimmune processes, cause the onset and progression of the disease in certain individuals (e.g., trauma to the erect penis). However, the animal and cell models may help to define the paracrine influences that processes not directly injuring the tunica albuginea may exert on the tunical fibroblasts and lead to PD, such as those that may occur after penile nerve damage subsequent to radical prostatectomy. But, the most important lesson from these models is that the study of a neglected condition, PD, that consistently fails to attract the attention of funding agencies may end up constituting a model for the extrapolation of novel therapeutic targets to other urogenital fibroses. It is not too speculative to assume that findings in PD may even be applicable to nonurological disorders in which chronic inflammation, fibrosis, and ossification are main pathophysiological determinants of the severity and consequences of the disease.

ACKNOWLEDGMENTS

The work conducted by us and our associates that is cited in this review has been essentially funded by National Institutes of Health grant R01DK-53069 and by grants from the Eli and Edythe Broad Foundation and from Bayer Corporation and in certain aspects by National Institute of Health grants G12RR-03026 and 5P20MD000545.

REFERENCES

1. Gonzalez-Cadavid NF, Rajfer J. New insights on the cellular and molecular pathology of Peyronie's disease. Nature Clin Pract Urol 2005; 2: 291–298.
2. Gholami SS, Gonzalez-Cadavid NF, Lin C-S, Rajfer J, Lue TF. Peyronie's disease: a review. J Urol 2002; 169: 1234–1241.
3. Mulhall JP, Creech SD, Boorjian SA, et al. Subjective and objective analysis of the prevalence of Peyronie's disease in a population of men presenting for prostate cancer screening. J Urol 2004; 171: 2350–2353.
4. Schwarzer U, Sommer F, Klotz T, Braun M, Reifenrath B, Engelmann U. The prevalence of Peyronie's disease: results of a large survey. BJU Int 2001; 88: 727–730.
5. Smith CJ, McMahon C, Shabsigh R. Peyronie's disease: the epidemiology, aetiology and clinical evaluation of deformity. BJU Int 2005; 95: 729–732.
6. Diegelmann RF, Evans MC. Wound healing: an overview of acute, fibrotic and delayed healing. Front Biosci 2004; 9: 283–289.
7. Gonzalez-Cadavid NF, Rajfer J. Therapy of erectile function: potential future treatments. Endocrine 2004; 23: 167–176.
8. Azadzoi KM, Schulman RN, Aviram M, Siroky MB. Oxidative stress in arteriogenic erectile dysfunction: prophylactic role of antioxidants. J Urol 2005; 174: 386–393.
9. Thurston AJ. Dupuytren's disease. J Bone Joint Surg Br 2003; 85: 469–477.
10. Brown RD, Ambler SK, Mitchell MD, Long CS. The cardiac fibroblast: therapeutic target in myocardial remodeling and failure. Annu Rev Pharmacol Toxicol 2005; 45: 657–687.
11. See F, Kompa A, Martin J, Lewis DA, Krum H. Fibrosis as a therapeutic target post-myocardial infarction. Curr Pharm Des 2005; 11: 477–487.
12. Moncrieff J, Lindsay MM, Dunn FG. Hypertensive heart disease and fibrosis. Curr Opin Cardiol 2004; 19: 326–331.
13. Lopez B, Gonzalez A, Diez J. Role of matrix metalloproteinases in hypertension-associated cardiac fibrosis. Curr Opin Nephrol Hypertens 2004; 13: 197–204.
14. Hirschberg R, Wang S. Proteinuria and growth factors in the development of tubulointerstitial injury and scarring in kidney disease. Curr Opin Nephrol Hypertens 2005; 14: 43–52.
15. Negri AL. Prevention of progressive fibrosis in chronic renal diseases: antifibrotic agents. J Nephrol 2004; 17: 496–503.
16. Susic D, Varagic J, Ahn J, Frohlich ED. Collagen cross-link breakers: a beginning of a new era in the treatment of cardiovascular changes associated with aging, diabetes, and hypertension. Curr Drug Targets Cardiovasc Haematol Disord 2004; 4: 97–101.
17. Ferrini MG, Davila H, Valente EG, Gonzalez-Cadavid NF, Rajfer J. Aging-related induction of inducible nitric oxide synthase (iNOS) is vasculo-protective in the arterial media. Cardiovascular Res 2004; 61: 796–805.
18. Lotersztajn S, Julien B, Teixeira-Clerc F, Grenard P, Mallat A. Hepatic fibrosis: molecular mechanisms and drug targets. Annu Rev Pharmacol Toxicol 2005; 45: 605–628.

19. Barnes PJ, Hansel TT. Prospects for new drugs for chronic obstructive pulmonary disease. Lancet 2004; 364: 985–996.
20. El-Sakka AI, Hassoba HM, Chui RM, Bhatnagar RS, Dahiya R, Lue TF. An animal model of Peyronie's-like condition associated with an increase of transforming growth factor β mRNA and protein expression. J Urol 1997; 158: 2284–2290.
21. El-Sakka AI, Hassan MU, Nunes L, Bhatnagar RS, Yen TS, Lue TF. Histological and ultrastructural alterations in an animal model of Peyronie's disease. Br J Urol 1998; 81: 445–452.
22. El-Sakka AI, Bakircioglu ME, Bhatnagar RS, Yen TS, Dahiya R, Lue TF. The effects of colchicine on a Peyronie's-like condition in an animal model. J Urol 1999; 161: 1980–1983.
23. Bivalacqua TJ, Champion HC, Leungwattanakij S, et al. Evaluation of nitric oxide synthase and arginase in the induction of a Peyronie's-like condition in the rat. J Androl 2001; 22: 497–506.
24. Ferrini MG, Vernet D, Magee TR, et al. Antifibrotic role of inducible nitric oxide synthase (iNOS). Nitric Oxide 2002; 6: 1–12.
25. Vernet D, Ferrini MG, Valente E, Magee TR, Bou-Gharios G, Rajfer J, Gonzalez-Cadavid NF. Effect of nitric oxide on fibroblast differentiation into myofibroblasts in cell cultures from the Peyronie's fibrotic plaque and in its rat model in vivo. Nitric Oxide 2002; 7: 262–276.
26. Valente EG, Vernet D, Ferrini MG, Qian A, Rajfer J, Gonzalez-Cadavid NF. PDE L-arginine and PDE inhibitors counteract fibrosis in the Peyronie's fibrotic plaque and related fibroblast cultures. Nitric Oxide 2003; 9: 229–244.
27. Ferrini MG, Kovanecz I, Nolazco G, Rajfer J, Gonzalez-Cadavid NF. Effects of long-term treatment with vardenafil on the development of the fibrotic plaque in a rat model of Peyronie's disease. BJU Int 2003; 97: 625–633.
28. Davila H, Ferrini M, Rajfer J, Gonzalez-Cadavid NF. Fibrin induction of a Peyronie's-like plaque in the rat penile tunica albuginea. A new model for Peyronie's disease. Br J Urol 2003; 91: 830–838.
29. Davila H, Magee TR, Rajfer J, Gonzalez-Cadavid NF. Peyronie's disease is associated with an increase of plasminogen activator inhibitor-1 in fibrotic plaque. Urology 2005; 65: 645–648.
30. Davila HH, Magee TR, Rajfer J, Gonzalez-Cadavid NF. Gene therapy with the inducible nitric oxide synthase (iNOS) cDNA regresses the fibrotic plaque in an animal model of Peyronie's disease. Biol Reprod 2004; 71: 1568–1577.
31. Mulhall JP, Thom J, Lubrano T, Shankey TV. Basic fibroblast growth factor expression in Peyronie's disease. J Urol 2001; 165: 419–423.
32. Mulhall JP, Anderson MS, Lubrano T, Shankey TV. Peyronie's disease cell culture models: phenotypic, genotypic and functional analyses. Int J Impot Res 2002; 14: 397–405.
33. Mulhall JP, Martin DJ, Lubrano T, Moser M, Kwon E, Wojcik E, Shankey TV. Peyronie's disease fibroblasts demonstrate tumorigenicity in the severe combined immunodeficient (SCID) mouse model. Int J Impot Res 2004; 16: 99–104.
34. Mulhall JP. Expanding the paradigm for plaque development in Peyronie's disease. Int J Impot Res 2003; 15(suppl 5): S93–S102.
35. Qian A, Meals R, Rajfer J, Gonzalez-Cadavid NF. Comparison of gene expression profiles between Peyronie's disease and Dupuytren's contracture. Urology 2004; 64: 399–404.
36. Vernet D, Qian A, Nolazco G, et al. Evidence that osteogenic progenitor cells in the human tunica albuginea may originate from stem cells. Implications for Peyronie's disease. Biol Reprod 2005; 73: 1199–1210.
37. Gonzalez-Cadavid NF, Rajfer J. Molecular and cellular aspects of the pathophysiology of Peyronie's disease. Drug Discovery Today. Disease Mech 2004; 1: 99–106.
38. Desmouliere A, Darby IA, Gabbiani G. Normal and pathologic soft tissue remodeling: role of the myofibroblast, with special emphasis on liver and kidney fibrosis. Lab Invest 2003; 83: 1689–1707.
39. Gabbiani G. The myofibroblast in wound healing and fibrocontractive diseases. J Pathol 2003; 200: 500–503.
40. Phan SH. The myofibroblast in pulmonary fibrosis. Chest 2002; 122: 286S–289S.
41. Sato M, Suzuki S, Senoo H. Hepatic stellate cells: unique characteristics in cell biology and phenotype. Cell Struct Funct 2003; 28: 105–112.
42. Kershenobich Stalnikowitz D, Weissbrod AB. Liver fibrosis and inflammation. A review. Ann Hepatol 2003; 2: 159–163.
43. Leask A, Abraham DJ. TGF-β signaling and the fibrotic response. FASEB J 2004; 18: 816–827.

44. Brunner G, Blakytny R. Extracellular regulation of TGF-β activity in wound repair: growth factor latency as a sensor mechanism for injury. Thromb Haemost 2004; 92: 253–261.

45. Wang W, Koka V, Lan HY. Transforming growth factor-β and Smad signalling in kidney diseases. Nephrology (Carlton) 2005; 10: 48–56.

46. Tsuchida K. Activins, myostatin and related TGF-β family members as novel therapeutic targets for endocrine, metabolic and immune disorders. Curr Drug Targets Immune Endocr Metabol Disord 2004; 4: 157–166.

47. Gonzalez-Cadavid NF, Bhasin S. Role of myostatin in metabolism. Curr Opin Clin Nutr Metabol Care 2004; 7: 451–457.

48. El-Sakka AI, Hassoba HM, Pillarisetty RJ, Dahiya R, Lue TF. Peyronie's disease is associated with an increase in transforming growth factor-beta protein expression. J Urol 1997; 158: 1391–1394.

49. Gelman J, Garban H, Shen R, et al. Transforming growth factor-1 (TGF-1) and penile growth in the rat during sexual maturation. J Androl 1998; 19: 50–57.

50. El-Sakka AI, Selph CA, Yen TS, Dahiya R, Lue TF. The effect of surgical trauma on rat tunica albuginea. J Urol 1998; 159: 1700–1707.

51. Somers KD, Sismour EN, Wright GL Jr, Devine CJ Jr, Gilbert DA, Horton CE. Isolation and characterization of collagen in Peyronie's disease. J Urol 1989; 141: 629–631.

52. Chiang PH, Chiang CP, Shen MR, Huang CH, Wang CJ, Huang IY, Shieh TY. Study of the changes in collagen of the tunica albuginea in venogenic impotence and Peyronie's disease. Eur Urol 1992; 21: 48–51.

53. Gentile V, Modesti A, La Pera G, et al. Ultrastructural and immunohistochemical characterization of the tunica albuginea in Peyronie's disease and veno-occlusive dysfunction. J Androl 1996; 17: 96–103.

54. Magee TR, Qian A, Rajfer J, Levine L, Gonzalez-Cadavid NF. Gene expression profiles in the Peyronie's disease plaque. Urology 2002; 59: 451–457.

55. Hertig A, Rondeau E. Plasminogen activator inhibitor type 1: the two faces of the same coin. Curr Opin Nephrol Hypertens 2004; 13: 39–44.

56. Idell S. Coagulation, fibrinolysis, and fibrin deposition in acute lung injury. Crit Care Med 2003; 31: S213–S220.

57. Kucharewicz I, Kowal K, Buczko W, Bodzenta-Lukaszyk A. The plasmin system in airway remodeling. Thromb Res 2003; 112: 1–7.

58. Ravanti L, Kahari VM. Matrix metalloproteinases in wound repair. Int J Mol Med 2000; 6: 391–407.

59. Brock G, Hsu GL, Nunes L, von Heyden B, Lue TF. The anatomy of the tunica albuginea in the normal penis and Peyronie's disease. J Urol 1997; 157: 276–281.

60. Davis CJ Jr. The microscopic pathology of Peyronie's disease. J Urol 1997; 157: 282–284.

61. Devine CJ Jr, Somers KD, Jordan SG, Schlossberg SM. Proposal: trauma as the cause of the Peyronie's lesion. J Urol 1997; 157: 285–290.

62. Van de Water L. Mechanisms by which fibrin and fibronectin appear in healing wounds: implications for Peyronie's disease. J Urol 1997; 157: 306–310.

63. Somers KD, Dawson DM. Fibrin deposition in Peyronie's disease plaque. J Urol 1997; 157: 311–315.

64. Ehrlich HP. Scar contracture: cellular and connective tissue aspects in Peyronie's disease. J Urol 1997; 157: 316–319.

65. Zargooshi J. Trauma as the cause of Peyronie's disease: penile fracture as a model of trauma. J Urol 2004; 172: 186–188.

66. Ciancio SJ, Kim ED. Penile fibrotic changes after radical retropubic prostatectomy. BJU Int 2000; 85: 101–106.

67. Percy C, Pat B, Poronnik P, Gobe G. Role of oxidative stress in age-associated chronic kidney pathologies. Adv Chronic Kidney Dis 2005; 12: 78–83.

68. Gawrieh S, Opara EC, Koch TR. Oxidative stress in nonalcoholic fatty liver disease: pathogenesis and antioxidant therapies. J Investig Med 2004; 52: 506–514.

69. Tsutsui H. Novel pathophysiological insight and treatment strategies for heart failure—lessons from mice and patients. Circ J 2004; 68: 1095–1103.

70. Cheng ZJ, Vapaatalo H, Mervaala E. Angiotensin II and vascular inflammation. Med Sci Monit 2005; 11: RA194–RA205.

71. Sikka SC, Hellstrom WJ. Role of oxidative stress and antioxidants in Peyronie's disease. Int J Impot Res 2002; 14: 353–360.

72. Lieber CS. Alcoholic fatty liver: its pathogenesis and mechanism of progression to inflammation and fibrosis. Alcohol 2004; 34: 9–19.

73. Siwik DA, Colucci WS. Regulation of matrix metalloproteinases by cytokines and reactive oxygen/nitrogen species in the myocardium. Heart Fail Rev 2004; 9: 43–51.

74. Lin CS, Lin G, Wang Z, Maddah SA, Lue TF. Upregulation of monocyte chemoattractant protein 1 and effects of transforming growth factor-β 1 in Peyronie's disease. Biochem Biophys Res Commun 2002; 295: 1014–1019.

75. Wang Z, Lin G, Lue TF, Lin CS. Wogonin suppresses cellular proliferation and expression of monocyte chemoattractant protein 1 in Peyronie's plaque-derived cells. BJU Int 2003; 92: 753–757.

76. Lopez B, Gonzalez A, Diez J. Role of matrix metalloproteinases in hypertension-associated cardiac fibrosis. Curr Opin Nephrol Hypertens 2004; 13: 197–204.

77. Jacob MP. Extracellular matrix remodeling and matrix metalloproteinases in the vascular wall during aging and in pathological conditions. Biomed Pharmacother 2003; 57: 195–202.

78. Zieman SJ, Kass DA. Advanced glycation endproduct crosslinking in the cardiovascular system: potential therapeutic target for cardiovascular disease. Drugs 2004; 64: 459–470.

79. Susic D, Varagic J, Ahn J, Frohlich ED. Crosslink breakers: a new approach to cardiovascular therapy. Curr Opin Cardiol 2004; 19: 336–340.

80. Li YY, Feldman AM. Matrix metalloproteinases in the progression of heart failure: potential therapeutic implications. Drugs 2001; 61: 1239–1252.

81. Levine LA. Review of current nonsurgical management of Peyronie's disease. Int J Impot Res 2003; 15: S113–S120.

82. Gelbard MK, James K, Riach P, Dorey F. Collagenase versus placebo in the treatment of Peyronie's disease: a double-blind study. J Urol 1993; 149: 56–58.

83. Cole A. Increased endogenous inhibitors of collagenases within Peyronie's plaques may represent a scar remodeling disorder. J Urol 2005; 173: 255.

84. Ramadori G, Saile B. Mesenchymal cells in the liver—one cell type or two? Liver 2002; 22: 283–294.

85. Ariyan S, Enriquez R, Krizek TJ. Wound contraction and fibrocontractive disorders. Arch Surg 1978; 113: 1034–1046.

86. Somers KD, Dawson DM, Wright GL Jr, et al. Cell culture of Peyronie's disease plaque and normal penile tissue. J Urol 1982; 127: 585–588.

87. Bisson MA, McGrouther DA, Mudera V, Grobbelaar AO. The different characteristics of Dupuytren's disease fibroblasts derived from either nodule or cord: expression of α-smooth muscle actin and the response to stimulation by TGF-β$_1$. J Hand Surg [Br] 2003; 28: 351–356.

88. Hirano D, Takimoto Y, Yamamoto T, Hirakata H, Kawata N. Electron microscopic study of the penile plaques and adjacent corpora cavernosa in Peyronie's disease. Int J Urol 1997; 4: 274–278.

89. Ahuja SK, Sikka SC, Hellstrom WJ. Stimulation of collagen production in an in vitro model for Peyronie's disease. Int J Impot Res 1999; 11: 207–212.

90. Mody N, Parhami F, Sarafian TA, Demer LL. Oxidative stress modulates osteoblastic differentiation of vascular and bone cells. Free Radic Biol Med 2001; 31: 509–519.

91. Peng H, Huard J. Muscle-derived stem cells for musculoskeletal tissue regeneration and repair. Transpl Immunol 2004; 12: 311–319.

92. Zwaginga JJ, Doevendans P. Stem cell-derived angiogenic/vasculogenic cells: possible therapies for tissue repair and tissue engineering. Clin Exp Pharmacol Physiol 2003; 30: 9000–9008.

93. Andresen R, Wegner HE, Banzer D, Miller K. Ultrasound and soft-tissue radiography to monitor local interferon-alpha 2B treatment in Peyronie's disease. Acta Radiol 1996; 37: 352–356.

94. Hauck EW, Hackstein N, Vosshenrich R, et al. Diagnostic value of magnetic resonance imaging in Peyronie's disease—a comparison both with palpation and ultrasound in the evaluation of plaque formation. Eur Urol 2003; 43: 293–299.

95. Karpman E, Das S, Kurzrock EA. Penile calciphylaxis: analysis of risk factors and mortality. J Urol 2003; 169: 2206–2209.

96. Sartore S, Chiavegato A, Faggin E, et al. Contribution of adventitial fibroblasts to neointima formation and vascular remodeling: from innocent bystander to active participant. Circ Res 2001; 89: 1111–1121.

97. Schurch W. The myofibroblast in neoplasia. Curr Top Pathol 1999; 93: 135–148.

98. Bedossa P, Paradis V. Regression of hepatic fibrosis physiopathological aspects and clinical reality [in French]. Presse Med 2003; 32: 704–710.

99. Chatziantoniou C, Boffa JJ, Tharaux PL, Flamant M, Ronco P, Dussaule JC. Progression and regression in renal vascular and glomerular fibrosis. Int J Exp Pathol 2004; 85: 1–11.

100. Hu L, Sealey JE, Chen R, et al. Nitric oxide synthase inhibition accelerates the pressor response to low-dose angiotensin II, exacerbates target organ damage, and induces renin escape. Am J Hypertens 2004; 17: 395–403.

101. Rossi MA, Ramos SG, Prado CM. Chronic inhibition of nitric oxide synthase induces hypertension and cardiomyocyte mitochondrial and myocardial collagen remodelling in the absence of hypertrophy. J Hypertens 2003; 21: 993–1001.

102. Chang HR, Wu CY, Hsu YH, Chen HI. Reduction of ventricular hypertrophy and fibrosis in spontaneously hypertensive rats by L-arginine. Chin J Physiol 2005; 48: 15–22.

103. Wehling-Henricks M, Jordan MC, Roos KP, Deng B, Tidball JG. Cardiomyopathy in dystrophin-deficient hearts is prevented by expression of a neuronal nitric oxide synthase transgene in the myocardium. Hum Mol Genet 2005; 14: 1921–1933.

104. Smith RS Jr, Agata J, Xia CF, Chao L, Chao J. Human endothelial nitric oxide synthase gene delivery protects against cardiac remodeling and reduces oxidative stress after myocardial infarction. Life Sci 2005; 76: 2457–2471.

105. Gonzalez-Cadavid NF, Rajfer J. The pleiotropic effects of inducible nitric oxide synthase (iNOS) on the physiology and pathology of penile erection. Curr Pharm Des 2005; 11: 4041–4046.

106. Wang H, Chen XP, Qiu FZ. Increased hepatic expression of nitric oxide synthase type II in cirrhotic rats. World J Gastroenterol 2004; 10: 1923–1927.

107. Hochberg D, Johnson CW, Chen J, et al. Interstitial fibrosis of unilateral ureteral obstruction is exacerbated in kidneys of mice lacking the gene for inducible nitric oxide synthase. Lab Invest 2000; 80: 1721–1728.

108. Chen Y, Hozawa S, Sawamura S, et al. Deficiency of inducible nitric oxide synthase exacerbates hepatic fibrosis in mice fed high-fat diet. Biochem Biophys Res Commun 2005; 326: 45–51.

109. Kenyon NJ, Gohil K, Last JA. Susceptibility to ovalbumin-induced airway inflammation and fibrosis in inducible nitric oxide synthetase-deficient mice: mechanisms and consequences. Toxicol Appl Pharmacol 2003; 191: 2–11.

110. Peters H, Daig U, Martini S, et al. NO mediates antifibrotic actions of L-arginine supplementation following induction of anti-thy1 glomerulonephritis. Kidney Int 2003; 64: 509–518.

111. Huang JS, Chuang LY, Guh JY, et al. Effect of nitric oxide-cGMP-dependent protein kinase activation on advanced glycation end-product-induced proliferation in renal fibroblasts. J Am Soc Nephrol June 15, 2005 [Epub ahead of print].

112. Kukreja RC, Ockaili R, Salloum F, et al. Cardioprotection with phosphodiesterase-5 inhibition—a novel preconditioning strategy. J Mol Cell Cardiol 2004; 36: 165–173.

113. Schwartz EJ, Wong P, Graydon RJ. Sildenafil preserves intracorporeal smooth muscle after radical retro-pubic prostatectomy. J Urol 2004; 171: 771–774.

114. Wang Y, Kramer S, Loof T, et al. Stimulation of soluble guanylate cyclase slows progression in anti-thy1-induced chronic glomerulosclerosis. Kidney Int 2005; 68: 47–61.

115. Violi F, Cangemi R, Sabatino G, Pignatelli P. Vitamin E for the treatment of cardiovascular disease: is there a future? Ann NY Acad Sci 2004; 1031: 292–304.

116. Meydani M. Vitamin E modulation of cardiovascular disease. Ann NY Acad Sci 2004; 1031: 271–279.

117. McGowan TA, Zhu Y, Sharma K. Transforming growth factor-β: a clinical target for the treatment of diabetic nephropathy. Curr Diab Rep 2004; 4: 447–454.

118. Weis SM, Zimmerman SD, Shah M, et al. A role for decorin in the remodeling of myocardial infarction. Matrix Biol 2005; 24: 313–324.

119. Huijun W, Long C, Zhigang Z, Feng J, Muyi G. Ex vivo transfer of the decorin gene into rat glomerulus via a mesangial cell vector suppressed extracellular matrix accumulation in experimental glomerulonephritis. Exp Mol Pathol 2005; 78: 17–24.

120. Li T, Surendran K, Zawaideh MA, Mathew S, Hruska KA. Bone morphogenetic protein 7: a novel treatment for chronic renal and bone disease. Curr Opin Nephrol Hypertens 2004; 13: 417–422.

121. Prieto Castro RM, Leva Vallejo ME, et al. Combined treatment with vitamin E and colchicine in the early stages of Peyronie's disease. BJU Int 2003; 91: 522–524.

122. Chiao TB, Lee AJ. Role of pentoxifylline and vitamin E in attenuation of radiation-induced fibrosis. Ann Pharmacother 2005; 39: 516–522.

123. Lin SL, Chen YM, Chiang WC, Tsai TJ, Chen WY. Pentoxifylline: a potential therapy for chronic kidney disease. Nephrology (Carlton) 2004; 9: 198–204.

124. Riedl CR, Sternig P, Galle G, et al. Liposomal recombinant human superoxide dismutase for the treatment of Peyronie's disease: a randomized placebo-controlled double-blind prospective clinical study. Eur Urol Jun 24, 2005 [Epub ahead of print].

125. Bivalacqua TJ, Armstrong JS, Biggerstaff J, et al. Gene transfer of extracellular SOD to the penis reduces O2-* and improves erectile function in aged rats. Am J Physiol Heart Circ Physiol 2003; 284: H1408–H1421.

126. Artaza JN, Bhasin S, Magee TR, et al. Myostatin inhibits myogenesis and promotes adipogenesis in 10T(1/2) mesenchymal multipotent cells. Endocrinology 2005; 146: 3547–3557.

127. Cavasin MA, Rhaleb NE, Yang XP, Carretero OA. Prolyl oligopeptidase is involved in release of the antifibrotic peptide Ac-SDKP. Hypertension 2004; 43: 1140–1145.

4

The Clinical Implications of Basic Science Research in Peyronie's Disease

John P. Mulhall, MD

SUMMARY

Despite centuries of recognition, the condition that is Peyronie's disease remains a puzzle. Conventional wisdom suggests that trauma to the erect or semi-erect penis is the inciting event that sets off a cascade of events at the cellular level that results in localized fibrosis of the tunica albuginea. However, many questions remain unanswered at this juncture, among the most important of which are why do so few men manifest this condition? Why is there such an ethnic predilection? What are the cofactors that, along with penile trauma, lead to plaque development? Historically, cytokine overexpression, autoimmune, and genetic factors have been cited as contributors. This chapter endeavors to conduct an evidence-based assessment of the literature as it pertains to the pathophysiology of Peyronie's disease. Furthermore, an effort is made to evaluate contemporary literature pertaining to novel concepts in Peyronie's disease pathogenesis including nitric oxide synthase alterations, free radical generation, pathogen involvement, and animal model development. In conclusion, although plausible that the near future will see improved developments in our understanding of this condition, groundbreaking work will require research funding beyond that which is currently available.

Key Words: Peyronie's disease; fibroblasts; fibrin cell cycle dysregulation; cytokines; cytogenetics.

INTRODUCTION

In essence, Peyronie's disease (PD) remains a mystery. More than 250 years after the initial description in the medical literature, the condition remains a mystery. Despite valiant efforts at defining the condition and postulation regarding the pathophysiology, its exact etiology remains a mystery. Although conventional wisdom suggests that trauma to the erect or semierect penis is the inciting event that sets off a cascade of events at the cellular level that results in localized fibrosis of the tunica albuginea (Fig. 1), many questions remain unanswered, including the following: Why do so few men manifest this condition? Why does there appear to be such an ethnic predilection? Why is there such a variation in the biology of plaque development and disease progression? What are the cofactors that, along with penile trauma, lead to plaque development? (*See* Fig. 2.)

From: *Current Clinical Urology:*
Peyronie's Disease: A Guide to Clinical Management
Edited by: L. A. Levine © Humana Press Inc., Totowa, NJ

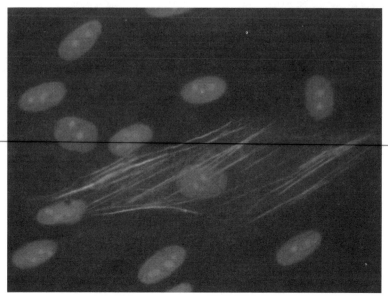

Fig. 1. Photomicrograph (400×) of a preparation of plaque-derived fibroblasts stained with smooth muscle α-actin (a marker for smooth muscle that stains green). Nuclei are counterstained with propidium iodide (red). This micrograph illustrates the fact that a proportion of PD plaque-derived fibroblasts (approx 20%) are myofibroblasts, which stain positively with smooth muscle antibodies. (*See* the companion DVD for color versions of the figure.)

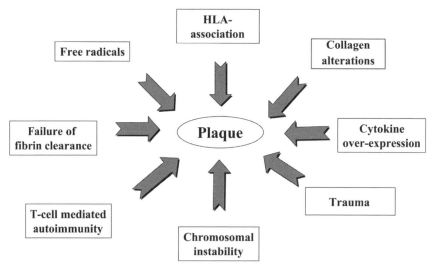

Fig. 2. Proposed mechanisms of plaque development in Peyronie's disease. This graphic illustrates what is probably a historical thought process concerning Peyronie's disease pathophysiology (*see* Fig. 3). Although there are data supporting the involvement of these factors in plaque development, this graphic fails to demonstrate adequately the interplay between the factors.

PD has been termed a *fibromatosis*. However, the exact definition of a fibromatosis is a condition characterized by the development of multiple fibrous tumors. Fibromatoses have a range of biological behaviors, from completely benign (osteosclerosis, Dupuytren's

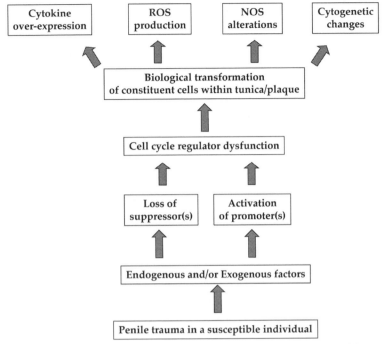

Fig. 3. Novel paradigm for plaque development in Peyronie's disease. This algorithm probably more closely represents the sequence of events in Peyronie's disease pathophysiology.

contracture) to aggressive with malignant potential (ovarian thecoma, desmoid tumor). Other than the coexistence in some men with Dupuytren's contracture, the presence of other fibrous tumors in men with PD has not been identified. Although Peyronie's disease has not been recognized as a condition with the potential for malignant transformation, it is interesting to note that, at the time of plaque incision and grafting surgery, plaque tissue is often adherent to the corporal smooth muscle, suggesting locally aggressive behavior of PD plaque.

MODELS FOR THE STUDY OF PEYRONIE'S DISEASE

The generation of a reliable, reproducible model for PD is a vital requirement for the advancement of our understanding of this disease process and is essential for the evaluation and development of novel therapeutic strategies. There are two types of models that have been investigated. Cell culture models have been used extensively in other areas of research and were first described in PD by Somers et al. in the late 1980s (1). The purpose of an in vitro model is to provide a model derived from the constituent cells of the tissue studied. The advantages of such a model include the ability to characterize the biology of the condition and the ability to manipulate the cells using a variety of agents, which may allow the development of new therapies. The major disadvantage is that such models may fail to represent the in vivo condition. The study of PD plaque-derived fibroblasts, for example, does not account for the complex in vivo environment in which the cells normally exist and function.

In PD, cell culture models have been used to study fibroblast growth characteristics (Fig. 3), cytogenetic changes, cell cycle regulator function, and cytokine expression (2–5).

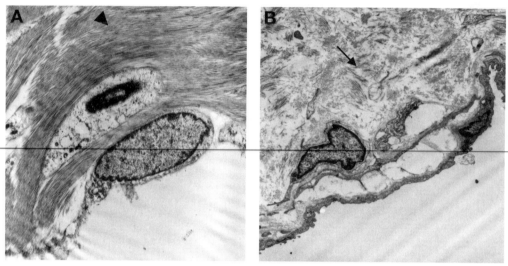

Fig. 4. Two photomicrographs stained for collagen. Panel **A** demonstrates the normal rat penis; the image on the right (**B**) demonstrates dysregulation and an overabundance of collagen in the rat penis injected with fibrin. Image courtesy of Jacob Rajfer, MD.

Another ex vivo model is the use of plaque tissue for experimental investigation. This model is useful for the study of the presence of proteins and messenger ribonucleic acid ribonucleic acid (RNA) within this tissue. It has also been utilized for microarray analysis, a contemporary strategy commonly used for hypothesis generation in basic science research *(6)*.

The second model that has been studied is an animal model. The purpose of developing an animal model is to precisely mimic the in vivo process. Through such a model, expansion of the understanding of the pathophysiology of PD may be possible. The potential advantages of such a model include the ability to assess therapeutic interventions prior to human exposure. For an animal model to be valid, however, it must adequately represent the condition studied. In PD, the most widely studied model has been developed by the University of California at San Francisco group and involves the injection of cytomodulin, a synthetic heptapeptide with transforming growth factor (TGF)-β-like activity, into the tunica albuginea of the rat *(7)*. This technique has been shown to replicate the pathology of PD that is profound fibrosis. The use of this specific agent arose from the finding the TFG-β was overexpressed in PD plaque tissue compared to control tunica *(8)*. Much experimentation is in progress on the penises of rats injected with cytomodulin (or more recently fibrin), and much hypothesis generation is also conducted based on this model. The potential deficiency of such an approach is that it may fail to take into account the upstream factors that lead to plaque development. Clearly, this model is representative of penile fibrosis but may not be an ideal model for the study of Peyronie's disease.

PROPOSED PATHOGENETIC MECHANISMS

The precise etiology or etiologies of PD remain uncertain. Historically, a number of factors have been cited as potential contributors to the pathogenesis of a PD plaque (Fig. 2). These include trauma to the penis in the erect or semierect state, overproduction

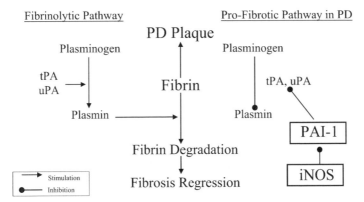

Fig. 5. A schematic illustrating a proposal for the interplay between fibrin, PAI-1 (plasminogen activator 1), and iNOS (inducible nitric oxide synthase). (*See* the companion DVD for color versions of the figure.) Image courtesy of Jacob Rajfer, MD.

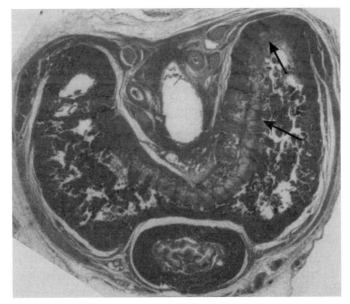

Fig. 6. Transverse section of a rat penis previously injected with cytomodulin (a synthetic heptapeptide with TGF-β properties. Note the extensive tunical changes (outlined by black arrows). Also note the intracorporal changes seen in this model not characteristic of Peyronie's disease. Image courtesy of Trinity Bivalacqua, MD.

of collagen and alterations in the type of collagen deposited in the tunica (Fig. 4), overproduction of cytokines that induce fibrosis, alterations in T-cell-mediated immunity and HLA associations, failure to degrade and clear fibrin from the tunica albuginea, free radicals, and chromosomal instability.

Trauma

RATIONALE

The concept introduced by Horton and Devine that trauma to the penis leads to PD continues to be accepted two decades after its introduction *(9–11)*. Trauma is believed to be the primary inciting event in the cascade of events that leads to PD plaque develop-

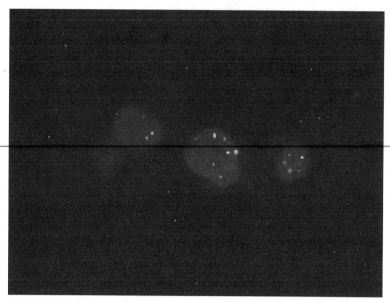

Fig. 7. Fluorescent *in situ* hybridization (FISH) photomicrograph (400×). Peyronie's disease plaque-derived fibroblast nuclei are stained with DAPI (blue); two probes are used to stain for chromosome 7 (red) and 8 (green). This FISH micrograph demonstrates trisomy for both chromosomes. (*See* the companion DVD for color versions of the figure.)

ment *(11)*. The torqueing stresses that occur during penetrative sexual relations are believed to result in delamination of the tunical fibers, resulting in microhemorrhages; acute, then chronic inflammation; and eventually scar formation. We certainly see men who have fractured their penis who later developed penile angulation, so this level of trauma leads to a form of PD, but it is unknown how we can be sure that repetitive torqueing of the penis leads to PD, especially when so few men develop the condition when presumably the majority of men having sexual intercourse torque the penis during this act.

DATA

The minority of patients give a history of a distinct traumatic episode. In my practice, this is less than 10% of patients, and in many the traumatic episode that is reported is likely not to be a major contributor to the development of plaque. In a questionnaire-based study, patients with PD and erectile dysfunction (ED) had an increased likelihood of having sustained penile trauma than patients without either PD or ED. In this analysis, however, there was no difference in trauma reporting between patients with PD and men with ED *(12)*. Although the trauma theory is attractive, there is a paucity of evidence-based analyses to evaluate its role in the genesis of PD plaque. Despite this, it can be easily appreciated that the penis may be torqued during sexual intercourse, and the location of the majority of plaques in dorsal and ventral locations is consistent with the ventrodorsal stresses that are inflicted on the penis during sexual intercourse.

CONCLUSIONS

It is likely that, although trauma is an important contributor, alone it is unlikely to produce PD; it needs to be combined with other biological factors to result in the profound fibrotic reaction that leads to plaque development.

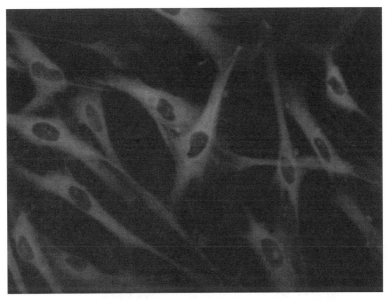

Fig. 8. Immunofluorescence photomicrograph (300×). This image demonstrates p53 (stained green with FITC) in plaque-derived fibroblasts. Note the sequestration of p53 within the cytoplasm of the cells and the absence of staining within the nuclei. This illustrates that p53 is stabilized and anchored within the cytoplasm. The mechanisms of this are unclear at this time. (*See* the companion DVD for color versions of the figure.)

Failure of Fibrin Degradation

RATIONALE

The concept that fibrin accumulation leads to profound tunical scarring was put forth by Somers and Dawson *(13)*. This was based on a pathological examination of plaque tissue from men with PD. It has been suggested that the avascular tunica albuginea fails to clear the fibrin deposited after intratunical microhemorrhages that occur on tunical delamination. Fibrin has been known to exert a profound desmoplastic reaction, and it is easy to see how such "fibrin trapping" might lead to plaque development (Fig. 5).

DATA

Somers and Dawson examined plaque tissue for collagen, elastin, and fibrin content. The findings in PD plaque tissue were compared to the findings in control tunica and Dupuytren's contracture tissue. Immunohistochemistry demonstrated that fibrin was present in 95% of the plaque tissue and was not seen in the control tissues. These findings were confirmed using immunoblotting techniques for fibrin *(13)*. These findings were also documented, although not as consistently, in Dupuytren's contracture tissue. Because of these pathological findings, the University of California at Los Angeles (UCLA) group has utilized fibrin injection into the rat tunica to develop a novel animal model.

CONCLUSIONS

Although the Somers and Dawson study *(13)* demonstrates the presence of fibrin in PD plaque tissue, it tells us little about its role or of the events that lead to fibrin deposition and, more important, the reason for the failure of fibrin degradation. At this time, the fibrin injection model in my opinion is a valiant effort but most probably does not represent PD.

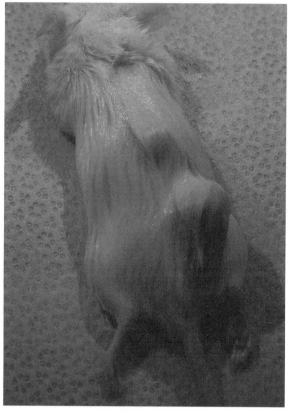

Fig. 9. Photograph of a severe combined immunodeficient (SCID) mouse inoculated with Peyronie's disease plaque-derived transformed fibroblasts. Note the two subcutaneous nodules present over the back and rump of the mouse.

Collagen Alterations

RATIONALE

Suggesting collagen changes as a source of PD is easy to understand as this is essentially scar formation with the tunica albuginea. This mechanism has been postulated as a contributor in other biologically similar conditions, such as proliferative scars.

DATA

Pathologically, collagen deposition is increased in the tunica albuginea. Furthermore, there is disorganization of the native collagen bundles and a reduction in elastin fiber presence with disorganization *(15)*. Using immunohistochemistry, Somers and Dawson demonstrated that plaque tissue had aberrantly stained collagen and disruption of elastin fibers in excess of 90% of specimens studied *(13)*. It has also been shown that there is a shift in the type of collagen deposited, from the predominant type I to type III *(16–18)*, although these findings have not been reported in a consistent fashion.

Regardless of the upstream events involved in the pathogenesis of PD, it is clear that the development of fibrosis follows a pathway similar to wound healing, except that the normal termination signals are altered, resulting in excessive deposition of extracellular matrix (ECM), which is predominantly collagen, and destruction of normal tissue architecture and function. Thus, the dysregulated wound-healing process serves as the conventional paradigm for the study of this condition.

Tissue injury initiates a complex cascade of events that involve the (1) activation of monocytes, macrophages, and platelets; (2) release of cytokines and growth factors; (3) fibroblast recruitment and proliferation; and (4) increased synthesis and decreased degradation of ECM. Great interest has been expressed in the study of factors involved in collagen degradation and synthesis, specifically matrix metalloproteinases (MMPs) and tissue inhibitors of metalloproteinases (TIMPs). There are several members of the collagenase (MMP) family, but it has been suggested that MMP-1, MMP-8, and MMP-13 are the most important for wound-healing purposes *(19,20)*.

Cole et al. have been analyzing MMP and TIMP profiles of tunica albuginea *(21)*. Latent collagenases have been present in tunica (plaque and periplaque) excised from young men but not in tunica albuginea from older men, suggesting that there may be an intrinsic defect in collagen degradation in the older population. TIMPs are proteins that inhibit MMP activity and thus may have a direct impact on collagen degradation. The TIMP family has four members (TIMP-1, -2, -3, and -4). Cole et al. and Cole and Levine demonstrated that TIMPs are present in plaque tissue in levels higher than in the perilesional tunica albuginea *(21,22)*. Thus, a combined decrease in collagenase activity in the tunica albuginea of older patients along with higher TIMP levels in plaque may contribute to the unsuccessful repair of Peyronie's plaque that may contribute to this scar remodeling disorder.

Conclusions

Although in normal wound healing an as-yet unidentified mechanism terminates ECM production when healing is complete, in PD the well-orchestrated control mechanisms of normal wound healing are lost, which results in the characteristic fibrosis. Whether the collagen alterations described are representative of PD or just a fibrotic response to injury is unclear at this time. Future strategies may benefit from addressing collagen degradation, particularly manipulation of MMPs or TIMPs. At the time of writing this chapter, industry had expressed some interest in the development of collagenase for intralesional injections. Trials have yet to commence.

Genetic Predisposition

Rationale

Most authorities agree that the majority of men suffering from PD are Caucasian. Thus, it is easy to see why interest exists in the concept that perhaps there is a familial or genetic predisposition to this condition. Although familial clustering is uncommon in my practice, a less-than-open discussion within the males of a family may account for such low reporting.

Data

Some reports have suggested either familial clustering or autosomal-dominant transmission of this condition *(23)*. In 1982, Chilton et al. conducted a retrospective review of 408 patients and found a familial incidence in 1.9% of patients. In this study, there was also a 15.3% incidence of Dupuytren's contracture in patients with PD. The authors thus stated that there was a 17% incidence of genetic causes of PD. This study has not been replicated in the modern era; therefore, it is uncertain what role genetics plays in this condition.

From a population genetics standpoint, there are a number of reports assessing HLA linkage (24–29). Nachsteim and Rearden analyzed serum of 31 men with PD for class II HLA antigens and compared the findings to 19 aged-matched urological patients as well as 75 organ donor cadavers believed to be representative of the general population (24). Using polymerase chain reaction (PCR) technology, the frequency of HLA-DQ5 was greater in patients with PD compared to controls (61 vs 19%), suggesting a role for an autoimmune component in this disorder.

Ralph et al. performed tissue-typing in 51 patients with documented PD and found a significant association between PD and HLA-B27 (26). However, no significant association was found with other HLA-B group antigens or HLA-Cw7, HLA-DR3, or HLA-DQ2. These last findings confirmed earlier work by Leffel et al. (30). It is thus conceivable that penile trauma in a patient with a predisposing HLA type may be required for the development of a tunical plaque. Could the ethnic difference in the predilection for PD be accounted for by such a simple explanation? It is likely that large cohorts of PD patients of multiethnic origin would need to undergo HLA typing to answer this question.

Schiavino et al. demonstrated that in patients with PD, 76% had at least one abnormal immunological test. 48% had an abnormality in T cell-mediated immunity and 38% had markers of auto-immune disease (29,31). Stewart et al. showed an increase in levels of antielastin serum antibodies in men with PD (31). Ralph et al. studied the sera of 100 men with PD for circulating antibodies. Circulating antipenis antibodies were not demonstrated in serum. Plaque tissue was also assessed and demonstrated the deposition of immunoglobulin M antibodies as well as T lymphocytes within the subtunical space (26). Thus, it appears that there are some features of autoimmunity present in a consistent fashion; in particular, it appears that cell-mediated immunity is altered in this condition. It is probable that this does not represent an intrinsic deficiency in the immune system of patients with PD; rather, it is a local phenomenon confined to the tunica albuginea.

CONCLUSIONS

In my opinion, disbelief that there is not some genetic predisposition to PD is difficult. It is likely that, where funding is available, further analysis of genetics and HLA typing in particular will occur. Absent from the literature is a single population pedigree analysis in PD sufferers. This is a classic example of the disinterest level in this condition on behalf of grant-funding agencies.

Infection

RATIONALE

In medicine, when a disease etiology cannot be explained, an infectious etiology is often postulated. Clearly, the tunica does not demonstrate any signs of a bacterial infection, but the issue remains unanswered (much in the way that modern theory pertaining to chronic pelvic pain disorder and even prostate cancer is unanswered), such that viral involvement has been postulated.

DATA

There has been minimal exploration of the role of pathogens in this condition. Ralph et al. analyzed fecal, urine, and urethral samples for the presence of bacteria, including *Yersinia, Salmonella, Shigella, Campylobacter, Gonococcus,* and *Chlamydia (26).* Serum titers were also assessed for antibacterial antibodies. All specimen cultures were negative, and patients with PD failed to show any elevation of serum titers for anti-*Klebsiella*, anti-*Proteus,* or anti-*Escherichia coli* antibodies.

Evidence supports a role for infectious agents in the development of atherosclerosis as well as the development of arterial restenosis following coronary artery angioplasty, conditions that biologically involve fibroblasts and fibrosis *(32–36)*. In the latter condition, endoluminal trauma, such as that which occurs during balloon angioplasty, is believed to reactivate the implicated pathogens. This reactivation leads to hyperplastic growth of the fibroblasts within the arterial wall and subsequent fibrosis and arterial occlusion. The altered cell growth and the association with trauma make pathogen-associated arterial disease a potential model for the study of PD.

For years, seroepidemiological evidence has supported a link between cytomegalovirus (CMV) and atherosclerosis. Elevated CMV antibody titers are more common in patients undergoing surgery for atherosclerotic disease when compared to matched control patients. CMV has also been implicated in the development of postangioplasty restenosis, carotid artery intimal thickening, and accelerated atherosclerosis in patients with cardiac transplant. It has proven difficult to culture CMV (and herpesviridae in general) from atheromata. However, failure to culture virus particles does not preclude their involvement in the genesis of atherosclerosis. Indeed, there is excellent documentation supporting a role for the herpesviridae in triggering diseases without persisting in an infectious form in the affected tissue. This has been termed the *hit-and-run* mechanism. Although CMV infiltrates endothelial cells and smooth muscle cells, it is well recognized that CMV has a particularly high affinity for fibroblasts. Preliminary work in our laboratory has identified CMV deoxyribonucleic acid (DNA) in some of our PD plaque-derived fibroblasts using nested PCR techniques. Confirmation of these early results in all of our cell cultures will be required to confirm this as a possible contributor to the pathogenesis of the condition. If confirmed that CMV is present in PD fibroblasts, further work will be required to define whether it represents an innocent bystander or if it plays a significant role in the genesis of plaque.

More recent work has also implicated the pathogen *Chlamydia pneumoniae* in the pathogenesis of atherosclerosis *(37)*. Although the evidence linking *C. pneumoniae* to atherogenesis is not as strong as that implicating CMV, there is evidence using a variety of techniques, including immunocytochemistry. The association of CMV and *C. pneumoniae* with atherosclerotic arterial disease may represent a model for PD because trauma to the semi-erect penis is believed to be the inciting event in the pathogenesis of PD, and CMV in particular is reactivated by trauma. Figure 3 outlines a novel paradigm for the pathophysiology of PD. Penile trauma in a susceptible individual leads to activation of endogenous factors within the tunica albuginea that initiates a series of events that may include loss of suppressor genes or upregulation of promoter genes that eventuate in aberration in cell cycle regulator function. These changes result in biological transformation of the fibroblasts within the tunica albuginea and lead to further alterations, including nitric oxide synthase (NOS) changes, cytogenetic instability, free-radical generation, and fibrogenic cytokine over-production. The conglomeration of these factors finally leads to unregulated ECM deposition, which develops into a plaque. Is it possible that trauma to tunica albuginea that is infiltrated with a dormant pathogen in a genetically predisposed individual (HLA associated) is the combination of factors that leads to plaque development?

CONCLUSIONS

Using PCR, we have conducted screening for a number of DNA viruses, in particular herpes simplex virus (HSV) 1, HSV-2, HSV-7, Epstein-Barr virus, human papillomavirus, CMV, and BK and JC viruses. All have been negative or only inconsistently positive. Thus, there is no convincing data supporting viral involvement in PD, but it may be that our technology is not sensitive enough to assess for prior viral infiltration of the tunica albuginea.

Free Radicals

RATIONALE

Where there is trauma, inflammation, and fibrosis, you will find the quest for free radicals. Free radicals include reactive oxygen species (ROS) and reactive nitrogen intermediates (RNIs). The generation of free radicals has been postulated in PD tissue *(38)*. ROS are free radicals derived from oxygen and are highly oxidant in nature. ROS include superoxide anion (O^-), hydrogen peroxide (H_2O_2), and hydroxyl anion (OH^-). RNIs include nitric oxide (NO) and peroxynitrite ($OONO^-$). The presence of these free radicals is called a state of *oxidative stress*. The current understanding of the role of oxidative stress in PD is incomplete. Finally, there exist some data to support the use of antioxidants (vitamin E, superoxide dismutase) in the treatment of PD; however, as with much of the data regarding medical therapy for PD, the results are mixed *(39,40)*.

DATA

Much of the discussion regarding free radicals in PD is based on the documented cellular response and the finding of round cells in PD plaque tissue on histological sections. There are data to support the presence of peroxynitrite overexpression in cavernosal tissue of men with PD as well as peroxynitrite overproduction in the rat model of PD. No data exist to date, however, to demonstrate that free radicals play a direct role in PD plaque tissue itself. Sikka and Hellstrom suggested that ROS and RNIs function through the intermediary nuclear factor (NF)-κB by upregulating genes involved in fibrogenesis as well as the gene for NOS *(38)*.

CONCLUSIONS

Currently, the exact role of free radicals in PD remains ill defined. Despite this, exploration into anti-free-radical therapies is occurring in a number of other disease states. Therefore, a more in-depth elucidation of their role in PD may aid in the development of therapeutics for the condition.

Cytokines

RATIONALE

Since the early observations of Alexis Carrel, who noted that substances within embryonic juices affected cell proliferation, cytokines have been identified as ubiquitous. Cytokines are subdivided into proinflammatory (such as the interleukins), antifibrotic (such as the interferons), and profibrotic *(41,42)*. The profibrotic or fibrogenic cytokines include tumor necrosis factor-α, TGF-β (Fig. 6), fibroblast growth factor (FGF), and platelet-derived growth factor (PDGF) families. The last function by increasing collagen production by fibroblasts as well as increasing fibroblast proliferation rates.

DATA

A number of workers have demonstrated the overexpression of cytokines in PD *(5, 8)*. Lue and associates evaluated the role of TGF-β in PD *(10)*. The protein expression of growth factors TGF-β_1, TGF-β_2, and TGF-β_3 was determined with Western blotting using a chemiluminescence detection system. They demonstrated that there was an increased expression of TGF-β_2 by PD tissue compared to control tunical tissue. They excised control tissue from men without PD at the time of penile prosthesis implantation. No significant increase in expression of TGF-β_2 or TGF-β_3 was demonstrated. TGF-β_1 protein expression was detected in 26 out of 30 tissue specimens from patients with PD and in only 1 tissue specimen from a patient in the control group. Histological examination of the 4 patients with PD without TGF-β_1 protein expression showed relatively healthy tunica with minimal ultrastructural changes. The authors contended that this finding supported the hypothesis that TGF-β_1 is involved in the pathogenesis of PD.

We have analyzed supernatants from cell culture for levels of basic fibroblast growth factor (bFGF) using an enzyme-linked immunosorbent assay (ELISA) *(5)*. ELISA analysis demonstrated that plaque-derived fibroblasts produced fourfold more bFGF than foreskin-derived fibroblasts. As bFGF is a fibrogenic cytokine inducing the production of ECM by fibroblasts and is mitogenic for fibroblasts, the demonstration of its overexpression by PD plaque-derived fibroblasts suggests a role for this cytokine in the pathogenesis of PD. The University of California at San Francisco group demonstrated overexpression of monocyte chemoattractant protein 1 in plaque and normal tunica tissue from men with PD compared to control cells *(43)*. Furthermore, they have shown that monocyte chemoattractant protein 1 is upregulated when cells are treated with TGF-β. Thus, there is robust evidence to support a role for a number of fibrogenic cytokines in the pathogenesis of PD.

CONCLUSIONS

Manipulation of fibrogenic cytokine production has been explored experimentally in other conditions and represents a potential strategy in PD *(44)*.

Cytogenetic Alterations

RATIONALE

It has been appreciated for a long time that the development of plaque involves two contemporaneous events: the overexpression of ECM (collagen) and cellular fibroblast proliferation. PD plaque-derived fibroblasts exhibit greater cell proliferation rates than normal tunical cells.

DATA

Because previous experiments by others in PD and the associated Dupuytren's contracture have indicated macroscopic changes in specific chromosomes, exploration of cytogenetic alterations has been conducted in PD cultured fibroblasts. Cytogenetic studies of fibroblasts grown from the related fibromatosis Dupuytren's contracture have also revealed chromosomal instability in the majority of fibroblasts from the fibrotic palmar fascia, specifically an increase in the number of copies of chromosomes 7 and 8, as well as deletions of the Y chromosomes. A number of studies have demonstrated that the disease process occurring in Dupuytren's contracture involved marked chromosome instability, particularly trisomy of chromosomes 7 and 8 *(45,46)*.

Somers et al. examined, using karyotyping, cell cultures derived from PD plaque tissue, adjacent tunica, dermis, and lymphocytes in patients with PD and compared the results to cell cultures established from the tunica albuginea of control patients. Chromosomal abnormalities were detected in 7 of 12 PD patients (58%). Thus, the similarity in cytogenetic findings between PD and Dupuytren's contracture suggests the potential for a common pathway for the fibrosis that occurs in both of these conditions. Regardless of the inciting event, the pathological fibrosis that ensues is the result of the normal wound-healing process gone awry.

We have undertaken studies of numerical changes in specific chromosomes using fluorescent *in situ* hybridization (FISH; Fig. 7) *(47)*. For these studies, we used probes to chromosomes 7, 8, 17, 18, X, and Y. These specific chromosomes were selected based on chromosomes that were aneusomic in Dupuytren's contracture *(45,46)*. On FISH microscopy, we demonstrated consistent aneusomies in PD plaque-derived fibroblasts compared to normal chromosomal complement in control fibroblasts. One of the other interesting findings is that these chromosomal aberrations are present in plaque-derived fibroblasts at very early passages; thus, it is probable that these alterations are present at the commencement of cell culture and do not represent culture artifact. The presence of aneusomies in early passage plaque-derived cells, combined with the absence of any cytogenetic instability in either foreskin or normal tunica-derived fibroblasts, suggests that chromosomal instability in PD plaque-derived fibroblasts is not the result of culture artifact and is therefore likely to be significant.

We have furthermore demonstrated in men with PD that fibroblasts derived from tunica extracted from an area remote from the actual plaque also demonstrate cytogenetic changes, suggesting that PD may be a field defect of the tunica albuginea. This would suggest that the tunica of men with PD itself is predisposed to the development of this condition. The cytogenetic changes, however, are at the cellular level and are not systemic alterations. It is again likely that these alterations are the result of upstream events that result in chromosomal instability.

Other workers have explored cytogenetic changes in PD fibroblasts. Yamanaka et al. assessed DNA isolated from PD plaque tissue for loss of heterozygosity (LOH) and microsatellite alterations (MSIs) *(48)*. Using PCR technology, chromosomes 3, 8, and 9 were selected, and 20 different polymorphic markers were used to assess for MSI and LOH. Of the patients, 40% demonstrated MSI or LOH on at least one locus. These data confirm that cytogenetic instability is prevalent in PD tissue, and that it is probably more widespread throughout the plaque-derived fibroblast genome than previously demonstrated.

CONCLUSIONS

The therapeutic implications of these cytogenetic changes are not readily appreciable. It is probable that these data will more likely explain the biology of PD plaque-derived fibroblasts, which may in turn help us elucidate future pharmacological interventions.

Cell Cycle Dysregulation

Besides increased deposition of collagen, PD is characterized by cellular overproliferation. p53 is intrinsically involved in cell cycle regulation, apoptosis, and DNA damage repair pathways. Aberrant p53 function leading to cell proliferation and immortalization has been implicated in benign and malignant proliferative disorders *(49)*. Absence, alteration, or loss of function of this protein may allow damaged cells, normally halted from passage through the cell cycle, to pass and proliferate, resulting in unregulated cell replication (Fig. 8). Using immunofluorescence, we have demonstrated cellular p53 protein expression in PD plaque-derived fibroblasts but not in control fibroblasts *(4)*. The difference in p53 expression between each individual plaque-derived cell culture and foreskin cells was highly statistically significant. The data clearly demonstrate the presence of p53 in plaque fibroblasts; foreskin fibroblasts demonstrated only a background level of immunofluorescence, indicating no detectable p53. Immunoblotting confirmed detectable levels of p53 in the PD plaque-derived fibroblasts *(50)*.

On flow cytometric analysis, the response of neonatal foreskin fibroblasts to irradiation was characterized by an expected increase in the percent of both G_1 and G_2/M populations, with a concomitant decrease in percentage of S-phase cells, demonstrating the presence of functioning cell cycle checkpoints. In contrast to these findings, plaque fibroblasts showed little change in cell cycle compartments following 5-Gy γ-irradiation, indicating that the p53 pathway is nonfunctional in plaque fibroblasts; thus, there is a lack of functioning cell cycle checkpoints in these cells *(4)*. These data represent the first indication that there is an abnormality in the p53 pathway in plaque-derived fibroblasts. This supports previous findings from analyses of p53 function in other fibromatoses *(51,52)*. The implications of p53 abnormalities in PD are unknown but potentially far-reaching.

In a confirmatory study, high-passage PD plaque-derived fibroblasts were injected into mice with severe combined immunodeficiency (SCID) and demonstrated tumorigenicity (Fig. 9) *(53)*. This finding illustrates that fibroblasts derived from PD plaque are biologically transformed, which in turn suggests that these cells have an altered genome, supporting a potential role for upregulation of proto-oncogenes, downregulation of suppressor genes, or inclusion of exogenous DNA into the cellular genome. Biologically transformed fibroblasts have higher proliferation rates, produce more collagen, and demonstrate chromosomal instability, all of which have been demonstrated in our cell culture model of PD.

The UCLA group has used microarray technology to assess for genes that are upregulated in plaque tissue extracted from men with PD *(6)*. This approach has been successfully applied to other disease entities, including prostate disease, renal cell carcinoma, colon cancer, aging, and multiple sclerosis. mRNA levels were compared between plaque and normal tunica tissue using two distinct gene chips (Clontech and Affymetrix). This group found several genes that were upregulated and a small number that were downregulated. In summary, the finding indicated that genes involved in matrix production (procollagenase IV) and cell proliferation (c-myc, protomysoisn-β) were upregulated, and those involved in matrix degradation (elastase IIB) were downregulated. The utilization of gene chips has allowed the development of "disease-related profiles," which will further our understanding of the biology of this condition and may permit the development of novel therapeutics.

CONCLUSIONS

These data, although intriguing and representing elegant work, much like the cytokine data do little to explain the nature of PD and more likely explain the downstream events that occur once the PD cascade has been initiated. It is interesting that PD plaque-derived fibroblasts seem to act in such a dysregulated fashion and are tumorigenic in SCID mouse models, suggesting perhaps an inherent defect in these cells. This may in turn explain why some men are susceptible to this condition and others are not.

NOS and PD

NOS and PD

A great deal of interest has arisen in the role of NO and NOS in the pathophysiology of PD. Both no and nos are well known to andrologists because of the role they play in erectile function. NOS has three varieties: neuronal (NOS-I), endothelial (NOS-III), and inducible (NOS-II) or iNOS (58). The last is produced by smooth muscle cells and macrophages, among other cell types. The production of iNOS is stimulated by cytokines (interleukin-1, TNF-β), interferon, endotoxin, and NF-κB (55). At supraphysiological levels, NO resulting from iNOS upregulation starts to play a role as an oxidant generator. Peroxynitrite is a potent free radical and a poor vasorelaxant and can be generated from excess NO. The role of iNOS in wound healing is confusing. Under certain circumstances, it promotes wound healing; under others, it may be fibrogenic and destructive. Recent data suggest that mice deficient in iNOS experienced delayed wound healing. On the other hand, iNOS may play a role in fibrogenesis; for example, inhibition of iNOS decreases fibrosis in an animal model of collagen-induced arthritis. Bivalacqua et al. demonstrated increased levels of iNOS protein and decreased levels of endothelial NOS protein in the cavernosal tissue of men with PD (55).

Vernet et al. explored the impact of NO on fibroblast differentiation in the rat model of PD (56). Myofibroblasts are present in PD plaque and represent a distinct population of cells in cells cultured from PD plaque tissue. These workers found that the myofibroblast population was increased in human PD plaque tissue as well as rat tunica after TGF-β injection when compared to control tunica. Furthermore, chemical inhibition of iNOS resulted in an increase in myofibroblast number, suggesting that iNOS may play some role in limiting the myofibroblast population in an effort to reduce tunical scarring and contraction.

Thus, although defining the contribution of iNOS and NO in the genesis of PD is in its embryonic stages and much work remains to be done, preliminary data indicate that there is probably a role for these factors in the pathophysiology of PD. The UCLA group has been interested in plasminogen activator inhibitor 1 (PAI-1). This factor is an inhibitor of fibrin clearance. Using a rat fibrin model of PD (14) (see Chapter 13), they have demonstrated that (1) PAI-1 levels are elevated in the fibrin-injected animals compared to the saline-injected animals, and that (2) PAI-1 levels are higher in PD cells and tissue compared to "normal" tunica albuginea using both immunohistochemistry and reverse transcriptase PCR (57).

CONCLUSIONS

NO and NOS have long been targets for ED treatment, and it is possible that their manipulation in PD, for example through gene therapy or small interfering RNA interference technologies, may translate into an avenue worth exploring therapeutically.

THE FUTURE

Although we are at point in time of the greatest basic science interest in this condition, we remain at a point far away from therapeutics that may be of benefit to patients. In my opinion, the greatest deficiency for the testing of novel therapeutics is the absence of an animal model that clearly and definitively represents PD (as opposed to penile fibrosis). In the words of the PD research pioneer Tom Lue: "Urologists are left with no research funding, no institutional support and no patient advocates in helping the fight against the disease. Nevertheless, armed with our scientific curiosity, innovative minds and sincerity to serve our patients we will eventually prevail" (58).

REFERENCES

1. Somers KD, Dawson DM, Wright GL Jr, et al. Cell culture of Peyronie's disease plaque and normal penile tissue. J Urol 1982; 127: 585–588.
2. Anderson MS, Shankey TV, Lubrano T, Mulhall JP. Inhibition of Peyronie's plaque fibroblast proliferation by biologic agents. Int J Impot Res 2000; 12(suppl 3): S25–S31.
3. Mulhall JP, Thom J, Lubrano T, Shankey TV. Cytogenetic evidence in support of Peyronie's disease being a tunical field defect process. J Urol 2000; 163: 747A.
4. Mulhall JP, Branch J, Lubrano T, Shankey TV. Perturbation of cell cycle regulators in Peyronie's disease. Int J Impot Res 2001; 13: S21–S28.
5. Mulhall JP, Thom J, Lubrano T, Shankey TV. Basic fibroblast growth factor expression in Peyronie's disease. J Urol 2001; 165: 419–423.
6. Gonzalez-Cadavid NF, et al. Gene expression in Peyronie's disease. Int J Impot Res 2002; 14: 361–374.
7. El-Sakka AI, Hassoba HM, Chui RM, Bhatnagar RS, Dahiya R, Lue TF. An animal model of Peyronie's-like condition associated with an increase of TGF-β mRNA and protein expression. J Urol 1997; 158: 2284–2290.
8. El-Sakka AI, Hassoba HM, Pillarisetty RJ, Nunes L, Dahiya R, Lue TF. Peyronie's disease is associated with an increase in transforming growth factor β protein expression. J Urol 1997; 158: 1391–1397.
9. Devine CJJ, Somers RD, Lagoda LE. Peyronie's disease: pathophysiology. Prog Clin Biol Res 1991; 370: 355–358.
10. Devine CJJ, Angemeir RW. Anatomy of the penis and male perineum. AUA Update 1993; 12.
11. Devine CJJ, Somers KD, Jordan GH, Scholssberg SM. Proposal: trauma as the cause of Peyronie's lesion. J Urol 1997; 157: 285–290.
12. Jarow JP, Lowe FC. Penile trauma: an etiologic factor in Peyronie's disease and erectile dysfunction. J Urol 1997; 158: 1388–1390.
13. Somers KD, Dawson DM. Fibrin deposition in Peyronie's disease plaque. J Urol 1997; 157: 311.
14. Davila HH, Ferrini MG, Rajfer J, et al. Fibrin as an inducer of fibrosis in the tunica albuginea of the rat: a new animal model of Peyronie's disease. BJU Int 2003; 91: 830–838.
15. Akkus E, et al. Structural alterations in the tunica albuginea of the penis: impact of Peyronie's disease, aging and impotence. Br J Urol 1997; 79: 47–53.
16. Bitsch M, Kromann-Andersen B, Schou J, et al. The elasticity and the tensile strength of tunica albuginea of the corpora cavernosa. J Urol 1990; 143: 642–645.
17. Chiang PH, Chiang CP, Shen MR, et al. Study of the changes in collagen of the tunica albuginea in venogenic impotence and Peyronie's disease. Eur Urol 1992; 21: 48–51.
18. Dini G, Grappone C, Del Rosso M, et al. Intracellular collagen in fibroblasts of Peyronie's disease. J Submicrosc Cytol 1986; 18: 605–611.
19. Aurich M, Poole AR, Reiner A, et al. Matrix homeostasis in aging normal human ankle cartilage. Arthritis Rheum 2002; 46: 2903.
20. Aurich M, Squires GR, Reiner A, et al. Differential matrix degradation and turnover in early cartilage lesions of human knee and ankle joints. Arthritis Rheum 2005; 52: 112.
21. Cole AA, CS-Szabo G, Levine LA. Decreased collagenase in the tunica albuginea of older patients could contribute to the progression of Peyronie's plaque. J Urol 2004; 171: 4(suppl), abstract 1247.
22. Cole AA, Levine LA. Increased endogenous inhibitors of collagenases within Peyronie's plaques may represent a scar remodeling disorder. J Urol 2005; 173(suppl), abstract 944.
23. Chilton CP, Castle WM, Westwood CA, Pryor JP. Factors associated in the etiology of Peyronie's disease. Br J Urol 1982; 54: 748.
24. Nachsteim DA, Rearden A. Peyronie's disease is associated with an HLA class II antigen HLA-DQ5, implying an autoimmune etiology. J Urol 1996; 156: 1330.
25. Ralph DJ, Mirakian R, Pryor JP, Bottazzo GF. The immunological features of Peyronie's disease. J Urol 1996; 155: 159–162.
26. Ralph DJ, Schwartz G, Moore W, Pryor JP, Ebringer A, Bottazzo GF. The genetic and bacteriological aspects of Peyronie's disease. J Urol 1997; 157: 291–294.
27. Rompel R, Mueller-Eckhardt G, Schroeder-Printzen I, et al. HLA antigens in Peyronie's disease. Urol Int 1994; 52: 34–37.
28. Rompel R, Weidner W, Mueller-Eckhardt G. HLA association of idiopathic Peyronie's disease: an indication of autoimmune phenomena in etiopathogenesis? Tissue Antigens 1991; 38: 104–106.

29. Schiavino D, Sasso F, Nucera E. Immunologic findings in Peyronie's disease: a controlled study. Urology 1997; 50: 764–768.
30. Leffell MS, Devine CJ Jr, Horton CE, et al. Non-association of Peyronie's disease with HLA B7 cross-reactive antigens. J Urol 1982; 127: 1223–1224.
31. Stewart S, Malto M, Sandberg L, et al. Increased serum levels of anti-elastin antibodies in patients with Peyronie's disease. J Urol 1994; 152: 105–106.
32. Libby P, Egan D, Skarlatos S. Roles of infectious agents in atherosclerosis and restenosis: an assessment of the evidence and need for future research. Circulation 1997; 96: 4095–4103.
33. Sambiase NV, Higuchi ML, Nuovo G, et al. CMV and transplant-related coronary atherosclerosis: an immunohistochemical, in-situ hybridization and PCR in situ study. Mod Pathol 2000; 13: 173–179.
34. Tanaka K, Zou JP, Takeda K, et al. Effects of human CMV immediate early proteins on p53-mediated apoptosis in coronary artery smooth muscle cells. Circulation 1999; 99: 1656–1659.
35. Yamashiroya HM, Ghosh L, Yang R, Robertson AL. Herpesviridae in the coronary arteries and aorta of young trauma victims. Am J Pathol 1988; 130: 71–79.
36. Zhou YF, Leon MB, Waclawiw MA, et al. Association between prior CMV infection and the risk of restenosis after coronary atherectomy. N Engl J Med 1996; 335: 624–630.
36. Stewart S, et al. Increased serum levels of anti-elastin antibodies in patients with Peyronie's disease. J Urol 1994; 152: 105–106.
37. Wong YK, Dawkins KD, Ward ME. Circulating Chlamydia pneumoniae DNA as a predictor of coronary artery disease. J Am Coll Cardiol 1999; 34: 1435–1439.
38. Sikka SC, Helstrom WJG. Role of oxidative stress and antioxidants in Peyronie's disease. Int J Impot Res 2002; 14: 353–360.
39. Ludwig G. Evaluation of conservative therapeutic approaches to Peyronie's disease (fibrotic induration of the penis). Urol Int 1991; 47: 236–239.
40. Primus G. Orgotein in the treatment of plastic induration of the penis (Peyronie's disease). Int Urol Nephrol 1993; 25: 169–172.
41. Kovacs EJ. Fibrogenic cytokines: the role of immune mediators in the development of fibrosis. Immunol Today 1991; 12: 17–23.
42. Kovacs EJ, Dipietro LA. Fibrogenic cytokines and connective tissue production. FASEB J 1994; 8: 854–861.
43. Lin CS, Lin G, Wang Z, et al. Upregulation of monocyte chemoattractant protein 1 and effects of transforming growth factor-β 1 in Peyronie's disease. Biochem Biophys Res Commun 2002; 295: 1014–1019.
44. Miyajima A, Chen J, Lawrence C, et al. Antibody to transforming growth factor-beta ameliorates tubular apoptosis in unilateral ureteral obstruction. Kidney Int 2000; 58: 2301–2313.
45. Bowser-Riley S, Bain AD, Noble J, et al. Chromosome abnormalities in Dupuytren's disease. Lancet 1975; 2: 1282–1283.
46. Sergovich FR, Botz JS, McFarlane RM. Nonrandom cytogenetic abnormalities in Dupuytren's disease. N Engl J Med 1983; 308: 162–163.
47. Mulhall JP, Nicholson B, Pierpaoli S, Lubrano T, Shankey TV. Chromosomal instability is demonstrated by fibroblasts from the tunica of men with Peyronie's disease. Int J Impot Res 2004; 16: 288.
48. Yamanaka M, Ribeiro-Filho L, El-Sakka A, et al. Genetic instability in Peyronie's disease. J Urol 2001; 165: 201.
49. Levine AJ. p53, the cellular gatekeeper for growth and division. Cell 1997; 88: 323–331.
50. Martin DJ, Lubrano T, Shankey TV, Choubey D, Mulhall JP. Immunoblot analysis of p53 and cyclin D in Peyronie's disease. Int J Impot Res 2002.
51. Moffatt EJ, Kerns BJ, Madden JM, et al. Prognostic factors for fibromatoses: a correlation of proliferation index, estrogen receptor, p53, retinoblastoma, and src gene products and clinical features with outcome. J Surg Oncol 1997; 65: 117–122.
52. Yokoi T, Tsuzuki T, Yatabe Y, et al. Solitary fibrous tumour: significance of p53 and CD34 immunoreactivity in its malignant transformation. Histopathology 1998; 32: 423–432.
53. Mulhall JP, Martin DJ, Lubrano T, et al. Peyronie's disease fibroblasts demonstrate tumorigenicity in the severe combined immunodeficiency (SCID) mouse model. Int J Impot Res 2004; 16: 99.
54. Burnett AL. Nitric oxide regulation of penile erection: biology and therapeutic implications. J Androl 2002; 23: S20–S26.

55. Bivalacqua TJ, Champion HC, Leungwattanakij S, et al. Evaluation of nitric oxide synthase and arginase in the induction of a Peyronie's-like condition in the rat. J Androl 2001; 22: 497–506.

56. Vernet D, Ferrini MG, Valente EG, et al. Effect of nitric oxide on the differentiation of fibroblasts into myofibroblasts in the Peyronie's fibrotic plaque and in its rat model. Nitric Oxide 2002; 7: 262–276.

57. Davila HH, Magee TR, Zuniga FI, et al. Peyronie's disease associated with increase in plasminogen activator inhibitor in fibrotic plaque. Urology 2005; 65: 645.

58. Lue TF. Peyronie's disease: an anatomically based hypothesis and beyond. Int J Impot Res 2002; 14: 411.

5

Evaluation of the Man
With Peyronie's Disease

Jason M. Greenfield, MD and Laurence A. Levine, MD

SUMMARY

The proper evaluation of the male patient with Peyronie's disease (PD) involves a focused medical history as well as a detailed sexual history. Coupled with an extensive history of the disease, these components are crucial to the subjective assessment. The two main components of the objective assessment include the physical exam focusing on the penis, and evaluation of the patient at maximum erection with (preferred) or without duplex ultrasound. The most important component of the physical exam is assessment of the penis for length, deformity, and plaque. Erectile capacity is one of the most important parameters in the assessment of the man with PD. Duplex ultrasonography after injection with a vasoactive agent is the recommended means for evaluation of vascular flow parameters and erectile response, and it allows objective measurement of deformity in the erect state. The association between PD and erectile dysfunction has been firmly established. The patient's response to pharmacological agents both before and after development of PD may factor into decisions regarding the direction of future therapy for both problems. Evaluation of the male with PD varies across clinical studies, and no standard currently exists. This chapter provides a framework for obtaining the subjective and objective information for the man presenting with PD.

Key Words: Duplex ultrasonography; erectile dysfunction; hinge-effect; penile curvature; penile deformity; penile shortening; Peyronie's disease.

INTRODUCTION

Despite increasing knowledge about Peyronie's disease (PD), no standardized approach to the evaluation of the man with PD currently exists. Although numerous clinical trials of therapies are performed internationally each year, results are difficult to interpret because of lack of uniformity in the reporting of results. A validated questionnaire has yet to be established. In addition, the subjective and objective data on which the patient assessment should focus, and the methods of obtaining such data, have yet to be agreed on. If true strides are to be made in the management of PD, then homogeny must be established among researchers of this disease. The aim of this chapter is twofold. First, we review the subjective and objective parameters currently employed in the evaluation of

From: *Current Clinical Urology:*
Peyronie's Disease: A Guide to Clinical Management
Edited by: L. A. Levine © Humana Press Inc., Totowa, NJ

the man with PD. Second, we suggest an algorithm and patient questionnaire to aid in patient assessment and treatment.

SUBJECTIVE ASSESSMENT

The initial evaluation of the man with PD begins with the patient interview. A detailed history should be taken that includes the duration and onset of the disease, inciting event (if any), and the presenting signs and symptoms (pain, deformity, erectile function). While recording the patient's subjective curvature deformity, the degree as well as the direction of the curve should be noted. Although curvature is the most common presenting complaint, pain, other deformities of the shaft, and erectile dysfunction (ED) can be significantly distressing to the patient or may even be the primary concern. Regarding penile deformities other than curvature, patients may also admit to complaints of shaft narrowing, indentation, hinging, distal softening, and penile shortening. Prior therapies to which the patient has been exposed will also provide insight into the history of the patient's disease. It is common for the man presenting with PD to have undergone a trial of at least one oral therapy for PD before reaching the office.

Duration of disease is an especially important point to elicit in the patient interview. When planning treatment for the patient's disease, stability of the deformity is critical to establish before surgical intervention is considered. Lack of change in the patient's deformity as well as the duration of that stability should be investigated and recorded as part of the patient's history.

Pain is another critical point in the patient interview. The pain each patient experiences can vary greatly between subjects. Patients may experience pain with touch, erection, or intercourse. Pain may have resolved, be persistent, or acutely worsening, which may also yield information about the stability of the disease. It also is helpful to elicit the factors involved with the discomfort, including local inflammation or torque on the penis occurring during coitus but not with erection alone.

A detailed general medical and sexual history is also indicated. The medical history should focus on identifying a history of trauma as well as a personal or family history of wound-healing disorders, including Dupuytren's contracture. It is also important to identify vascular risk factors for ED, including hypertension, diabetes, hyperlipidemia, and smoking history. In terms of erectile function, baseline subjective rigidity should be assessed. Patients may grade their erections on a numerical scale (e.g., a 4-point scale) (1). Particular questions that can prove helpful in describing the extent of ED include, "Are your erections adequate for penetration?" as well as, "If your penis had no deformity, would your current rigidity be adequate for vaginal penetration and completion of intercourse?"

Sexual function may be assessed using a validated questionnaire. One such questionnaire is the International Index of Erectile Function (2). Wincze et al. proposed an additional questionnaire that they called the Erection Quality Scale (3). It is critical for the questionnaire to be done both before and after any therapy is instituted for PD. Consistency across clinical trials in terms of utilizing validated questionnaires (not to mention the same questionnaire) is severely lacking. In fact, in a review of 68 articles focusing on PD, only 6% of the studies used any form of validated questionnaire (4).

A strong relationship between PD and ED has been well established (5). A study by Kadioglu et al. investigated the two diseases and their presentation in the outpatient setting. Of 448 patients with PD, 16% were detected during a diagnostic workup for ED (6). This represents a significant proportion of patients with an initial complaint of ED having PD as an incidental finding.

Previous therapies used by the patient for ED may provide insight not only into the severity of ED but also into the cause of PD development in that individual. Examples of PD developing with the use of intracavernosal and injection therapies as well as commercial vacuum constriction devices are present in the literature (7,8). Although trauma is not identified as an inciting factor in all patients who present with PD, it should be investigated in all patients who present with Peyronie's. We suggest the use of a patient questionnaire for all new patients presenting with PD to aid in the evaluation (Fig. 1).

OBJECTIVE ASSESSMENT

The first portion of the objective evaluation of the man with PD should be the physical exam. In addition to focusing on the genitourinary exam, attention should also be paid to the patient's hands for evidence of Dupuytren's contracture. Obviously, examination of the penis is critical.

Penile length should first be measured. Although no standard exists for measuring penile length, it is our opinion that the best and most consistent manner in which to perform this is by measuring the distance dorsally from corona to pubis with the penis on full stretch. It is important that pressure is applied to the suprapubic fat pad for an accurate measurement. Measurements done ventrally or with erection are difficult to reproduce.

Objective evaluation is recommended to include routine penile duplex ultrasound with pharmacological stimulation, usually with an injectable agent, to induce a full erection similar to or better than that which the patient would normally experience during sexual arousal. This modality will allow for obtaining an objective measure of vascular flow parameters during erection and curvature as well as assess plaque characteristics and erectile response to intracavernosal injection. Although dynamic penile ultrasound is a desirable study as it can provide a variety of useful information, the key objective measure to obtain is curvature. Therefore, if this modality is not available, direct physical evaluation of the erect penis using oral or injectable agents may be used.

Curvature is perhaps the most important parameter in the assessment. Despite the fact that penile curvature is the hallmark of PD, there is no consensus on how to measure curvature objectively. The subjective assessment given by the patient is not sufficient as the only means of reporting the deformity as discrepancy commonly exists between subjective and objective measurements. The most reliable method of reporting curvature seems to be measurement with a protractor or goniometer by the physician or technician at the time of maximum erection. A commonly utilized and reported technique in the literature is the use of photography, either by the patient or physician. Conclusions and measurements of the patient's deformity are then drawn from the photographs. This technique is not recommended because of its propensity for error and inconsistency. Vacuum-induced erections generally cause the shaft to appear straighter than it would normally and are therefore unsuitable for the objective assessment of curvature. This seems to be caused by extratunical girth created by the vacuum, which can mask curvature or indentation.

As mentioned, both the degree and the direction of curvature are important to note during the exam. First, to assess changes after treatment properly, these parameters must be identified and compared to their pretreatment state. Direction of curvature has multiple implications. If a surgical straightening is considered, for example, in a patient with a ventral curve, then plications may need to be placed along the dorsum of the penis,

PEYRONIE'S DISEASE PATIENT QUESTIONNAIRE

Date: _____

Name: _____   Age: _____   Marital Status: _____

PLEASE CIRCLE THE MOST ACCURATE ANSWER OR FILL IN THE BLANKS

I. History

1. When did you first notice the presence of Peyronie's disease? _____

2. Please number the order (1,2,3) in which the following symptoms occurred(if at all)
    (Pain)   (Lump)   (Curvature or Bend)

3. Did the penile deformity occur: (Suddenly)   (Gradually)

4. Do you recall (Pain), (Injury) or (bending) of your penis during intercourse before developing Peyronie's disease? ( ) No   ( ) Yes, Please describe (i.e., Mis-thrust, Female on top):_____
_____

5. Do you recall any other injury to your Penis?   ( ) No   ( ) Yes (When did this occur and what was the nature of your injury?) _____

6. Have you been treated for Peyronie's disease prior to this visit? ( ) No   ( ) Yes (Circle the treatment you received):   (Vitamin E)   (Potaba)   (Colchicine)   (Tamoxifen) (Injections: Verapamil, Interferon, steroids)   (Anti-inflammatory medication)
    (Other): _____
    Did you note any benefit from this therapy? ( ) No   ( ) Yes: What? _____

7. Are you currently undergoing treatment for Peyronie's disease? ( ) No   ( ) Yes (What treatment are you currently receiving?) _____

8. Do you or a family member have a history of: (Dupuytren's contracture) (Lederhose disease) (Any unusual scarring disorders) ( ) No ( ) Yes (Who?): _____

9. Has your penile curvature worsened over time?   ( ) No   ( ) Yes: Is it stable now? (How long?)
_____

10. Would you describe your penile curvature as: ( ) Up ( ) Down ( ) Left ( ) Right
Can you estimate the degree of curve? (Right angle is 90°, straight is 0°) _____

11. Have you noticed any shrinking or loss of length of your penis? ( ) No   ( ) Yes (Estimate how much in inches) _____

12. Have you noticed any other deformity?   ( ) No   ( ) Yes: (Circle all that apply)
(Hinge effect at head)   (Hinge effect at base)   (Narrowing of shaft): Left   Right
(All around like hourglass) - where on shaft   –   (base)   (mid)   (end of shaft);
(Softening of penis beyond lump/scar or curve)

THE FOLLOWING QUESTIONS ASK YOU TO GRADE THE QUALITY OF YOUR ERECTIONS – PLEASE CIRCLE THE NUMBER THAT BEST DESCRIBES THE QUALITY OF YOUR ERECTIONS
Use the following numbers (0-3) as a guide to describe the rigidity (hardness) of your penile erection when you are sexually aroused:
(0) No Erection   (1) Partial Erection not hard enough for penetration
(2) Partial Erection hard enough for penetration   (3) Full, rigid erection.

13. Prior to developing Peyronie's disease, would you grade your erection as:
        (0)   (1)   (2)   (3)

14. How would you grade your erection over the past month?
        (0)   (1)   (2)   (3)

Fig. 1. Peyronie's disease patient questionnaire.

15. Do you have any difficulty now in maintaining your erection after penetration? ( ) No   ( ) Yes

16. Do you currently have an erection in the morning before you urinate?
( ) No   ( ) Yes (How often?)
   (0)   (1)   (2)   (3)

17. Do you currently ever awaken at night and notice an erection?
( ) No   ( ) Yes (How often?)
   (0)   (1)   (2)   (3)

18. At present time, are you capable of having sexual intercourse?
( ) No   ( ) Yes

19. What is your sexual partner preference?
(Women)   (Men)   (Both)

20. Currently do you experience pain in your penis during sexual activity?
( ) No   ( ) Yes

21. Have you experienced pain in your penis at any time while you've had Peyronie's disease? ( ) Yes
( ) No   (At first but now gone)   (From start till now)

22. Does your partner experience pain during sexual intercourse due to the penile deformity?
( ) No   ( ) Yes

23. Do you have difficulty with penetration due to (Circle all that applies):
(Curvature)   (Hinge effect)   (Lack of firmness).

24. Has the presence of Peyronie's disease has effected your relationship with your sexual partner?
( ) No   ( ) Yes

25. Do you feel the presence of Peyronie's disease has affected your emotional status?
( ) No   ( ) Yes

26. Do you consider your current sexual desire/libido: (Normal)   (Low)   (High)

27. Have you noticed any change in the sensation of your penis since developing Peyronie's disease?
( ) No   ( ) Yes   (Decreased sensation) (Numbness)   (painful sensation).

28. Are you able to ejaculate? ( ) No   ( ) Yes (By what method-circle all that apply)
(Intercourse)   (Masturbation)   (Oral sex)

29. Are you troubled by rapid ejaculation? ( ) No   ( ) Yes   (Recently- only occasionally)
(Consistently throughout lifetime)   (Occasionally throughout lifetime)   (Recently – almost always)

30. Do you currently smoke? ( ) No   ( ) Yes: (Cigarettes) (Cigars) (Pipes) How much and long? (Per
day/week/month_____) (For_____Years/Months)

31. Have you smoked tobacco in the past? ( ) No   ( ) Yes   (How much :_____) (For how long
:_____)   (When did you quit_____)

32. Do you currently consume alcoholic beverages? ( ) No   ( ) Yes: (wine) (Beer) (Other)   How much:
(Rarely)   (_____Drinks per day)   (_____Drinks per week)   (_____Drinks per month).

33. Have you in the past consumed alcoholic beverages?   ( ) No   ( ) Yes: (wine) (Beer) (Other)
How much: (Rarely) (_____Drinks per day)   (_____Drinks per week) (_____Drinks per
month)
When did you stop:_____   (Have a history of alcoholism)

34. Are you presently taking medication prescribed by any doctor?   ( ) No ( ) Yes
(Please list all – Include aspirin, etc.):_____

35. Do you have a history of any of the following (even if under control with medicine)?   (Circle all that apply):
(Diabetes)   (High blood pressure)   (Elevated cholesterol)   (Coronary heart disease)
(severe straddle injury)   (Back trauma/ Surgery)
(Any other vascular disease; if yes, what :_____)

where injury to nerves may occur. Our investigation into penile shortening following tunica albuginea plication for penile curvature demonstrated that a ventral curve, with or without a lateral component, predisposes the patient to the greatest risk of significant penile shortening. Finally, degree of curvature also can guide the surgeon into whether plaque incision or excision with grafting may be necessary. It has been recommended that this more complex technique be considered for the man with a curvature greater than 60°, significant hourglass deformity causing hinge effect, and full erectile capacity (9).

Penile deformity may be noted on physical exam, especially during pharmacologically induced erection. Although it may be noted as an important complaint during the patient interview, there is currently no validated objective measurement of narrowing of the penile shaft. Techniques that may be considered include measuring shaft circumference with a flexible ruler or string during erection. Points of maximum and minimum circumference should be noted. Axial stability and hinging of the penis can only be assessed during an erection.

The existence of a palpable plaque and its characteristics should also be noted. In some patients, identification of a discrete plaque may be difficult. Some patients with PD may also exhibit hypertrophy of the septum between the paired corpora cavernosa. It is unclear at this time whether hypertrophic tissue is an extension of the plaque contributing to the deformity. Characteristics of the plaque that may be noted on physical exam may include plaque size, location, tenderness to palpation, and texture (calcification). Interestingly, plaque size has been commonly reported in clinical trials as a marker for successful treatment. However, plaque size in itself has yet to be proven as a reliable indicator of a reduction in penile deformity and patient satisfaction.

Part of the problem is that plaque size is difficult to measure or estimate. Plaques may have extensions in multiple directions that are difficult to identify by physical exam or other imaging modalities. The typical plaque is not discrete or uniform in thickness. Length, width, and depth of the plaque may all be variable. Estimating size with a ruler or caliper is likely the best technique but probably offers little significance in terms of assessing treatment options or treatment outcome. The presence of plaque calcification is best determined with a xeroradiograph or ultrasound. Although the implications of the presence of calcifications have yet to be fully elucidated, it has definite value in deciding on treatment options, especially in the case of nonsurgical treatment. This is because extensive platelike calcification rarely responds to medical therapy, including injections, whereas "stippled" calcification may not interfere with potential treatment benefit.

Although the exact characteristics of the penile plaque may offer little benefit, its presence in the man who is not presenting with PD as a chief complaint may be. For example, in a study, 534 men who presented to a urologist's office for prostate cancer screening underwent physical exam for evidence of a palpable penile plaque (10). Forty-eight patients (9%) were identified with plaque. In addition, these men with PD were also found to have significantly lower reported scores on the Sexual Health Inventory for Men questionnaire. This study adds to the suggestion that PD is not an uncommon finding in the patient presenting to the urologist's office with a complaint other than PD and should be considered to be a routine part of the general genitourinary exam.

The benefit of various imaging modalities in the evaluation of the man with PD has yet to be firmly established. In 1998, Andresen et al. examined various imaging modalities in 20 patients with PD (11). All patients underwent autophotography as well as ultrasound, plain x-ray using the two-plane technique similar to mammography, computed tomography (CT), and magnetic resonance imaging (MRI). Penile deviation was best assessed using plain x-ray in mammography technique. Of the 12 patients with calcified plaques, the calcification was noted in all patients with each imaging technique with the exception of MRI, which only identified 9 patients (75%). The imaging modalities able to identify thickening of the tunica albuginea were ultrasound, CT, and MRI (87.5, 25, and 75%, respectively). The only imaging modality that was able to identify periplaque inflammation was MRI coupled with gadolinium diethylenetriaminepentaacetic acid (gd-DTPA).

The final component of the objective assessment that must be addressed is erectile capacity. Again, this parameter is assessed both during the patient interview and during the objective assessment with duplex ultrasound and vasoactive injection. However, it is critical to realize that this assessment is important to the evaluation of the patient both before and after treatment. During the assessment of the pharmacologically induced erection, the patient's response should be noted with a numerical scale as well as the amount/number of doses required to achieve maximum erection. How the rigidity compares to the erection "at home" should also be graded independently by the patient (i.e., better, same, worse than at home). Objective estimates of erectile capacity may offer benefit, especially during counseling and decision making for further treatment (9,12). We recommend the use of a standard form for all patients undergoing dynamic duplex ultrasonography; an example is included in this chapter (Fig. 2).

CONCLUSIONS

Subjective and objective evaluations of the male with PD vary across clinical studies, and no standard currently exists. The subjective parameters elicited during the patient interview may vary, and a standard questionnaire has yet to be agreed on universally. A focused medical history as well as a detailed sexual history and history of the disease are crucial to the subjective assessment. The presence and description of curvature, pain, shaft deformity, and ED are all crucial points to be investigated. These areas must be investigated at each patient visit and are especially important to document before and after therapy is instituted. Assessing for the presence of PD in the patient presenting to the urologist's office with a seemingly unrelated chief complaint should also be considered, especially in the case of a patient with ED.

The two main components of the objective assessment are physical exam and evaluation of the patient at maximum erection with (preferred) or without dynamic duplex ultrasound. The physical exam should include a focused general exam with special attention to the hands as well as a comprehensive genitourinary exam. The most important component of the physical exam is assessment of the penis for length, deformity, and plaque. Penile length should be measured with the penis on full stretch and by measuring along the dorsal shaft from pubis to corona as this is the most consistently reproducible method. Deformities and curvature are best assessed during maximum erection. Direction and degree of curvature should be noted and are most consistently measured with a protractor or goniometer by the physician or technician performing the study. Plaque can be assessed both by physical exam or duplex ultrasonography. The value of plaque size in the evaluation has yet to be established. Other studies, such as plain x-ray, CT, and MRI, yield additional expense without proven benefit.

Erectile capacity is one of the most important parameters in the assessment of the man with PD. Duplex ultrasonography after injection with a vasoactive agent is the recommended means for evaluation of vascular flow parameters and erectile response. The

PENILE DUPLEX ULTRASOUND REPORT

Personal Information and Health History:

Name: _____   Date: _____

Age: _____   Physician: _____

HTN: _____ DM: _____ Smoker: _____ ETOH: _____

Cardiac Hx: _____ Other: _____

Medications: _____

Erectile Dysfunction: Peyronie's Disease:

Procedure Data:

Injected drug: (Papaverine / PGE1 / Tri-mix) Dose: _____ Re dosing:_____

Deep Cavernous Arterial Diameter

                         LEFT: RIGHT:

Before Injection: _____mm   _____mm

After Injection: _____mm   _____mm

Flow Velocity Information:

Initial Response ≤ 5 minutes (Tumescence phase)

           Peak Systolic (cm/sec)   End Diastolic (cm/sec)   RI

LEFT _____   _____   _____

RIGHT_____   _____   _____

Post Stimulation – Manual +/- Visual   (Rigidity Phase)

LEFT _____   _____   _____

RIGHT_____   _____   _____

Other Data:

Procedure Response   **Erectile Response**

        Hematoma _____   Maximum Rigidity by technician/MD (0 – 10 scale) _____

        Dizziness _____   Initial Response _____/_____

        Pain   _____   Maximum Response _____/_____

        Pulsatility (0 – 4 scale) _____   Reversal (necessary +/-; drug to reverse/dose) _____

                                      Plaque dimensions _____ L _____ W _____ D _____

                                      Curve (by protractor at max erection) L _____ R _____ Dorsal/Ventral ___

Findings: a) calcification   **Compared to Home Erection (by patient):**
          b) narrowing/indention – location _____   (same / better / worse)
          c) circumference – at base _____ at narrowed area _____
                    proximal to corona _____
          d) hinge effect
          e) dorsal artery perforators

Impression:

_____
_____
_____
_____
_____

Fig. 2. Penile duplex ultrasound report.

association between PD and ED has been firmly established. The patient's response to pharmacological agents both before and after development of PD may factor into decisions regarding the direction of future therapy for both diseases.

Examples of documentation that may be used in the subjective and objective assessment of the patient with PD are included in this chapter. Consistency in this evaluation across practicing urologists is crucial for promoting and furthering our knowledge of this disease.

REFERENCES

1. Levine LA, Estrada CR. Human cadaveric pericardial graft for the surgical correction of Peyronie's disease. J Urol 2003; 170: 2359–2362.
2. Rosen RC, et al. The International Index of Erectile Function (IIEF): a multidimensional scale for assessment of erectile dysfunction. Urology 1997; 49: 822–830.
3. Wincze J, et al. Erection Quality Scale: initial scale development and validation. Urology 2004; 64: 351–356.
4. Levine LA, Greenfield JM. Establishing a standardized evaluation of the man with Peyronie's disease. Int J Impot Res 2003; 15(suppl 5): S103–S112.
5. Weidner W, Schroeder-Printzen I, Weiske WH, Vosshenrich R. Sexual dysfunction in Peyronie's disease: an analysis of 222 patients without previous local plaque therapy. J Urol 1997; 157: 325–328.
6. Kadioglu A, et al. Incidentally diagnosed Peyronie's disease in men presenting with erectile dysfunction. Int J Impot Res 2004; 16: 540–543.
7. Kim JH, Carson CC. Development of Peyronie's disease with the use of a vacuum constriction device. J Urol 1993; 149: 1314.
8. Hakim LS, et al. Vacuum erection associated impotence and Peyronie's disease. J Urol 1996; 155: 534–535.
9. Levine LA, Lenting EL. A surgical algorithm for the treatment of Peyronie's disease. J Urol 1997; 158: 2149–2152.
10. Mulhall JP, et al. Subjective and objective analysis of the prevalence of Peyronie's disease in a population of men presenting for prostate cancer screening. J Urol 2004; 171: 2350–2353.
11. Andresen R, Wegner HE, Miller K, Banzer D. Imaging modalities in Peyronie's disease. An intrapersonal comparison of ultrasound sonography, x-ray in mammography technique, computerized tomography, and nuclear magnetic resonance in 20 patients. Eur Urol 1998; 34: 128–134.
12. Levine LA, Greenfield JM, Estrada CR. Erectile dysfunction following surgical correction of Peyronie's disease and a pilot study of the use of sildenafil citrate rehabilitation for postoperative erectile Dysfunction. J Sex Med 2005; 2: 241–247.

6 Oral Treatment of Peyronie's Disease

Claudio Teloken, MD, PhD, Tulio Graziottin, MD, and Patrick E. Teloken, MS

SUMMARY

This chapter reviews the possible effectiveness of oral agents as an option for treatment of Peyronie's disease (PD). We present the rationale for use of these drugs and base our recommendations on levels of published evidence and the report by the International Consultation on Urological Diseases. A definitive and ideal medical therapy for PD has yet to be established and will not be until we completely understand the trigger mechanism and the maintenance process of fibrosis in the tunica albuginea. Several oral substances have been proposed with promises of success; however, these agents appear to lack robust scientific support for their benefit. Until new evidence is available, the indications for oral treatment in PD are recent onset of disease, painful plaque, and unstable plaque. An early trial of inexpensive, safe, and well-tolerated oral therapy may be offered with limited enthusiasm for a positive outcome.

Key Words: Conservative management; medical treatment; oral treatment; Peyronie's disease.

Peyronie's disease (PD) has been challenging researchers since its description in 1743. PD is possibly a malfunction of the scarring process in the tunica albuginea, resulting in fibrosis and calcification of the tunica. The result of this process in some patients is penile bending, pain, and nodule formation. The usual course of PD has two distinct clinical phases: (1) early phase, in which the plaque is new, still in formation, and inflammation is noticeable; (2) late phase, in which plaque is relatively stable. Fibrosis predominates, and some cases progresses toward calcification.

Despite progress in the research for a precise etiology of PD, we still do not completely understand the trigger mechanism and the maintenance process of fibrosis in the tunica. The consequence of this limitation is the absence of an ideal medical treatment for PD. Several new approaches have been proposed to ameliorate the disease, although a definitive medical therapy for PD has yet to be established.

From: *Current Clinical Urology:*
Peyronie's Disease: A Guide to Clinical Management
Edited by: L. A. Levine © Humana Press Inc., Totowa, NJ

Table 1
Levels of Evidence and Grades of Recommendation Utilized in This Chapter

Level of evidence	Commentary
1	Usually meta-analysis of RCT or good-quality RCT
2	Low-quality RCT (<80% follow-up) or meta-analysis of good-quality prospective cohort studies
3	Good-quality retrospective case-control studies with appropriately matched control
	Good-quality case series
4	Expert opinion

Grades of recommendation	
A Highly recommended	Based on level 1 studies, exceptionally level 2 high-rated studies
B Recommended	Based on consistent level 2 or 3 studies or majority evidence from RCT
C Optional	Based on level 4 or majority evidence from level 2 or 3 studies
D Not recommended	No evidence or conflicting results; no recommendation is possible

RCT, randomized controlled trials. (Adapted from ref. 3.)

Until new evidence is presented, the indications for oral treatment in PD are as follows: (1) recent onset of disease; (2) pain in the plaque; (3) nonstable plaque; and (4) contraindication to surgery. Because the early stage of disease is reputed to respond better than well-established plaques, an early trial of inexpensive, safe, and well-tolerated oral therapy is often initially recommended (1). However, in a case without symptoms and palpable plaque, there is no scientific agreement that any intervention is necessary other than observation.

Oral treatment for PD requires more robust evidence of effectiveness given by randomized controlled trials (RCTs) (2). In this chapter, the levels of evidence and recommendations are based on the International Consultation on Urological Diseases (Table 1) (3).

PROCARBAZINE

Pharmacology

Procarbazine hydrochloride, a methyl hydrazine derivative, is primarily an antineoplastic agent (4). There is evidence that the drug may act by inhibiting the synthesis of proteins, RNA, and DNA. In addition, procarbazine may directly damage the DNA. Procarbazine is rapidly and completely absorbed following oral administration, metabolized primarily in the liver and kidneys, and excreted in the urine. The main toxic effect of the drug is bone marrow suppression, resulting in leukopenia, anemia, and thrombocytopenia. Hematological, gastrointestinal, neurological, cardiovascular, ophthalmic,

Table 2
Procarbazine vs Vitamin E:
Randomized, Single-Blind, Crossover Study (7)

	Improvement	
	50 mg procarbazine twice daily, 3 mo	*200 mg vitamin E three times daily, 3 mo*
Curvature	9%	37%
Curvature resolution	0	6.45%
No change	86.3%	61.2%
Curvature worsening	4.5%	0

respiratory, genitourinary, musculoskeletal, and endocrine adverse effects may occur (5). Nausea and vomiting are the most commonly reported side effects. Because of its action in mitosis and meiosis, azoospermia and infertility are potential side effects of the drug.

Because procarbazine hydrochloride possesses some monoamine oxidase (MAO) inhibitory activity, sympathomimetic drugs (including those in nose drops and cough preparations), local anesthetics, tricyclic antidepressants (e.g., amitriptyline hydrochloride, imipramine hydrochloride), and other drugs and foods with known high tyramine content such as cheese, bananas, yogurt, tea, coffee, wine and cola drinks, and cigarettes should be avoided. Procarbazine is contraindicated in patients with known hypersensitivity to the drug or inadequate marrow reserve.

Rationale for Use in Peyronie's Disease

Procarbazine inhibits the proliferation of rapidly dividing fibroblasts (6).

Scientific Evidence

Procarbazine was first utilized for the treatment of PD in the 1970s (2). In an open-label crossover study, 34 men were randomly assigned to receive procarbazine (20 mg twice daily) or vitamin E (200 mg three times daily) for 3 mo and after the other drug (Table 2) (7). Pain, deformity, lump, ease of penetration, and intercourse were assessed. Vitamin E was superior to procarbazine; however, because there was no placebo group, we cannot state that procarbazine has no effect in PD. Moreover, only 67% of patients completed the study. Procarbazine is probably not useful in PD because side effects are frequent (grade C).

VITAMIN E

Pharmacology

Vitamin E, a fat-soluble vitamin, is present in many foods, and wheat germ is a rich source of this substance. Vitamin E is metabolized in the liver and excreted in bile. The exact biological function of vitamin E in humans is still under investigation. Vitamin E has antioxidant properties, it is involved in the digestion and metabolism of polyunsaturated fat, in the reduction of platelet aggregation and blood clot formation, in the promotion of normal growth, in the development of muscle tissue, and in the synthesis of prostaglandin (8).

Table 3
Vitamin E vs Placebo:
Randomized, Double-Blind Crossover Study *(10)*

	N	Improvement	
		200 mg vitamin E three times daily, 3 mo	*Placebo*
Pain	14	5[a] (35.7%)	1 (7.1%)
Curvature	38	3 (7.89%)	0
Erection quality	39	0	3 (7.69%)
Penetration	35	3 (8.57%)	5 (14,2%)
Ability to have sex	35	5 (14.2%)	3 (8.57%)

[a]Two additional patients improved but stopped attending.

Vitamin E increases hypoprothombinemic response to oral anticoagulants, especially in doses higher than 400 IU/d. Thus, care should be taken when used concomitantly with oral anticoagulants.

Usual dosage in PD is 800–1000 IU/d *(5)*.

Rationale for Use in Peyronie's Disease

The antioxidant activity of the drug could have some benefit in PD.

Scientific Evidence

Scott and Scardino proposed the use of vitamin E in 1948 *(9)*. A randomized, double-blind, crossover, placebo-controlled trial was published in 1983 *(10)*. Sixty men received randomly vitamin E (200 mg) or placebo three times daily for 3 mo each (Table 3). Patients were evaluated monthly based on the severity of symptoms (pain, deformity, quality of erection, capacity of penetration, and coitus). Only 40 patients completed the study (67%), and vitamin E was not different from placebo with the possible exception of the improvement of pain. Despite lack of scientific evidence of its action in PD, vitamin E is inexpensive, safe, and widely utilized (grade C).

PARA-AMINOBENZOATE POTASSIUM

Pharmacology

Para-aminobenzoate (Potaba™) is considered a member of the vitamin B complex. Small amounts are found in cereal, eggs, milk, and meats. Detectable amounts are normally present in human blood, spinal fluid, urine, and sweat. Para-aminobenzoate is a component of several important biological systems, and it participates in a number of fundamental biological processes *(4)*. It has been suggested that Potaba exerts an antifibrotic effect by means of an unknown mechanism. It has been postulated that fibrosis results from an imbalance of serotonin and MAO mechanisms at the tissue level. Fibrosis is believed to occur when an excessive serotonin effect is sustained over a period of time. This could be the result of too much serotonin or too little MAO activity. Aminobenzoate potassium increases oxygen utilization at the tissue level. It has been suggested that this increased oxygen utilization could enhance the degradation of serotonin by

Table 4
Potaba Trial in PD:
Randomized, Double-Blind, Placebo-Controlled *(13)*

	3 g Potaba four times daily, 12 mo		Placebo	
	N	*Improvement*	*N*	*Improvement*
Pain	8	6 (75%)[a]	14	6 (43%)
Curvature	20	2 (10%)	21	3 (14%)
Plaque size	20	10 (50%)	21	7 (33%)
Ability to have sex	20	6 (30%)	21	3 (14%)

[a]Statistically significant difference.

enhancing MAO activity or other activities that decrease the tissue concentration of serotonin *(4)*.

Based on a review of this drug by the National Academy of Sciences–National Research Council, the Food and Drug Administration has classified the indications as follows: potassium aminobenzoate is possibly effective in the treatment of scleroderma, dermatomyositis, morphea, linear scleroderma, pemphigus, and Peyronie's disease.

Although infrequent, adverse reactions include anorexia, nausea, fever, and rash; they subside with the suspension of the drug. Desensitization can be accomplished and treatment resumed as necessary. Potaba should not be administered to patients taking sulfonamides, and care should be taken in patients with renal disease.

The average adult daily dose of Potaba is 12 g, usually given in four to six divided doses. Tablets must be taken with an adequate amount of liquid to prevent gastrointestinal upset *(5)*.

Rationale for Use in Peyronie's Disease

Because fibrosis of the tunica albuginea is a component of PD, Potaba could reduce fibrosis by increasing the oxygen supply at the tissue level and enhancing MAO activity.

Scientific Evidence

Zarafonetis and Horrax utilized Potaba in 1959 *(11)*. Initially, a small, blinded study suggested it to be efficacious *(12)*.

A multicenter RCT with 60 men compared 12 mo of treatment with 4 g Potaba three times a day and placebo. The final report of this study never was published; however, a preliminary report of the outcome for 41 men showed no benefit of the active treatment except for the possible improvement in pain (Table 4) *(13)* (level 2).

Another RCT published in the form of an abstract demonstrated less worsening of symptoms in the treatment group and no difference in improvement of pain *(14)*.

Weidner et al. performed an RCT comparing Potaba 12 g/d to placebo in 103 men with PD for less than 12 mo, noncalcified plaques, and without previous treatment. After 12 mo of therapy, no relevant difference in the improvement of preexisting penile deviation was found. However, Potaba exerted a significant protective effect with regard to new development or deterioration of penile curvature *(15)* (level 2).

Potassium para-aminobenzoate appears to be useful for stabilizing the disorder and preventing progression of penile curvature.

Nonetheless, treatment with Potaba is costly and its high rate of side effects probably limit its use in PD (grade C).

TAMOXIFEN

Pharmacology

Tamoxifen citrate, a triphenylethylene derivative, is a nonsteroidal agent that has demonstrated potent antiestrogenic properties in animals. The antiestrogenic effects may be related to its ability to compete with estrogen for binding sites in target tissues such as breast. Tamoxifen inhibits the induction of rat mammary carcinoma and exerts its anti-tumor effects by binding to the estrogen receptors *(4)*.

Tamoxifen is extensively metabolized after oral administration. Fecal excretion is the primary route of elimination.

Decreases in platelet counts, leukopenia, neutropenia, and pancytopenia have been occasionally reported. Alterations in hepatic enzymes and increase in serum concentrations of thyroxine (T_4) were observed in a few patients. Elevated thyroxine is possibly a result of an increase in thyroid-binding globulin; however, clinical hyperthyroidism has not been reported. Infrequent cases of hyperlipidemia have been reported *(5)*.

Loss of libido and impotence have been reported in some male patients. In oligosper-mic men who were receiving tamoxifen therapy, increased luteinizing hormone, folli-cle-stimulating hormone, testosterone, and estrogen concentrations were reported. Because tamoxifen and its metabolites are potent inhibitors of cytochrome P450 mixed-function oxidases, there is a potential for interaction with medications that require mixed-function oxidases for activation *(4)*.

When tamoxifen citrate is used in combination with coumarin-type anticoagulants, a significant increase in anticoagulant effect may occur, and careful monitoring of the patient's prothrombin time is recommended. In vitro studies showed interactions with erythromycin, cyclosporin, nifedipine, and diltiazem. However, the clinical significance of these in vitro studies is unknown.

Appropriate studies of the relationship of age to the effects of tamoxifen have not been performed in the geriatric population.

Rationale for Use in Peyronie's Disease

Tamoxifen is a synthetic nonsteroidal antiestrogen that inhibits keloid fibroblast pro-liferation and collagen production because of decreasing in vitro transforming growth factor-β production *(16,17)*.

Scientific Evidence

In the initial study of the use of tamoxifen in PD in 1992, Ralph and coworkers utilized the drug (20 mg twice daily) without controls in 36 men *(18)*. Improvements in pain (16 of 20 patients), erectile deformity (11 of 31 patients), and plaque shrinkage (12 of 35 patients) were reported. Patients with a history of disease of less than 4 mo obtained better response. On the other hand, Teloken and coworkers, in a double-blinded controlled report utilized tamoxifen (20 mg twice daily) in 25 patients in the late stage of disease (mean 20 mo). The authors did not demonstrate any therapeutic advantage of tamoxifen over placebo (Table 5) (level 2 evidence) *(19)* (grade C).

Table 5
Tamoxifen vs Placebo:
Randomized, Double-Blind, Placebo-Controlled *(19)*

	20 mg tamoxifen twice daily, 3 mo		Placebo	
	N	*Improvement*	*N*	*Improvement*
Pain	6	4 (66%)	4	3 (75%)
Curvature	13	6 (46%)	12	5 (42%)
Plaque size	13	4 (31%)	12	3 (25%)

COLCHICINE

Pharmacology

Colchicine, a phenanthrene derivative, is an antigout drug obtained from species of *Colchicum* and apparently exerts its effect by reducing the inflammatory response and diminishing phagocytosis. Following oral administration, this agent is absorbed from the gastrointestinal tract and is partially metabolized in the liver. The drug and its metabolites reenter the intestinal tract via biliary secretions, and the unchanged drug may be reabsorbed from the intestine. Plasma concentrations of colchicine and its metabolites decline at 1–2 h after ingestion and then increase, probably as a result of reabsorption of unchanged drug. After reabsorption, it is rapidly removed from the plasma, distributed into various tissues and concentrated in leukocytes. The drug and its metabolites are also distributed into other tissues, including kidneys, liver, spleen, and intestinal tract but appear to be absent in heart, skeletal muscle, and brain *(8)*.

Colchicine is contraindicated in patients who have serious gastrointestinal, hepatic, or cardiac disorders, and reduction in dosage is indicated if weakness, anorexia, nausea, vomiting, or diarrhea occurs. Colchicine should not be given in the presence of combined renal and hepatic disease. Daily dosage of oral colchicine should not exceed 0.6 mg in patients with serum creatinine concentrations of 1.6 mg/dL or greater or creatinine clearances of 50 mL/min or less; some patients can be adequately treated with 0.6 mg every other day *(4)*.

Colchicine has been shown to induce reversible malabsorption of vitamin B_{12}, apparently by altering the function of ileal mucosa.

Adverse reactions to colchicine appear to be a function of dosage. The possibility of increased colchicine toxicity in the presence of hepatic dysfunction should be considered. The appearance of peripheral neuritis, muscular weakness, nausea, vomiting, abdominal pain, diarrhea, urticaria, aplastic anemia, agranulocytosis, thrombocytopenia, dermatitis, purpura, or alopecia may require reduction of dosage or discontinuation of the drug. Because geriatric patients may have decreased renal function and because patients with renal impairment appear to be at increased risk of colchicine-induced toxicity, assessment of renal function should be performed in any aging patient for whom therapy is contemplated and initial dosage should be reduced and appropriate precautions initiated accordingly *(8)*.

Colchicine is inexpensive and reasonably well tolerated, but approximately one-third of patients will have diarrhea. If used in patients in the early stage, the dosage is 0.6 mg three times a day with meals. According to most authors, the higher daily dose should not exceed 2.4 mg.

Rationale for Use in Peyronie's Disease

Four mechanisms of action have been identified (6):

1. Colchicine binds to tubulin and causes it to depolymerize and subsequently inhibits mobility and adhesion of leukocytes.
2. It inhibits cell mitosis by disrupting the spindle fibers.
3. It blocks the lipoxygenase pathway of arachidonic acid metabolism, thus diminishing chemotaxis and inflammatory response.
4. It interferes with the transcellular movement of protocollagen.

By these means, colchine has antifibrotic, antimitotic, and anti-inflammatory activities.

Scientific Evidence

Dominguez-Malagon and coworkers utilized colchicine in three patients with fibromatoses, including one with PD (20). Early treatment with colchicine ameliorates a Peyronie-like condition in an animal model (21). In an uncontrolled pilot study, Akkus and coworkers demonstrated reduction of plaque size (12 of 24 patients), pain relief (7 of 9 patients), and improvement of penile curvature (7 of 19 patients) (22). Interestingly, some patients receiving high doses of colchicine for the treatment of familial Mediterranean fever developed PD (23).

In an uncontrolled study of 60 men with early disease (mean 5.7 mo) treated with 0.5 mg three times daily, colchicine improved the pain and ameliorated the deformity in 95 and 30% of the patients, respectively (24).

A single RCT studied 84 patients with noncalcified plaque (25). The mean disease duration was 15 mo, and patients received 0.5–2.5 mg of colchicine and placebo. Objective evaluation of the plaque and symptoms failed to demonstrate any action of colchicine (Table 6).

COLCHICINE PLUS VITAMIN E

Scientific Evidence

Prieto Castro and coworkers in a single-blind study compared the use of 1 mg colchicine twice daily plus 600 mg vitamin E twice daily vs 200 mg ibuprofen twice daily for 6 mo in patients with PD in the early stages (time from onset < 6 mo), penile curvature of less than 30°, and no erectile dysfunction (26). Plaque size and penile curvature significantly decreased in the group receiving colchicine plus vitamin E; however, pain relief was not different (Table 7) (level 2).

CARNITINE

Pharmacology

Levocarnitine (L-carnitine) is a naturally occurring substance required in mammalian energy metabolism. It has been shown to facilitate long-chain fatty acid entry into cellular mitochondria, thereby delivering substrate for oxidation and subsequent energy production. Fatty acids are utilized as an energy substrate in all tissues except the brain. In skeletal and cardiac muscle, fatty acids are the main substrate for energy production (4).

Table 6
Colchicine vs Placebo:
Randomized, Double-Blind, Placebo-Controlled *(25)*

	0.5–2.5 mg colchicine daily, 4 mo	*Placebo, 4 mo*
	Improvement	
Pain	60%	63.6%
Curvature change	17.1%	18.4%
Plaque size	10.5%	10%

Table 7
Vitamin E Plus Colchicine vs Ibuprofen: Randomized, Single-Blind *(26)*

	300 mg vitamin E twice daily plus 1 g colchicine twice daily, 6 mo	*200 mg ibuprofen twice daily, 6 mo*
	Improvement	
Pain	21 (91%)	15 (68%)
Curvature	6 (46%)[a]	4 (18%)
Plaque size change (cm)	−0.26[a]	+0.13

[a]Statistically significant difference.

Levocarnitine is indicated for treatment of primary systemic carnitine deficiency, a genetic impairment of normal biosynthesis or utilization from dietary sources; for the treatment of secondary carnitine deficiency resulting from an inborn error of metabolism; or for the prevention and treatment of carnitine deficiency in patients with end-stage renal disease supported on hemodialysis *(4)*.

Levocarnitine oral solution may be consumed alone or dissolved in drinks or other liquid foods to reduce taste fatigue. It should be consumed slowly, and doses should be spaced evenly throughout the day to maximize tolerance. Gastrointestinal reactions may result from too rapid consumption of the substance.

Various mild gastrointestinal complaints have been reported during the long-term administration of oral L-carnitine; these include transient nausea and vomiting, abdominal cramps, and diarrhea. Decreasing the dosage often diminishes or eliminates drug-related patient body odor or gastrointestinal symptoms when present. Tolerance should be monitored very closely during the first week of administration and after any dosage increases *(4)*.

The safety and efficacy of oral levocarnitine has not been evaluated in patients with renal insufficiency. Chronic administration of high doses of oral levocarnitine in patients with severely compromised renal function may result in accumulation of the potentially toxic metabolites *(5)*. In patients with preexisting seizure activity, an increase in seizure frequency or severity has been reported.

Table 8
Carnitine vs Tamoxifen: Randomized, Double-Blind *(27)*

	1 g carnitine twice daily, 3 mo	*20 mg tamoxifen twice daily, 3 mo*
	Improvement	
Pain	22 (92%)	15 (68%)
Curvature change	−7.5°	−0.5°
Plaque size change (mm^2)	−68.8	−26.9

Rationale for Use in Peyronie's Disease

It was suggested that carnitine restores cells when damaged by inflammation, probably because of inhibition of the toxic coenzyme acetyl-coenzyme A.

Scientific Evidence

The action of acetyl-L-carnitine was assessed in two RCTs. In the preliminary report, 48 patients (15 "acute" phase and 33 "chronic" phase) were randomly assigned to utilize 20 mg tamoxifen twice daily or 1 g acetyl-L-carnitine twice daily for 3 mo (Table 8) *(27)*. At 6 mo, acetyl-L-carnitine was significantly more effective than tamoxifen in reducing pain. Only acetyl-L-carnitine ameliorated penile bending; however, both drugs reduced plaque size. Tamoxifen induced significantly more side effects than acetyl-L-carnitine. However, patients in this study do not represent the typical patient with PD because they had mild degrees of curvature, and the mean duration of disease before seeking medical treatment was 5 wk.

In a second study utilizing ester-proprionyl-L-carnitine (acetyl-carnitine is no longer available), 75 men were randomly assigned in a double-blind design to receive weekly intraplaque verapamil (10-mg) injections plus ester-proprionyl-L-carnitine (1 mg twice daily) or tamoxifen (20 mg twice daily) alone for 3 mo *(28)*. The majority of the patients completed the trial (80%), but the amount of significant improvement in curvature and plaque size was 11.8° and 7.6 mm^2, respectively (level 2).

ONGOING TRIALS WITH ORAL DRUGS

Recently, many new drugs have been used in trials, however conclusive results are still wanted.

Fexofenadine (Allegra)

Fexofenadine HCl is an antihistamine with selective peripheral H_1-receptor antagonist activity. This drug is known to be substantially excreted by the kidney, and the risk of toxic reactions may be greater in patients with impaired renal function.

Gerald H. Jordan (personal experience) has utilized terfenadine (Seldane™) and more recently fexofenadine (Allegra™). Fexofenadine is utilized as a nonspecific antihistamine in doses of 60 mg twice a day in patients with unusual long and painful courses of symptomatic plaque. The medication is expensive, but well tolerated. Unfortunately, no definitive data are available yet.

Pentoxifylline

Pentoxifylline, a synthetic xanthine derivative, is a hemorrheologic agent. It is utilized for the treatment of intermittent claudication associated with peripheral vascular disease and for the management of acute and chronic cerebrovascular insufficiency. Although it has been shown to stimulate fibroblast apoptosis in an experimental model, the precise mechanism of action for pentoxifylline in management of PD remains unclear.

Anecdotally, an oral dose of 400 UI/d for 3 to 6 mo has been used. Overall, it is well tolerated.

Pentoxifylline Combined With Vitamin E

Studies involving pentoxifylline plus vitamin E demonstrated regression in radiation-induced fibrosis in uncontrolled studies *(29)*. Based on this, we are currently carrying out a prospective study using monotherapy or a combination of both drugs (400 IU pentoxifylline and 1000 IU vitamin E). Data are not available yet.

In radiation-induced fibrosis, the combination of both drugs was more effective than placebo monotherapy *(29)*. Gastrointestinal and nervous system effects are rarely reported.

CONCLUSION

A great number of oral medical treatments have been suggested and utilized in PD, however, few prospective clinical trials have been undertaken; so far, no drug has shown optimal results. Consequently, only limited advances in this particular field have been achieved. New drugs hold promise of success, although there is no consensus for the optimal design of a trial with oral therapy for PD, in part due to a lack of total understanding of the pathophysiological mechanism of the disease.

Every patient deserves a thorough discussion regarding possible risks and benefits of each oral agent. Patient preference has a significant role in the selection of specific oral therapy. With advances in the comprehension of the mechanisms of inflammation and scarring and the development of new agents, it is expected that more effective oral treatments for PD will become available.

REFERENCES

1. Mynderse LA, Monga M. Oral therapy for Peyronie's disease. Int J Impot Res 2002; 14: 340–344.
2. Pryor JP, Akkus E, Alter G, et al. Priapism, Peyronie's disease and penile reconstructive surgery. In: Second International Consultation on Sexual Dysfunction—Paris, France (Lue TF, Basson R, Rosen R, et al., eds.). Health Publications, 2004, pp. 383–408.
3. Evidence-based medicine: overview of the main steps for developing and grading guideline recommendations. In: Second International Consultation on Sexual Dysfunction—Paris, France (Lue TF, Basson R, Rosen R, et al., eds.). Health Publications, 2004, pp. 15–16.
4. USP DI Drug Information for the Health Care Professional. Thomson Micromedex; Greenwood Village, CO, 2005.
5. Mosby's Drug Consult. 15th ed. Mosby, St. Louis, MO, 2005.
6. Levine LA, Elterman L. Peyronie's disease and its medical management. In: Male Infertility and Sexual Dysfunction (Hellstrom WJ, ed.). Springer-Verlag, New York, 1997, pp. 474–480.
7. Morgan RJ, Pryor JP. Procarbazine (Natulan) in the treatment of Peyronie's disease. Br J Urol 1978; 50: 111.
8. AHFS Drug Information. American Society of Health-System Pharmacists, Bethesda, MD, 2005.
9. Scott W, Scardino P. A new concept in the treatment of Peyronie's disease. South Med J 1948; 41: 173–176.

10. Pryor J, Farrel CR. Controlled clinical trial of vitamin E in Peyronie's disease. Prog Reprod Biol Med 1983; 9: 41–45.

11. Zarafonetis CJ, Horrax TM. Treatment of Peyronie's disease with potassium para-aminobenzoate (Potaba). J Urol 1959; 81: 770–772.

12. Hasche-Klunder, R. [Treatment of Peyronie's disease with para-aminobenzoacidic potassium (POTABA) (author's trans.)]. Urologe A 1978; 17: 224–227.

13. Shah, PJR, Green NA, Adib RS, et al. A multicentre double blind controlled clinical trial of potassium paraaminobenzoate (Potaba) in Peyronie's disease. Prog Reprod Biol Med 1983; 9: 61–67.

14. Weidner W, Hauck EW, Schroeder-Printzen I, et al. Aminobenzoate potassium (Potaba) in the therapy of Peyronie's disease. Int J Impot Res 2000 (suppl); 50.

15. Weidner W, Hauck EW, Schnitker J. Potassium paraaminobenzoate (Potaba) in the treatment of Peyronie's disease: a prospective, placebo-controlled, randomized study. Eur Urol 2005; 47: 530–535.

16. Chau D, Mancoll JS, Lee S, et al. Tamoxifen downregulates TGF-β production in keloid fibroblasts. Ann Plast Surg 1998; 40: 490–493.

17. Mikulec AA, Hanasono MM, Lum J, et al. Effect of tamoxifen on transforming growth factor β_1 production by keloid and fetal fibroblasts. Arch Facial Plast Surg 2001; 3: 111.

18. Ralph DJ, Brooks MD, Bottazzo GF, et al. The treatment of Peyronie's disease with tamoxifen. Br J Urol 1992; 70: 648.

19. Teloken C, Rhoden EL, Grazziotin TM, et al. Tamoxifen vs placebo in the treatment of Peyronie's disease. J Urol 1999; 162: 2003–2005.

20. Dominguez-Malagon HR, Alfeiran-Ruiz A, Chavarria-Xicotencatl P, et al. Clinical and cellular effects of colchicine in fibromatosis. Cancer 1992; 69: 2478–2483.

21. El-Sakka AI, Bakircioglu ME, Bhatnagar RS, et al. The effects of colchicine on a Peyronie's-like condition in an animal model. J Urol 1999; 161: 1980–1983.

22. Akkus E, Carrier S, Rehman J, et al. Is colchicine effective in Peyronie's disease? A pilot study. Urology 1994; 44: 291–295.

23. Erdogru T, Usta MF, Ates M, et al. Development of Peyronie's disease during long-term colchicine treatment. Int Urol Nephrol 2003; 35: 207–208.

24. Kadioglu A, Tefekli A, Koksal T, et al. Treatment of Peyronie's disease with oral colchicine: long-term results and predictive parameters of successful outcome. Int J Impot Res 2000; 12: 169–175.

25. Safarinejad MR. Therapeutic effects of colchicine in the management of Peyronie's disease: a randomized double-blind, placebo-controlled study. Int J Impot Res 2004; 16: 238–243.

26. Prieto Castro RM, Leva Vallejo ME, Regueiro Lopez JC, et al. Combined treatment with vitamin E and colchicine in the early stages of Peyronie's disease. BJU Int 2003; 91: 522–524.

27. Biagiotti G, Cavallini G. Acetyl-L-carnitine vs tamoxifen in the oral therapy of Peyronie's disease: a preliminary report. BJU Int 2001; 88: 63–67.

28. Cavallini G, Biagiotti G, Koverech A, et al. Oral propionyl-L-carnitine and intraplaque verapamil in the therapy of advanced and resistant Peyronie's disease. BJU Int 2002; 89: 895–900.

29. Chiao TB, Lee AJ. Role of pentoxifylline and vitamin E in attenuation of radiation-induced fibrosis. Ann Pharmacother 2005; 39: 516–522.

7 Intralesional Treatment
of Peyronie's Disease

*Muammer Kendirci, MD, Landon Trost, MD
and Wayne J. G. Hellstrom, MD, FACS*

SUMMARY

Peyronie's disease (PD) is a pathological condition of the penis that is most likely
linked to the repetitive minor trauma that occurs during intercourse. The initial inflammatory process in some genetically susceptible individuals gives way to a subsequent
persistent low-level autoimmune response. At the cellular level, this disorder involves
increased deposition of collagen and glycosaminoglycans in the tunica albuginea of the
penis, which leads to fibrosis and eventual plaque formation. The fibrous plaque can
cause structural alterations in penile anatomy and sexual dysfunction. Experimental
research in PD has invoked a role for cytokines and fibroblast activity, which has motivated clinicians to explore a number of nonsurgical and minimally invasive treatment
options. With the experimental in vitro success of calcium channel blockers and interferons in counteracting the fibrotic process in PD, researchers have initiated a number
of clinical studies with these agents. Both intralesional verapamil and interferon α-2b
have demonstrated significant clinical benefits to men with PD regarding a decrease in
penile curvature and plaque size, reduction of penile pain on erection, and improved
sexual function. Intralesional injection therapy can be initiated in most cases of PD but
must be individualized to each man's presentation based on the onset and severity of the
disease, the patient's motivations, and realistic expectations from this therapy.

   Key Words: Collagenase; intralesional treatment; interferon; minimally invasive;
nonsurgical; Peyronie's disease; steroid; therapy; verapamil.

INTRODUCTION

Peyronie's disease (PD) is a localized connective tissue disorder characterized by an
inelastic, fibrous scar in the tunica albuginea of the penis (*1*). Most authorities believe that
PD is a result of repetitive trauma that occurs during intercourse, which in turn incites an
inflammatory process and subsequent low-level autoimmune response (*2*). This process
results in increased deposition of collagen and glycosaminoglycans, which eventually
leads to fibrosis of the tunica albuginea and plaque formation. The fibrous plaque often

From: *Current Clinical Urology:*
Peyronie's Disease: A Guide to Clinical Management
Edited by: L. A. Levine © Humana Press Inc., Totowa, NJ

Table 1
Proposed Mechanisms and Side Effects
of Various Agents Used in Intralesional Injection Therapy of PD

Drug	Mechanism of action	Side effects
Steroids	Anti-inflammatory, decreasing collagen synthesis	Local tissue atrophy, skin thinning, fibrosis
Collagenase	Collagen breakdown	No reported side effects
Orgotein	Anti-inflammatory, superoxide dismutase activity	Pain, swelling, stiffness, prickling or burning sensations, skin rashes, feeling of heaviness at the injection site
Interferon	Inhibition of fibroblast proliferation, stimulation of collagenase activity, inhibition of collagen production	Flulike symptoms, sinusitis, arthralgia, ecchymosis
Verapamil	Alters the balance of collagen synthesis and degradation	Penile bruising, ecchymosis, nausea, lightheadedness, pain

leads to alterations in penile anatomy and sexual dysfunction. Typical complaints of patients presenting with PD include a palpable penile plaque, pain on erection, and penile curvature.

The choice of a conservative treatment is a therapeutic dilemma. Oral treatment alternatives include vitamin E, potassium aminobenzoate (Potaba®), colchicine, tamoxifen, and L-carnitine. On the other hand, intralesional injection of various agents such as steroids, calcium channel blockers, clostridial collagenase, orgotein, and interferons (IFNs) have been promulgated as minimally invasive treatment options for PD (3) (Table 1).

STEROIDS

Because of their recognized anti-inflammatory effects, steroids were popular many years ago as an intralesional therapy for the treatment of PD. Bodner et al. first documented a decrease in plaque size and pain on erection using injections of the steroid dexamethasone (4). However, these authors reported that this treatment did not show any statistical difference from the natural history of the disease. Williams and Green used a long-acting glucocorticoid, triamcinolone hexacetonide, in 45 patients with PD and reported 36% complete or marked improvement in PD symptoms (5). Using 6–10 Dermo-jet percutaneous intraplaque injections of dexamethasone in 21 patients over 1–6 mo, Winter and Khanna reported a decrease in plaque size, reduction of pain on erection and discomfort during sexual intercourse, or a disappearance of all symptoms in a high percentage of their cases (6). They also reported a significant reduction in penile curvature. Although a few others reported some success with the use of intralesional steroids, side effects, such as local tissue atrophy, fibrosis, thinning of the skin, and immune suppression, the use of steroid injection therapy for PD has not garnered support from most authorities.

COLLAGENASE

The specific collagenolytic properties of clostridial filtrates were first described in the 1940s, and then Mandl et al. isolated the collagenolytic fraction and detailed the mode of purification in the 1950s *(7)*. In contrast to the vertebrate collagenases, which cleave the tropocollagen molecule into two fragments, the bacterial collagenases are known to act at many collagen sites along the peptide chain, clipping the short segments from each end *(8)*. An in vitro experimental study by Gelbard et al. investigated the effects of highly purified clostridial collagenase on various tissues, including Peyronie's plaque, tunica albuginea from patients undergoing penile prosthesis implantation, fresh human pericardium from cadavers, and human corpora cavernosa obtained at autopsy within 4 h of death *(9)*. Of importance, the clostridial collagenase-injected Peyronie's plaque fragment underwent considerable reduction in overall size and microscopically showed widespread fraying and dispersal of collagen bundles compared to the dense, compact collagen seen in the control tissue injected with saline. Dissolution of the plaque tissue occurred without diges-tion of elastic tissue, vascular smooth muscle, or the myelin sheaths of axons.

The theoretical benefit of intralesional collagenase on the alteration of the collagen content in PD plaques prompted the same researchers to design a pilot study in humans investigating the effects of intralesional purified clostridial collagenase in 31 men with PD *(10)*. The administered dose varied between 270 and 4800 units (mean 2328 units). β-Aminopropionitrile fumarate was administered to the last 25 patients as an adjuvant in an attempt to prevent recurrences by increasing the laxity of collagen formed at the site of the enzymatic wounding. Objective improvement in 65% of the study patients and pain resolution in 93% were reported, usually within 2 wk. Penile plaques either disap-peared or were altered significantly in 4 patients and decreased 20–100% in the remaining 16 patients. Objective relief of deformity using a vacuum-induced erection was docu-mented in 50% of 6 patients with small or impalpable plaques, 75% of 12 patients with moderate lesions, and 65% of 13 patients with large plaques. Side effects were pain at the injection site in 2 patients, ecchymosis in 21, and corporal rupture in 1.

The same group 8 yr later reported on the use of intralesional purified clostrial collagen-ase in 49 patients with PD in a prospective, randomized, placebo-controlled, double-blind study *(11)*. Patients were stratified into three groups based on disease severity (plaque size measurement using a caliper) and the degree of deformity during vacuum chamber photography, as well as using a modification of the Kelâmi classification. Category 1 patients were characterized as those with curvature of 30° or less or palpable plaque less than 2 cm in extent; category 2 patients displayed 30–60° angular deformity or 2- to 4-cm palpable plaque in maximal dimension; and category 3 patients were those with a penile curvature greater than 60° or more than 4 cm of palpable plaque. Treatment group patients in category 1 had 6,000 units, category 2 had 10,000 units, and category 3 had 14,000 units of total cumulative dose of purified clostrial collagenase (nucleolysin). A positive response for collagenase-injected patients was reported as 100% (3/3) in category 1, 36% (4 of 11) in category 2, and 13% (1 of 8) in category 3, whereas it was reported as 25% (1 of 4), 0% (0 of 13), and 0% (0 of 10) in the placebo patients for each category, respec-tively. Overall response was calculated as 36% (8 of 22) for the treatment arm and 4% (1 of 27) for the placebo arm ($p < 0.007$). Of importance, there were no significant side effects or allergic reactions reported. A multicenter, controlled study with intralesional collagenase is currently under initiation in the United States.

ORGOTEIN

The anti-inflammatory properties of orgotein were discovered in 1965 *(12)*. Orgotein, the pharmaceutical form of the bovine enzyme copper-zinc superoxide dismutase, is a metalloprotein compound with pronounced superoxide dismutase activity. Gustafson et al. injected orgotein into the indurated plaques of 22 patients with PD with long-standing and severe symptoms *(13)*. They reported marked improvement in sexual function without significant side effects. The main adverse reactions to orgotein were reported as pain, swelling, stiffness, prickling or burning sensations, skin rashes, and a feeling of heaviness at the injection site *(14)*. Currently, orgotein is not available for use in the United States, mainly because of off-label reports of toxicity.

VERAPAMIL

The rationale for the use of calcium channel blockers in the treatment of PD is based on successful in vitro data. Kelly showed that exocytosis of extracellular matrix molecules, including collagen, fibronectin, and glycosaminoglycans, were calcium-ion-dependent processes *(15)*. In addition, Aggeler et al. demonstrated that calcium antagonists induced a change in fibroblast cell morphology that caused an alteration in the protein secretory phenotype *(16)*. This change resulted in increased extracellular matrix collagenase activity as well as decreased collagen production and deposition. Verapamil, a calcium channel blocker, reduces intracellular calcium concentration, increases collagenase activity, and affects cytokine expression in the early phases of wound healing and inflammation *(17)*. Verapamil is known to inhibit in vitro fibroblast proliferation in plaques derived from patients with PD *(18)*.

The therapeutic serum levels of verapamil used for the treatment of hypertension and cardiac arrhythmias were calculated as $0.01–0.2 \mu M$ when administered orally *(19)*. However, the concentration of verapamil needed to retard extracellular matrix collagen synthesis in an in vitro study was in the $100\text{-}\mu M$ range. Therefore, intralesional application is obligatory to deliver sufficient levels of verapamil directly to the plaque.

In 1994, Levine et al. popularized the use of the calcium channel blocker verapamil by reporting on a dose-escalating trial in 14 men undergoing intralesional therapy for PD *(20)* (Table 2). The authors used biweekly injections of verapamil for 6 mo and increased the dose to 10 mg in a single setting. They documented pain resolution in 91% of patients, decrease in penile curvature in 42%, improvement in erectile function in 58%, and an increase in penile girth in 100% *(20)*.

With a similar dose of verapamil and treatment interval in 39 patients with PD, Arena et al. reported objective improvement in 50% of patients who had a diagnosis of PD for less than 1-yr duration but in only 10.2% of the patients who had the condition for more than 1 yr *(21)*. By contrast, an investigation of the efficacy of verapamil injection with steroid and placebo arms in a controlled study found no significant benefit in favor of verapamil *(22)*. This article has been criticized as injection was perilesional and not into the plaque. However, Rehman et al. performed a long-term single-blind study with verapamil injections in 14 patients using weekly injections for 6 mo *(23)*. They documented reduction in plaque volume in 57% of the verapamil group vs 28% in the placebo group. Furthermore, penile curvature improved from $37.7 \pm 9.3°$ to $29.5 \pm 7.3°$ in the verapamil-treated patients, but this difference was not significantly greater than placebo. These authors reported plaque softening and significant objective improvement in plaque-associated penile narrowing in all patients treated with verapamil. Subjective plaque-associated erectile dysfunction (diminished quality of erections) was improved in 42.87% of the verapamil group vs none in the control group. They concluded that intralesional verapamil was effective in patients with penile curvatures less than 30° and those with noncalcified plaques.

Table 2

Results of Verapamil Treatment Regarding Dose,
Number of Patients, Duration of Treatment, and Improvement Rates With Various Parameters

Reference	Patients (n =)	Dose (mg)	Duration	Pain relief	Decrease in curvature	Decrease in plaque size	Improved sexual function
20	14	10	Biweekly, 6 m	91%	42%	91%	58%
21	39	10	Biweekly, 6 m	91%	50% (PD < 1y) 10% (PD > 1y)	?	?
23	14 (Ver=7; Plc=7)	10	Weekly, 6 m	100% Ver. 100% Plc.	29% Ver. 0% Plc.	57% Ver. 28% Plc.	43% Ver. 0% Plc.
24	46	10	Biweekly, 6 m	97%	54%	97%	72%
25	156	10	Biweekly, 6 m	84%	60%	84%	83%

Plc, placebo; Ver, verapamil.

Subsequently, Levine reported affirmative results with intralesional verapamil regardless of disease severity and duration in an uncontrolled study of patients with PD (24). He employed 12 biweekly injections and documented a decrease in penile curvature in 54% and improvement in erectile function in 72% of PD patients. The author concluded that candidates with poorer prospects for success with verapamil injections include those with plaques larger than 5 cm³, extensive calcification, penile curvature greater than 90°, and no response after six injections.

As a follow-up, Levine and Estrada reported the results of a prospective, nonrandomized study of 156 patients with PD with a mean follow-up of 30.4 mo (25). They noted an objective improvement in penile curvature in 60% (10–75°, mean 25°), increase in girth in 83%, subjective increase in erectile rigidity distal to the plaque in 80%, and improved sexual function in 71% of the participants. Objective measures of curvature change were obtained at full erection using a protractor following intracorporal vasoactive injection by a blinded technician both before and following completion of the injection program. Side effects were noted only in 4% of the patients receiving verapamil and included minor complaints such as nausea, lightheadedness, penile pain, and ecchymosis. No cardiovascular events were reported. A major criticism of this and many studies using intralesional verapamil injections for the treatment of PD is the lack of a placebo arm.

In a related double-blind controlled study, Cavallini and colleagues investigated the effects of verapamil in men with advanced or recalcitrant PD (26). The authors divided 60 patients with PD into two groups: patients on intraplaque verapamil (10 mg/wk for 10 wk) and oral propionyly-L-carnitine (2 g/d for 3 mo) vs those on verapamil and oral tamoxifen (40 mg/d for 3 mo). These investigators documented significant reduction in penile curvature and plaque size and increase in sexual function in the verapamil and propionyly-L-carnitine groups, but they observed the same in the verapamil and tamoxifen group.

Mulhall et al. investigated the impact of intralesional verapamil injections on the progression and improvement of penile deformity in men with PD (27). Patients with a palpable plaque with penile curvature who presented within 12 mo after the onset of PD were included into this nonplacebo-controlled study. Intralesional verapamil was administered every 2 wk for a total of six injections, and the patients were evaluated at least 3 mo after the final injection. A curvature change equal to or greater than 5° was defined as an alteration (improvement or progression). After a mean 5.2 ± 1.8 mo of follow-up in 81 men with PD, intralesional injections of verapamil resulted in an improvement in 22% of the treated patients; 53% remained stable, and 25% worsened. The mean change in penile curvature in men who documented improvement (22 ± 15°) was higher in those with documented worsening (12 ± 7°). The investigators concluded that, compared to their previous natural history population (12% improving, 40% remaining stable, and 48% progressing over a 12-mo period), intralesional injection of verapamil is associated with a lower rate of deformity progression and slightly better improvement rate. A noted limitation of this study is that only six biweekly injections were given, which may not allow adequate time or drug exposure to effect change in scar tissue.

INTERFERONS

IFNs are low-molecularweight proteins that play an important role in the human immune system, mainly via antiproliferative and antitumorigenic effects (28). Duncan and partners first considered the therapeutic potential of IFN treatment for PD (29). These authors used human recombinant (hu-r) IFNs on cultured fibroblasts derived from excised PD plaques.

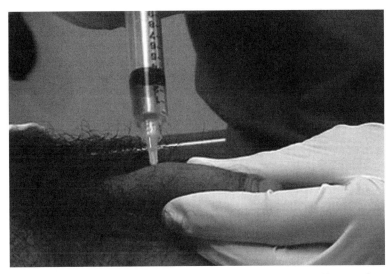

Fig. 1. Intralesional injection of IFN-α-2b into the Peyronie's disease plaque.

They cultured fibroblasts with hu-r-IFN-α2b, hu-r-IFN-βser17, and hu-r-IFN-γ, and noted a concentration-dependent inhibition of fibroblast proliferation and collagen production and an increase in collagenase production. Of note, hu-r-IFN-α and -β had no effect on fibroblast glycosaminoglycan or fibronectin production, and hu-r-IFN-γ caused a marked increase in production. These investigators demonstrated that IFNs, particularly IFN-α and -β, had important antifibrotic properties in relation to PD fibroblasts (i.e., hindering fibroblast production, decreasing collagen synthesis, and upregulating collagenase activity). They concluded that there was a scientific rationale for using IFNs to treat men suffering with PD.

A study by Ahuja and colleagues, using an in vitro model of corpora cavernosal-derived myofibroblasts, demonstrated that the presence of IFN-α-2b diminished collagen production *(30)*. It had already been established that IFNs can reduce collagen deposition and promote collagenaselike activities *(29)*. Dermatological studies have documented a short-term benefit of IFN-α-2b treatment in normalizing keloid fibroblast collagen, glycosaminoglycan, and collagenase production in vitro *(31)*. With these in vitro models of PD clearly supporting INF as a treatment concept, the next step was the initiation of pilot studies employing intralesional IFN (Fig. 1) in men with PD.

The first clinical report of intralesional IFN-α-2b treatment for PD appeared in an abstract by Benson et al. *(32)*. In 10 patients, the authors reported significant plaque softening, improvement in penile curvature, and resolution of penile pain. Wegner et al. subsequently reported on two studies using IFN-α-2b for PD *(33,34)*. In the first study, in 1995, they used 1×10^6 U INF-α-2b with five local injections into the plaques over 1 wk *(33)*. Patients were assessed 1–6 mo after the injections had been administered; a decrease in plaque size was noted in 28% of the men with noncalcified or minimally calcified plaques, and pain resolution occurred in all but 1 patient. However, there was adequate straightening of the penis in only 1 patient (from 18 to 10°) *(33)* (Table 3).

In another study using 3×10^6 U INF-α-2b in 30 patients, the same investigators reported no clinical benefit *(34)*. In their negative summary, they suggested that intralesional injection therapy of INF-α-2b was associated with intolerable side effects and was not

Table 3
Results of Intralesional Treatment With IFN-α-2b Regarding Dose, Number of Patients, Duration of Treatment, and Improvement Rates With Various Parameters

Reference	Patients (n =)	Dose (units)	Duration	Pain relief	Decrease in curvature	Decrease in plaque size	Improvement in sexual function	Plaque softening
33	25	1×10^6	Weekly, 5 wk	96%	4%	28%	?	?
34	30	3×10^6	Weekly, 3 wk	97%	3%	3%	?	?
35	10	1.5×10	3 times/wk, 3 wk	60%	60% (mean 20°)	33%	?	60%
36	21	1×10^6	Biweekly, 6 mo	90%	65%	85%	57%	100%
43	34	10×10^6	Biweekly, 14 wk	94%	47%	From 56.7 to 12.7 (mean, mm²)	79%	?
38	23	2×10^6	3 times/wk, 3 wk	100%	5%	0%	—	?
39	25	2×10^6	Biweekly, 6 wk	80%	67%	71%	5/7 patients	?
40	117 (IFN = 55; Plc = 62)	5×10^6	Biweekly, 12 wk	28.1% Plc, 67.7% IFN	8.8% Plc, 27.0% IFN (% mean decrease)	19.8% Plc, 54.6% IFN (% mean decrease, cm²)	5.96% Plc, 13.53% IFN (% mean increase in EF score)	11.1% Plc 33.3% IFN (% mean decrease)

The dose of IFN-α-2b is expressed as units. Plc, placebo.

[a]An additional three patients served as control with saline injection. No changes were observed in these placebo patients.

[b]Of 21 patients with PD, 7 were in the saline placebo arm. None of the men in the placebo group showed improvement after completion of intralesional injections.

[c]The injections were applied subcutaneously next to the plaque area. Patients who had erectile dysfunction at baseline were excluded from the study.

effective in men with PD. They asserted that surgery was the only option for men with PD. Besides an apparent negative bias, all of these early studies lacked a placebo arm.

In another study by Judge and Wisniewski, the effect of intralesional INF α-2b was studied in 13 men with severe PD of more than 12 mo duration *(35)*. Ten patients were placed in the study group, and 3 were included in a saline control group in which 1.5×10^6 U INF-α-2b was used three times a week over 3 wk. The investigators reported complete disappearance of pain on erection and a significant improvement in penile deformity in 6 of 10 patients. No changes were noted in the control (saline) patients. Although the objective improvement in deformity was relatively small (mean improvement of 20°), the authors concluded that patients with plaques smaller than 4 cm were likely to benefit from this treatment.

In another supportive study, Ahuja et al. in 1999 used intralesional INF-α-2b with 1×10^6 U biweekly for 6 mo in 21 patients and documented pain relief in 9 of 10 patients, subjective softening of the plaque in all patients, significant improvement in penile curvature in 65% of cases, and a decrease in penile plaque size in 85% of patients *(36)*. A major limitation again was the absence of a placebo control arm. These authors concluded that biweekly intralesional injections with IFN-α-2b into PD plaques produced significant improvements in penile curvature, diminished pain, and reduced plaque size.

Another study reported on intralesional injections with 4×10^6 U INF-α-2b once a week for 10 wk in patients with PD *(37)*. They showed decreased penile curvature in 39% of men and diminished plaque size in 38% of the participants. In still another small, nonrandomized, and prospective study of 23 patients using 2×10^6 U INF-α-2b three times a week for 3 wk, pain resolution was noted in 13 of 19 patients *(38)*. However, penile curvature improved in 1 patient, increased in 1 man, and remained unchanged in the remaining 21 patients. They did not perceive any significant change in plaque size and were not overly supportive of INF-α-2b therapy for the conservative treatment of PD, even though it appeared safe and well tolerated and lessened penile pain.

At our institution, in a placebo-controlled study, 21 patients (INF-α-2b in 14, placebo in 7 patients) were administered either 2×10^6 U IFN-α-2b or saline injections biweekly for 6 wk *(39)*. There was an improvement in penile curvature of 20° or more in 67% of men, pain relief in 80%, and subjective improvement in plaque size in 71% of the patients. In addition, we observed significant improvement in erectile function scores in 5 of 7 patients. No placebo patient documented improvement in penile curvature, plaque size, or pain relief.

These results motivated a group of PD researchers to conduct an evidence-based study on the use of IFN-α-2b for the minimally invasive treatment of PD. A prospective, multicenter, placebo-controlled, parallel study was conducted to determine the efficacy and safety of intralesional IFN-α-2b therapy in 117 consecutive PD patients with a mean age of 55 yr (62 in placebo, 55 in IFN-α-2b group) *(40)*. Saline 10 mL for control and INF-α-2b of 5×10^6 U for the study group were administered with six injections biweekly for a total of 12 wk. Objective evaluation of penile curvature was performed in the erect state utilizing a protractor (Bracco Diagnostics, Princeton, NJ), and plaque size was measured using a caliper (Schering, Kenilworth, NJ). Plaque density was assessed as grade 0 to grade 3. A subgroup of patients received an intracavernosal injection with 10–15 μg of prostaglandin E_1 combined with visual sexual stimulation to evaluate penile blood flow with penile duplex Doppler ultrasound at baseline and after completion of injections.

Of 117 patients, 103 (88%) completed the study. Penile curvature decreased from $49.9 \pm 2.4°$ to $36.4 \pm 2.1°$ in the IFN-α-2b group and from $50.9 \pm 2.5°$ to $46.4 \pm 2.1°$ in the placebo group. Pain resolution was documented as 28.1% in the placebo group and 67.7% in the IFN-α-2b group. The decrease in plaque size and plaque density in the IFN-α-2b group was significantly greater than in the placebo group. Although the improvements in International Index of Erectile Function scores in the IFN-α-2b group appeared better than in the placebo group, there was no significant difference between groups after injections. However, the mean peak systolic cavernosal artery velocity values with penile duplex Doppler ultrasound showed a statistically significant improvement in IFN-α-2b-treated patients after treatment compared to baseline.

Side effects frequently encountered in patients after intralesional IFN-α-2b injections such as sinusitis; flulike symptoms including fever, chills, and arthralgia; and minor penile swelling with ecchymosis were effectively treated with over-the-counter nonsteroidal anti-inflammatory agents and did not last for more than 48 h. This prospective, multicenter, placebo-controlled, parallel study demonstrated that intralesional IFN-α-2b appears safe and effective as a minimally invasive treatment alternative in PD after or with oral treatment and before surgery is considered.

There are a number of unanswered issues regarding INF-α-2b use in intralesional therapy of PD. The effective dose regimen for delivering IFN-α-2b has not been established. In clinical studies for PD, the doses ranged from 1×10^6 to 10×10^6 units. In the most recent prospective, placebo-controlled, multicenter study, IFN-α-2b 5×10^6 units was used *(40)*. Another issue is the frequency of injections. Given the fact that the half-life of intralesional IFN-α-2b is only 2 h, all application frequencies available in the literature seem appropriate. However, if each intralesional injection incites an augmented inflammatory process after each application, a period of 2 wk or more between each injection would seem more suitable before the inflammatory process completely disappeared. In addition, the site and method of intralesional injection are other issues. Most studies recommended injecting IFN-α-2b directly into the PD plaque after a circular anesthetic block has been administered to the penis. Some researchers administer the agent subcutaneously alongside (and not into) the plaque, which may explain their reported lack of efficacy.

Review of the *Physician's Desk Reference* revealed that administration of IFN-α-2b can be associated with a number of side effects, including constitutional symptoms (i.e., flulike symptoms), ecchymosis, arthralgia, and elevated liver enzyme levels *(41)*. The incidence and severity of these adverse events are clearly dose related, and the majority of adverse events occur more in conjunction with high dosage and long durations of therapy. Low-dose regimens (e.g., 1 to 5×10^6 units) have a much lower incidence and severity of complaints *(41)*. The flulike symptoms associated with IFN-α-2b therapy, although extremely common, are quite manageable using a nonsteroidal anti-inflammatory drug or antipyretic.

CONCLUSIONS

PD is a well-recognized urological condition with a number of anatomical and functional consequences involving the penis. Although surgical correction is ultimately successful in the majority of cases, most men with PD initially seek less-invasive therapeutic alternatives. Oral treatment modalities, such as vitamin E, para-aminobenzoic acid, and colchicine are recommended by many urologists to all men who present in the acute phase of the disease, despite the lack of any controlled studies documenting benefit *(42)*.

Intralesional therapies for PD have been under investigation since the 1990s. Calcium channel blockers used in intralesional injection therapy of PD have exhibited no significant adverse effects and are generally well tolerated. The need remains for a long-term prospective, multicenter, placebo-controlled study to confirm the efficacy of this treatment.

IFNs have been documented to have beneficial effects in a number of smaller studies with low numbers of PD participants. A randomized, prospective, placebo-controlled, multicenter study with IFN-α-2b demonstrated objective improvement in penile curvature, plaque size and density, and pain reduction. A notable drawback of IFNs is the associated flulike symptoms.

Basic research in PD will further elucidate the pathophysiology of PD and help identify new targets for intervention. In the meantime, the goals of any treatment modality are to improve patients' quality of life. Intralesional therapy for PD with verapamil or IFN-α-2b can serve as an intermediate (minimally invasive) form of therapy. Accumulated data show reduction of pain, normalization of penile anatomy, and erectile function with this modality of treatment.

REFERENCES

1. Smith BH. Peyronie's disease. Am J Clin Pathol 1966; 45: 670–678.
2. Jarow JP, Lowe FC. Penile trauma: an etiologic factor in Peyronie's disease and erectile dysfunction. J Urol 1997; 158: 1388–1390.
3. Hellstrom WJ, Bivalacqua TJ. Peyronie's disease: etiology, medical, and surgical therapy. J Androl 2000; 21: 347–354.
4. Bodner H, Howard AH, Kaplan JH. Peyronie's disease: cortisone-hyaluronidase-hydrocortisone therapy. J Urol 1954; 72: 400–403.
5. Williams G, Green NA. The non-surgical treatment of Peyronie's disease. Br J Urol 1980; 52: 392–395.
6. Winter CC, Khanna R. Peyronie's disease: results with dermo-jet injection of dexamethasone. J Urol 1975; 114: 898–900.
7. Mandl I, Zipper H, Ferguson LT. *Clostridium histolyticum* collagenase: its purification and properties. Arch Biochem Biophys 1958; 74: 465–475.
8. Gross J. Collagen biology: structure, degradation, and disease. Harvey Lect 1974; 68: 351–432.
9. Gelbard MK, Walsh R, Kaufman JJ. Collagenase for Peyronie's disease experimental studies. Urol Res 1982; 10: 135–140.
10. Gelbard MK, Lindner A, Kaufman JJ. The use of collagenase in the treatment of Peyronie's disease. J Urol 1985; 134: 280–283.
11. Gelbard MK, James K, Riach P, Dorey F. Collagenase vs placebo in the treatment of Peyronie's disease: a double-blind study. J Urol 1993; 149: 56–58.
12. Huskisson EC, Scott J. Orgotein in osteoarthritis of the knee joint. Eur J Rheumatol Inflamm 1981; 4: 212–218.
13. Gustafson H, Johansson B, Edsmyr F. Peyronie's disease: experience of local treatment with Orgotein. Eur Urol 1981; 7: 346–348.
14. Uthman I, Raynauld JP, Haraoui B. Intra-articular therapy in osteoarthritis. Postgrad Med J 2003; 79: 449–453.
15. Kelly RB. Pathways of protein secretion in eukaryotes. Science 1985; 230: 25–32.
16. Aggeler J, Frisch SM, Werb Z. Changes in cell shape correlate with collagenase gene expression in rabbit synovial fibroblasts. J Cell Biol 1984; 98: 1662–1671.
17. Roth M, Eickelberg O, Kohler E, Erne P, Block LH. Ca^{2+} channel blockers modulate metabolism of collagens within the extracellular matrix. Proc Natl Acad Sci USA 1996; 93: 5478–5482.
18. Mulhall JP, Anderson MS, Lubrano T, Shankey TV. Peyronie's disease cell culture models: phenotypic, genotypic and functional analyses. Int J Impot Res 2002; 14: 397–405.
19. Lee RC, Ping JA. Calcium antagonists retard extracellular matrix production in connective tissue equivalent. J Surg Res 1990; 49: 463–466.
20. Levine LA, Merrick PF, Lee RC. Intralesional verapamil injection for the treatment of Peyronie's disease. J Urol 1994; 151: 1522–1524.
21. Arena F, Peracchia G, Di Stefano C, Passari A, Larosa M, Cortellini P. [Clinical effects of verapamil in the treatment of Peyronie's disease]. Acta Biomed Ateneo Parmense 1995; 66: 269–272.

22. Teloken C. Objective evaluation of non-surgical approach for Peyronie's disease. J Urol 1996; 155: 633A. Abstract 1290.
23. Rehman J, Benet A, Melman A. Use of intralesional verapamil to dissolve Peyronie's disease plaque: a long-term single-blind study. Urology 1998; 51: 620–626.
24. Levine LA. Treatment of Peyronie's disease with intralesional verapamil injection. J Urol 1997; 158: 1395–1399.
25. Levine LA, Estrada CR. Intralesional verapamil for the treatment of Peyronie's disease: a review. Int J Impot Res 2002; 14: 324–328.
26. Cavallini G, Biagiotti G, Koverech A, Vitali G. Oral propionyl-l-carnitine and intraplaque verapamil in the therapy of advanced and resistant Peyronie's disease. BJU Int 2002; 89: 895–900.
27. Mulhall JP, Guhring P, Depierro C. Intralesional verapamil prevents progression of Peyronie's disease. J Urol 2005; 173(4 suppl): 253, A936.
28. Stuart-Harris RC, Lauchlan R, Day R. The clinical application of the interferons: a review. NSW Therapeutic Assessment Group. Med J Aust 1992; 156: 869–872.
29. Duncan MR, Berman B, Nseyo UO. Regulation of the proliferation and biosynthetic activities of cultured human Peyronie's disease fibroblasts by interferons-α, -β and -γ. Scand J Urol Nephrol 1991; 25: 89–94.
30. Ahuja SK, Sikka SC, Hellstrom WJ. Stimulation of collagen production in an in vitro model for Peyronie's disease. Int J Impot Res 1999; 11: 207–212.
31. Berman B, Duncan MR. Short-term keloid treatment in vivo with human interferon α-2b results in a selective and persistent normalization of keloidal fibroblast collagen, glycosaminoglycan, and collagenase production in vitro. J Am Acad Dermatol 1989; 21(4 pt 1): 694–702.
32. Benson RC, Knoll LD, Furlow WL. Inteferon-alpha-2b in the treatment of Peyronie's disease. J Urol 1991; 145: 342A.
33. Wegner HE, Andresen R, Knipsel HH, Miller K. Treatment of Peyronie's disease with local interferon-α 2b. Eur Urol 1995; 28: 236–240.
34. Wegner HE, Andresen R, Knispel HH, Miller K. Local interferon-α 2b is not an effective treatment in early-stage Peyronie's disease. Eur Urol 1997; 32: 190–193.
35. Judge IS, Wisniewski ZS. Intralesional interferon in the treatment of Peyronie's disease: a pilot study. Br J Urol 1997; 79: 40–42.
36. Ahuja S, Bivalacqua TJ, Case J, Vincent M, Sikka SC, Hellstrom WJ. A pilot study demonstrating clinical benefit from intralesional interferon alpha 2B in the treatment of Peyronie's disease. J Androl 1999; 20: 444–448.
37. Novak TE, Bryan W, Templeton L, Sikka S, Hellstrom WJ. Combined intralesional interferon α 2B and oral vitamin E in the treatment of Peyronie's disease. J La State Med Soc 2001; 153: 358–363.
38. Brake M, Loertzer H, Horsch R, Keller H. Treatment of Peyronie's disease with local interferon-α 2b. BJU Int 2001; 87: 654–657.
39. Dang G, Matern R, Bivalacqua TJ, Sikka S, Hellstrom WJ. Intralesional interferon-α-2B injections for the treatment of Peyronie's disease. South Med J 2004; 97: 42–46.
40. Hellstrom WJ, Kendirci M, Matern R, et al. Single-blind, multicenter, placebo-controlled, parallel study to assess the safety and efficacy of intralesional interferon α-2b for minimally invasive treatment for Peyronie's disease. J Urol 2006; 176(1): 394–398.
41. Kirkwood JM, Bender C, Agarwala S, et al. Mechanisms and management of toxicities associated with high-dose interferon α-2b therapy. J Clin Oncol 2002; 20: 3703–3718.
42. LaRochelle JC, Levine LA. Survey of primary care physicians and urologists regarding Peyronie's Disease. J Urol 2005; 173(4 suppl): 254, A941.
43. Astorga R, Cantero O, Contreras D, et al. Intralesional recombinant interferon α-2b in Peyronie's disease. Arch Esp Urol 2000; 53: 665–671.

8 Topical Therapy

Iontophoresis and Electromotive Drug Administration

Savino M. Di Stasi, MD, PhD,
Antonella Giannantoni, MD, PhD,
Emmanuele A. Jannini, MD,
Giuseppe Vespasiani, MD, Luigi Storti, MD,
Francesco Attisani, MD, and Robert L. Stephen, MD

SUMMARY

Electromotive drug administration (EMDA) is a method of increasing the transport of drugs across barriers by means of an electric current. In patients with Peyronie's disease, EMDA of verapamil into the tunica albuginea provides measurable drug levels in plaque tissue. Four clinical studies using different methods showed that EMDA of verapamil and dexamethasone is a safe and effective treatment for Peyronie's disease, reducing plaque volume, penile deviation, and pain, and can contribute to the improvement in erectile capacity and sexual function.

Key Words: Electromotive drug administration; iontophoresis; Peyronie's disease.

INTRODUCTION

Induratio penis plastica (IPP), commonly known as Peyronie's disease, is a wound-healing disorder characterized by areas of inflammation followed by fibrosis (scarring) along the shaft of the penis *(1)*. The lesions may be single or multiple; they are situated within the tunica albuginea and have the appearance of hardened plaques.

Although Peyronie's disease does not cause major health problems and is certainly not life-threatening, for many individuals it significantly impairs quality of life as a source of major distress. In fact, there is frequently pain, angulation (bending) of the penis, and erectile dysfunction (ED) with further psychosexual and psychorelational problems.

The natural history of the disease is not encouraging. In a small proportion (<10%) of patients, plaques become smaller in size and occasionally disappear completely. However, in the majority of subjects there is a "roller coaster" course with intermittent flare-up in which frequently the plaques become calcified/hardened to a chalky, bonelike consistency that becomes a permanent feature of the penile landscape.

From: *Current Clinical Urology:*
Peyronie's Disease: A Guide to Clinical Management
Edited by: L. A. Levine © Humana Press Inc., Totowa, NJ

Occasionally, IPP is associated with some other diseases, notably the fibrous scarring of Dupuytren of the palm. More frequently, IPP follows some type of penile trauma such as sexual accidents, surgery, or repeated intrapenile injections. But, in many cases, the etiology of IPP cannot be related to any known cause. The presence of many different therapeutic approaches to IPP demonstrates that it is a field vital and crucial in urology and the therapies are often ineffective *(2)*. Surgery is aimed to correct the deformity, but it is not a minor procedure, and full disclosure of side effects causes a substantial proportion of patients to decline treatment. There is also the problem of either an ongoing or a recurrent disease process that leads to failure. Systemic drug administration frequently results in a negative benefits–risks ratio in which side effects exceed the therapeutic benefit.

A classical strategy is to localize drug administration directly into and around the plaque. This provides high concentrations at the site of disease with minimal systemic effects. In a large, uncontrolled clinical study, Levine et al. demonstrated significant improvement in patients following intralesional injection of verapamil *(3)*. However, multiple intralesional injections may be uncomfortable and, although rare, may be harmful.

Another approach is transdermal diffusive drug delivery. A report described that, if verapamil cream is directly applied on the penis skin, no detectable levels of the drug can be found in the underlying tunica *(4)*. On the basis of anecdotal reports suggesting that iontophoretic delivery of steroids is beneficial in some patients with IPP *(5–7)*, transdermal electromotive administration of verapamil has been studied, resulting in detectable drug levels in approx 70% of tunica specimens tested *(8)*. Furthermore, four clinical studies with different drug and treatment regimens using electromotive delivery of verapamil in combination with dexamethasone demonstrated objective improvement in patients with Peyronie's disease *(9–12)*.

ELECTROMOTIVE DRUG ADMINISTRATION

Basic Principles

Various electrokinetic phenomena can be recruited to accelerate drug administration across biological membranes and into the underlying tissues: iontophoresis, electroosmosis/electrophoresis, and electroporation.

Iontophoresis describes the accelerated transport of ions (into tissue) by means of an electric current passed through a solution containing the ions i to be administered *(13)* at a rate defined by Faraday's law:

$$Ji = I(tr)/z \; F \; mol/s$$

where I is the current (amperes), tr is the proportion of applied current carried by I, and z is the valency; F is the Faraday constant *(14)*. Usually, iontophoresis is associated with increased transport of water that will carry any nonionized solutes present, a phenomenon often termed *electroosmosis*, a form of "solvent drag." Drug transport rate Dd/dt is the algebraic sum of that induced by passive diffusion (PD) and by electromotive drug administration (EMDA) $(Dd/dt = PD + EMDA)$, but when dealing with a membrane of low permeability such as the skin, EMDA is so dominant that, for all practical purposes, it may be considered the sole force manipulating drug transport. Thus, administration rates not only are markedly increased but also are controllable simply by varying the current intensity.

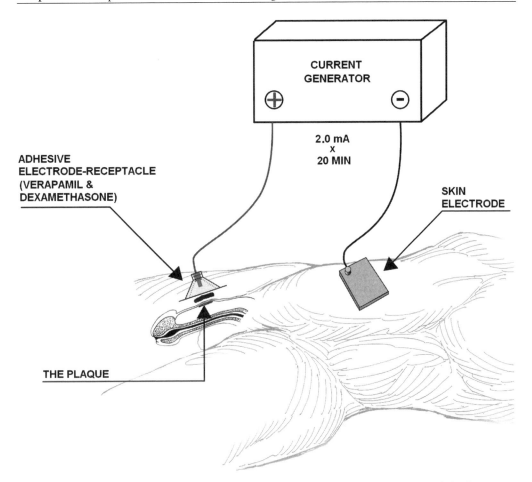

Fig. 1. Schematic illustration of the components of EMDA system for Peyronie's disease.

Electroosmosis/electrophoresis is used to describe the current-induced convective flow of water in association with ions, which can accelerate the transport of ionized molecules down coulombic gradients, nonionized polar molecules *(13)*, and ionized molecules against their coulombic gradients *(15)*.

Electroporation implies increasing the permeability of biological membranes under the influence of an electric field, which promotes increased transport rates down concentration gradients *(16)*.

Because of the multiple electrokinetic forces involved, the term EMDA was coined to describe accelerated drug transport rates down concentration gradients *(17)*.

Technology, Methodology, and Drugs

The EMDA drug delivery system is composed of three basic components: a battery (current generator), a 5-mL adhesive electrode receptacle, and a skin dispersive (grounding) electrode (Figs. 1 and 2).

The EMDA technique is easily described. During treatment, a small battery-powered current source (9 V) is attached by an electrical lead to a 5-mL adhesive electrode receptacle (anode) sited to the penile skin overlying the plaque. A second lead is attached to

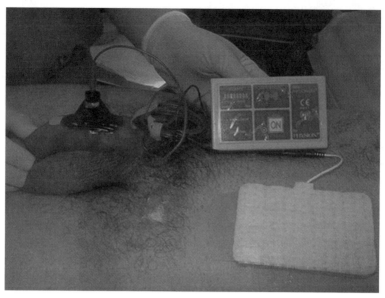

Fig. 2. EMDA apparatus in position for treatment with the reservoir sited over the plaque and the grounding pad secured to the skin on the left lower quadrant.

a dispersive electrode (cathode) placed on the skin of the lower abdomen to close the electrical circuit. The receptacle is filled with a solution of the required drug, the electrical current is turned on for a specified length of time, and the drug is driven into and around the plaque.

Two medications have been selected, dexamethasone and verapamil. Dexamethasone is a potent anti-inflammatory drug, and in the formulation provided, dexamethasone sodium phosphate, it is readily transported by electric current. This drug certainly reduces inflammation associated with the plaque and may even help to reduce plaque size. When verapamil is administered by EMDA, local concentrations in the plaque may be effective with very low systemic concentrations, resulting in virtually no reported systemic side effects. The mechanism of action is similar to the injection of drug into the plaques, but with two important differences: (1) because the volume of fluid administered is small, there is no associated pain; and (2) because the skin is not breached or broken with a needle, there is no risk of infection.

There are certain medical conditions that preclude the use of EMDA: (1) patients with pacemakers or other electrically sensitive equipment are excluded because the applied electric current could derange the functioning of such equipment; (2) known allergies to either of the two drugs (this is most unlikely because allergies to verapamil are rare, and they are almost unheard of with dexamethasone); (3) damage to the skin at and around the site of the plaques (including infection, rash, abrasion, or superficial scars) must be treated and eliminated before applying EMDA, or burns to the skin could result.

Experimental and Clinical Studies

In 1967, the first study of iontophoresis using C21 esterified glucocorticoids for the treatment of Peyronie's disease was described (5). A sodium carbonate solution at pH 8.5 was used as a buffer solution; 0.3 cc hydrocortone phosphate was added. The direct current source was obtained from a Teca CH-3 variable-pulse generator. Initial treatment did not exceed 4 mA for 6 min to determine skin tolerance safely. The average treatment consisted of two 6-min doses at 4–8 mA with an average of 12 treatments three times a week. That study included 12 patients ranging in age from 37 to 68 yr. The duration of disease ranged from 3 mo to 6 yr. Of the 12 patients, 9 complained of pain on intercourse. In all of these, there was complete resolution of pain after the treatment was completed. In 8, there was a loss of rigidity of the penile shaft with or without angular deformities: 4 patients had complete return of rigidity, 3 improved, and 1 was unchanged. In all 12 patients, the plaques became softer but did not disappear. In 5 patients, there were definite signs of regression of the lesion.

The efficacy of iontophoresis using a combination of dexamethasone, lidocaine, and verapamil as first-line nonsurgical treatment for Peyronie's disease was reported by Riedl et al. *(9)*. In this uncontrolled prospective study, 100 unselected patients with Peyronie's disease were treated with three weekly courses of iontophoresis. The drug mixture was administered by an electrical current of 5 mA placed in a self-adhesive receptacle fixed to the penile skin overlying the plaque. Plaques were measured with a measuring tape or ultrasound if not easily palpable. When possible, penile deviation was documented by photographs. Resolution of pain was observed in 96% of patients, reduction in plaque size in 53%, and improvement of penile deviation in 37%. Impaired sexual function was improved in 19 of 43 patients (44%). The benefit of iontophoresis therapy was more pronounced in patients with a short history of disease. These results confirm that the success of conservative therapy is an inverse function of disease duration. Improvement rates in plaque and deviation status decreased from 63.6 and 36.4%, respectively, for lesions of less than 3 mo in duration vs 26.9 and 27%, respectively, for disease duration of more than 1 yr. These data represent cogent argument for early initiation of medical therapy and suggest that the best results are achieved when disease progression is not likely to occur.

The purpose of the third study was to clarify the actual therapeutic potential of a new transdermal drug delivery system (EMDA) for selected patients with Peyronie's disease *(10)*. Montorsi and associates treated 40 men with Peyronie's disease by EMDA using orgotein, dexamethasone, and lidocaine in a double-blinded, placebo-controlled, partial crossover study. They also reported on another 25 men who were treated in an uncontrolled study with verapamil and dexamethasone. Sessions used 3 mA current for 20 min three times a week, with assessment at 1 and 3 mo after the initiation of therapy. The authors reported disappearance of penile pain in 100% of men, significant improvement or disappearance of penile plaque in 90% (two-drug group) and 79% (three-drug group), improvement in penile deformity in 88% (two-drug group) and 62% (three-drug group), and improved penile rigidity in more than 80% in both groups. The benefit of this therapy appears to be more pronounced in patients with a shorter duration of disease. The main advantage of this treatment is that this administration is painless. Neither group reported adverse effects. The authors concluded the following:

> Overall, the combination of verapamil-dexamethasone achieved better clinical results than the three-drug combination. Electromotive drug administration is a novel technique capable of safely achieving satisfactory results in selected patients with Peyronie's disease not only in terms of improvement of patient's symptoms but also due to the reduced need for penile surgery.

In 2003, Levine et al. *(8)* reported on the use of EMDA to transport verapamil into the tunica albuginea. This noncontrolled, nonrandomized, single-blinded study used either verapamil at 10 mg alone or verapamil with epinephrine for 20 min in men with Peyronie's disease who then immediately underwent plaque excision. The levels of verapamil in the excised tunica were compared with levels in the tunica from men who either had no EMDA treatment or had intralesional injection of verapamil. These authors found detectable levels of verapamil in 10 (71.4%) of 14 men treated with topical verapamil delivered by EMDA. They found EMDA to be a safe technique that is capable of transporting verapamil into the tunica. Epinephrine, which was used to decrease vascular dispersion, did not increase tunical concentrations.

In 2003, Di Stasi et al. *(11)* reported results from their prospective, nonblinded study of 49 men. The study involved treatments with verapamil at 5 mg and dexamethasone at 8 mg with EMDA, four times a week for 6 consecutive weeks. During each session, the drug mixture was administered from a receptacle fixed to the skin overlying the plaques, using 2.4-mA pulsed current for 20 min. Plaque size and penile deviation were evaluated by dynamic penile duplex ultrasonography, x-ray, and photographs; pain, erectile function, and capacity for vaginal penetration were assessed using a specific questionnaire. Vital signs and side effects were also recorded. Pain resolved in 88%; curvature disappeared in 10% and improved greater than 50% in 35%; plaque disappeared in 8% and was noted to be at least 50% smaller in another 14%; ED was completely resolved in 42% and improved in another 17%; and vaginal penetration was possible after treatment in 68% and improved in another 5%. The treatment was very well tolerated with the exception of transient skin erythema at the site of the penile and dispersive electrodes. The authors found that results were better in men with smaller, noncalcified plaques.

The most recent trial from this group was published in 2004 in the *Journal of Urology* *(12)*. Patients with Peyronie's disease were randomly assigned to a study group (47 patients) and a control group (49 patients). For each treatment session, an electrode receptacle was sited over the plaque and filled with either 5 mg verapamil and 8 mg dexamethasone (study group) or 2% lidocaine (control group); 2.4 mA electric current was applied for 20 min. Each participant received four sessions per week for 6 consecutive weeks. The authors found a significant decrease in plaque volume, a significant improvement in penile deviation, and significant relief of erectile pain in the study group compared with the control group. Indeed, although no patient in the control group exhibited complete resolution of either the plaque or the penile deviation, the plaque resolved completely in 5 (14%) of the study patients. Penile deviation also completely resolved in 5 (14%) of study patients. Erectile activity was regained in 11% of the control group compared with 51% in the study group. Although transient erythema was reported at the sites of the electrodes in all patients, no other adverse effects were reported. Overall, the authors concluded as follows: "Intraplaque electromotive [administration of] verapamil and dexamethasone induce substantial objective improvement in Peyronie's disease compared to electromotive lidocaine administration."

In 2005, Greenfield and associates reported on their experience with a placebo-controlled, double-blind trial of 10 mg verapamil vs saline EMDA *(18)*. The Physion Mini-Physionizer (Physion, Mirandola, Italy) device was used to deliver 2 mA to the plaque two or three times per week for 12 wk. Objective measures of deformity performed following papaverine injection to induce maximum erection before and 1 mo after treatment revealed improvement of curvature in 65% (mean 9°; range 5–30°) of those receiving verapamil vs 58% of those exposed to saline (mean 7°; range 5–30°). These results suggest that a directly applied electric current alone may result in a positive change to the Peyronie's plaque. This is not surprising as there is abundant support for this in the dermatological literature, indicating the salutary effects of electric field therapy on healing wounds *(19)*. Further studies will be necessary to confirm the benefit of combination therapy, such as using EMDA with verapamil and dexamethasone.

DISCUSSION

Until recently, Peyronie's disease was relegated to an obscure niche in urology. This is surprising because 3–5% of men are affected by the disease. However, this is rapidly changing: Most of the major urological meetings devote special sessions to Peyronie's disease, and attendance is increasing.

In spite of increased interest, the etiology and pathophysiology of Peyronie's disease are still unclear. The pathology is strongly indicative of abnormal wound healing that gives rise to fibrosis within the tunica albuginea *(1)*, and the large number of treatments currently available attest to the fact that none is uniformly successful *(2)*. Surgical correction of the deformity is designed to correct advanced deformity, but it is not a minor procedure, and full disclosure of side effects causes a substantial proportion of patients to refuse this treatment. Oral systemic drug administration frequently results in more side effects than therapeutic benefit.

Intraplaque injections ameliorate the symptoms *(2)* but are invasive, and it is almost impossible to achieve even drug distribution by injecting into the hardened tissue of a plaque.

Electromotive administration of verapamil and dexamethasone is a safe and effective treatment for Peyronie's disease, reducing plaque volume, penile deviation, and pain, and can contribute to the subjective improvement in erectile capacity and sexual function. Furthermore, this method of localized drug administration has some distinct advantages; it is painless, theoretically results in an even distribution of drug throughout the plaque, and has no risk of infection and a minimal risk of systemic side effects from the drugs. There is always a risk of thermal damage to the skin, although this was not reported in the published clinical studies.

Initially, various drugs (lidocaine, orgotein, dexamethasone) were used during EMDA of Peyronie's plaques on a trial-and-error basis. However, with increasing experience the combination of dexamethasone and verapamil has been selected for drug mechanism or action rationale, absence of toxicity, relatively low cost, and effectiveness.

Employment of verapamil for the treatment of Peyronie's disease has a solid scientific basis *(20,21)*, and its accelerated electromotive delivery is a consequence of electrical repulsion between the anode and positively charged verapamil ions *(22)*. The use of dexamethasone rests on previous case reports *(5,7)* and the effectiveness of the combination of verapamil and dexamethasone in four clinical studies *(9–12)*. Its mode of electromotive administration is unusual. Supplied as the ester, dexamethasone bears a weak negative charge with electrical attraction toward the anode that is superseded by an electroosmotic flow of water accompanying the flux of positively charged ions (verapamil) away from the anode and transporting dexamethasone against its coulombic gradient, known as *solvent drag (16)*. Electric current readily accelerates transdermal administration of lidocaine *(22)*. This agent was used in the control group because, like verapamil, it is a vasodilator, and its local anesthetic action provides pain relief during and immediately after treatment.

Although noninvasive intraplaque administration of "anti-collagen"/anti-inflammatory agents resulted in significant improvement in patients with Peyronie's disease, there were some unexplained features. About 30% of the study group showed a poor or absent objective response, yet their disease had no distinguishing characteristics from the responders, and the reduction in measurable plaque volume of responders was prompt, which was not the case in patients treated with intralesional injections *(3)*. This may be caused by variable levels of drug delivery to the plaque or the unique plaque characteristics of each individual.

At the 2003 annual meeting of the American Urological Association, two investigators reported on prospective controlled studies for treatment of the disease *(23,24)*. One described intralesional electromotive administration of verapamil, the other intralesional injections of interferon, and both reported objective improvement of curvature in their control arms using 0.9% NaCl as placebo: 50% of patients in the electromotive group and 39% in the injection group, which easily exceed spontaneous remission rates of 29, 13, and 7% reported for the natural history of the disease *(20–22)*. It can be (and was) argued that the patient population in the electromotive study is as yet too small, but the same restriction does not apply to the injection study, which had an adequate number.

These unexpected findings elicited a suggestion that energetic interference—electric current or multiple injections—somehow arrested or reversed the disease process *(23)*. If so, this does not explain the results in our lidocaine control group, who demonstrated no significant improvement. Obviously, these and other studies must be pursued with particular attention directed toward placebo agents. A localized pharmacological action caused by NaCl *per se* is almost impossible to conceive. But, an agent such as lidocaine exhibits membrane-stabilizing properties, which may interfere with energy delivery or the tissue-remodeling process. There are other possibilities, and at present, the only firm conclusion to be drawn is that investigators dealing with Peyronie's disease must recognize the need for further investigation into a complex disorder.

CONCLUSIONS

Transdermal electromotive administration of verapamil and dexamethasone for Peyronie's disease is a safe and effective treatment. Results appear better when treatments are applied shortly after disease onset (acute phase), but there have also been benefits repeated in mature lesions.

ACKNOWLEDGMENT

Robert L. Stephen leaves us with the memory of an inspiring teacher, scientist, colleague, and friend. We sorely miss him.

REFERENCES

1. Gholami SS, Lue TF. Peyronie's disease. Urol Clin North Am 2001; 28: 377–390.
2. Hellstrom WJ, Bivalacqua TJ. Peyronie's disease: etiology, medical, and surgical therapy. J Androl 2000; 21: 347–354.
3. Levine LA, Goldman KE, Greenfield JM. Experience with intraplaque injection of verapamil for Peyronie's disease. J Urol 2002; 168: 621–625.
4. Martin DJ, Badwan K, Parker M, Mulhall JP. Transdermal application of verapamil gel to the penile shaft fails to infiltrate the tunica albuginea. J Urol 2002; 168: 2483–2485.
5. Rothfeld SH, Murray W. The treatment of Peyronie's disease by iontophoresis of C21 esterified glucocorticoids. J Urol 1967; 97: 874–875.
6. Kahn J. Use of iontophoresis in Peyronie's disease. A case report. Phys Ther 1982; 62: 995–996.
7. Fishman IJ, Wong HY, Griffith DP. Case report. Iontophoretic delivery of steroids in the treatment of Peyronie's disease: case reports of three successful outcomes. Minim Invasive Ther 1994; 3: 121–122.

8. Levine LA, Estrada CR, Shou W, Cole A. Tunica albuginea tissue analysis after electromotive drug administration. J Urol 2003; 169: 1775–1778.
9. Riedl CR, Plas E, Engelhardt P, Daha K, Pflüger H. Iontophoresis for treatment of Peyronie's disease. J Urol 2000; 163: 95–99.
10. Montorsi F, Salonia A, Guazzino G, et al. Transdermal electromotive multi-drug administration for Peyronie's disease: preliminary results. J Androl 2000; 21: 85–90.
11. Di Stasi SM, Giannantoni A, Capelli G, et al. Transdermal electromotive administration of verapamil and dexamethasone for Peyronie's disease. BJU Int 2003; 91: 825–829.
12. Di Stasi SM, Giannantoni A, Stephen R, et al. Prospective, randomized study using transdermal electromotive administration of verapamil and dexamethasone for Peyronie's disease. J Urol 2004; 171: 1605–1608.
13. Bellantone NH, Rim S, Francoeur ML, Rosadi B. Enhanced percutaneous absorption via iontophoresis. Evaluation of an in vitro system and transport of model compounds. Int J Pharm 1986; 30: 63–72.
14. Banga AK, Chien YW. Iontophoretic delivery of drugs: fundamentals, developments and biomedical applications. J Controlled Release 1988; 7: 1–24.
15. Glass JM, Stephen RL, Jacobson CJ. The quality and distribution of radiolabeled dexamethasone delivered to tissue by iontophoresis. Int J Dermatol 1980; 19: 519–525.
16. Prausnitz MR, Bose VG, Langer R, Weaver JC. Electroporation of mammalian skin: mechanism to enhance transdermal drug delivery. Proc Natl Acad Sci USA 1993; 90: 10,504–10,508.
17. Stephen RL, Miotti D, Bettoglio R, Rossi C, Bonezzi C. Electromotive administration of a new morphine formulation: morphine citrate. Artif Organs 1994; 18: 461–465.
18. Greenfield JM, Shah SJ, Levine LA. Verapamil vs saline in electromotive drug administration (EMDA) for Peyronie's disease: a double-blind placebo-controlled trial. Presented at the Fall 2005 meeting of the Sexual Medicine Society of North America, New York City.
19. Ojigwa JC, Isseroff RR. Electrical stimulation of wound healing. J Invest Dermatol 2002; 36: 1–12.
20. Roth M, Eickelberg O, Kohler E, Erne P, Block LH. Ca^{2+} channel blockers modulate metabolism of collagens within the extracellular matrix. Proc Natl Acad Sci USA 1996; 93: 5478–5482.
21. Anderson MS, Shankey TV, Lubrano T, Mulhall JP. Inhibition of Peyronie's plaque fibroblast proliferation by biologic agents. Int J Impot Res 2000; 3(suppl): S25.
22. Petelenz TJ, Buttke JA, Bonds C, et al. Iontophoresis of dexamethasone: laboratory studies. J Controlled Release 1992; 7: 141–145.
23. Levine LA, Sevier VL. A double-blind, placebo-controlled trial of electromotive drug administration (EMDA) using verapamil vs saline for Peyronie's disease: preliminary results. J Urol 2003; 169(suppl): 274. Abstract 1066.
24. Hellstrom W, Eichelberg C, Pryor JL, et al. A single-blind, multi-center, placebo-controlled study to assess the safety and efficacy of intralesional interferon α-2b in the non-surgical treatment of Peyronie's disease. J Urol 2003; 169(suppl): 274. Abstract 1065.

9 Topical Therapy for Peyronie's Disease

Ultrasound, Laser, Gels/Creams/Solutions

Paul F. Engelhardt, MD *and* Claus R. Riedl, MD

SUMMARY

Topical therapy for Peyronie's disease has been offered since the time of de la Peyronie. It would seem that, given the readily palpable location of a Peyronie's plaque, direct application to the skin over the plaque would be a reasonable treatment option. Unfortunately, owing to the barrier effect of the skin and the vascularity of the underlying tissue layers, getting adequate levels of a topically applied agent to the underlying plaque has proved to be challenging. This chapter reviews the treatments that have been used as topical agents for Peyronie's disease with particular focus on energy transfer methods to enhance drug penetration either alone or in combination with topical agents, including steroids, β-aminopropionitrile, verapamil creams, and liposomal superoxide dismutase gel. Clearly, the development of an easily applied therapy that has evidence of benefit for the patient with Peyronie's disease would be much appreciated. For this to occur, further study of the pathogenesis of this disorder will be necessary to allow development of such topical agents.

Key Words: Liposomal superoxide dismutase; Peyronie's disease; topical laser; topical therapy; topical ultrasound; verapamil cream.

INTRODUCTION

The subdermal, easily palpable location of Peyronie's cavernosal plaques has made local therapy a principal option since the definition of this penile disease. François de la Peyronie treated his patients, as reported in his initial disease description, with mercury and, most exotically, the holy water of the French thermal spa Barèges, which resulted in the first reported complete remission *(1)*. In the 1800s, iodine, arsenic, and camphor were used, based on the understanding of that epoch that regarded Peyronie's disease (PD) as a consequence of venereal infection (which was a frequent medical problem at that time) *(2,3)*.

Topical therapies include not only ointments and gels, but also physical devices that deliver energy to the plaques with the perspectives of possible resolution of induration and remodeling of cavernosal deformation. In 1943, Wesson was the first to report on

From: *Current Clinical Urology:*
Peyronie's Disease: A Guide to Clinical Management
Edited by: L. A. Levine © Humana Press Inc., Totowa, NJ

the use of shortwave diathermy for PD therapy *(4)*. However, despite the ostensible accessibility of the plaques, topical regimens have failed to demonstrate significant efficacy in general. This has led to more refined methods for drug or energy application to the plaques, like electromotive drug administration and extracorporeal shockwave therapy.

Similar to other conservative treatment regimens, topical therapies are mainly (if not exclusively) beneficial in the early inflammatory and painful stage of PD *(5,6)*. Nonoperative therapies are mainly symptom directed and should be regarded as analgesic as well as preventive against disease progression. However, because the number of controlled investigations commenting on these statements is sparse, they cannot be supported without discussion. Although improvement has been reported with a multitude of conservative therapies, predictability and consistency of results vary considerably.

LASER AND ULTRASOUND THERAPY

Laser and ultrasound therapy for PD have never been established as a standard treatment option. No reports on laser therapy are available in the literature written in English. Regimens (single vs combination therapy) vary, as do the lasers and ultrasound devices used for therapy.

Felipetto et al. compared local combination therapy with laser and ultrasound to plaque injections with orgotein in 68 patients and stated that the first is at least as effective as and significantly better tolerated than the second *(7)*.

Mazo used a helium-neon laser-based device called Ulamag to treat 713 patients with PD between 1981 and 1988 and observed excellent results in 16% and good results in 75% of his patients, as judged by decrease of plaque size and hardness as well as disappearance of pain and resumption of sexual life. Complete cure was obtained only in patients with initial-stage disease *(8)*.

As early as 1961, Dugois cited a series of 20 cases of PD that were treated with a minimum of 20 sessions of local ultrasound and showed a high rate of improvement that was even accelerated in conjunction with α-chymotrypsin injections *(9)*. Liakhovitskii treated 67 patients with ultrasound and noted a high rate of response, with absence or marked decrease of pain after 20–25 treatments in 52 patients *(10)*. An improvement of curvature or plaque size was observed to a lesser degree.

In 1967, Heslop et al. reported on nine patients treated with ultrasound therapy. They applied a dose of up to 3 W/cm^2 for 10 min and performed 6–42 sessions (average 16 sessions). Although the clinical assessment suggested a good outcome after therapy, with two patients cured and five improved, the subjective evaluation of the patients seemed to be unsatisfactory regarding restitution of sexual function. The authors critically stated that ultrasound in their hands was not any more effective than other methods described in the literature, but with its simplicity bears some advantage over more invasive and expensive therapies. They commented that pain was usually relieved after a course of six treatments, and that once pain ceased, they saw little advantage in continuing the treatment *(11)*.

Frank and Scott reported in 1971 on the efficacy of ultrasonic treatment for symptomatic PD *(12)*. There were 25 patients treated five times per week for 5 min with 1.5 W/cm^2. The total number of treatments varied individually. Subjective improvement was noted by 23 of 25 patients regarding overall sexual function, and a decrease in plaque size occurred in 19 of 25 patients. The authors hypothesized that heat production at tissue interfaces might be the mechanism responsible for the good results observed.

Miller and Ardizzone combined ultrasound with a hydrocortisone ointment used as a conducting vehicle *(13)*. They suggested that the steroid drug is transported into the tissue by the ultrasound energy. Therapy was standardized for 10 treatments in daily intervals with a dose of 1.5 W/cm^2 and a treatment time of 5 min. This treatment course was repeated after 6–8 wk on the patient's request, resulting in up to six courses for 3 patients. Of the patients, 19/25 were regarded as improved, with most of the patients showing a decrease in plaque size *(14)* and pain *(9)* and only 4 an improvement of penile deviation.

No morbidity was described from proper application of the various ultrasound devices used by these authors.

LOCAL MEDICAL THERAPY

Although local therapies with gels and ointments have certainly been widely used for PD throughout centuries, mostly without rationale and documentation, there are few reports on these therapeutic attempts. Whether this is because of the lack of success is not known.

In 1977, Gärtner and Heise reported good success with local application of a solution containing prednisolone (0.125) and dimethyl sulfoxide (90.0, completed with aqua ad 100.0) *(15)*. This solution was put on the penile lesions with a brush (about 0.1 mL) twice a day and continued for 3 mo, eventually followed by retreatment after a 4-wk break. All 10 patients had painful lesions before therapy, and pain resolved in 5 patients and improved in the remaining ones. No definable change of plaques and deviation was observed. No side effects occurred except mild dermatitis at initiation of therapy. The authors admitted that this treatment was not very successful from an objective point of view but appreciably relieved subjective symptoms in patients with PD.

Gelbard et al. treated nine patients with a 4-wk course of β-aminopropionitrile free base as the pure liquid *(16)*. The drug was applied topically over the plaque twice daily in a dosage of 15–20 µL/cm^2 and formed a thin film over the area of the lesion. β-Aminopropionitrile prevents crosslinking of collagen by irreversible inhibition of lysyl oxidase, and this mechanism was considered beneficial for PD tunical changes. However, only three of nine patients reported subjective improvement of pain, and another two reported reduction of penile bending, whereas no objective change of PD symptoms was observed. The authors stated that outcome was unimpressive but that this kind of therapy had a rational basis and might lead to more successful approaches.

VERAPAMIL GEL/CREAM

Local therapy with verapamil, a calcium antagonist normally used for treatment of cardiac arrhythmias and hypertension, was introduced as an intralesional injection therapy by Levine et al. in 1994 *(14)*. The rationale for using this drug is that production and secretion of the major plaque components collagen, fibronectin, and glycosaminoglycans is a calcium-dependent process that can be reduced by calcium antagonists *(17–19)*. Similarly, the proteolytic activity of collagenase is increased with consecutive enhancement of tissue remodeling *(20,21)*.

Several reports of various investigators (including only one controlled study) suggested that intralesional verapamil injections are effective in reducing PD symptoms and tissue changes in an appreciable proportion of patients *(22)*. The same has been postulated for the broadly advertised topical verapamil creams that are produced in patented formulations but not Food and Drug Administration approved. In 2001, Fitch and Easterling reported on a four-arm controlled study of 57 patients with PD comparing the efficacy of topical verapamil gel, trifluoperazine, magnesium sulfate, and placebo for a treatment period of 3 mo *(23)*. Verapamil proved to be more effective than the other drugs, with an improvement of curvature in 91.7% of patients (vs 14.3–26.7% for the other three groups), a decrease of plaque volume in 91.7% (37.5–70%), pain resolution in 100%, and an improvement of erectile function in 71%. Interestingly, a larger set of data from the same authors but dated 1 yr earlier (2000) has been released on the Internet; this report presents the outcome of 608 patients treated with 40 mg verapamil gel twice daily for 1–16 mo *(24)*. Improvement rates were lower than in the first report.

These favorable reports with verapamil gel have never been published in peer-reviewed journals and are heavily contradicted by a study by Martin et al. published in 2002 *(25)*: In eight men undergoing penile prosthesis implantation, verapamil gel was applied to the penile skin for 12 h, followed by tunical biopsy during the planned procedure and verapamil assessment in the tunical tissue and urine by high-power laser diode. In contrast to small amounts of verapamil found in urine, no verapamil was detected in any of the tunica specimens examined. The authors stated that, based on these findings, the use of transdermal verapamil for PD has no scientific basis.

In addition to these findings, Lee and Ping found in 1990 that the effect of verapamil on collagen synthesis and collagenase activity is dose dependent, and that adequate local amounts of verapamil can only be obtained by injection to avoid systemic side effects *(19)*. Thus, it is questionable whether transdermal formulations of verapamil could ever show any efficacy equivalent to intralesional injections or, more conveniently, electromotive drug administration, an electrokinetic procedure that has been shown to deliver verapamil in adequate quantities to tunical tissue *(26)*.

LIPOSOMAL SUPEROXIDE DISMUTASE GEL

Superoxide dismutase (SOD) is a potent radical-scavenging enzyme capable of interrupting inflammatory cascades by tissue deprivation of free oxygen radicals. In the 1980s, promising results were obtained with intralesional injection of bovine-type SOD in several small uncontrolled studies *(27–33)*. It was hypothesized that reduction or interruption of the inflammatory process in early PD could stop or even reverse the typical disease-related symptoms. Because of the withdrawal of bovine SOD from the market in 1993 as a consequence of severe allergic reactions, these early results have not been confirmed in controlled studies.

Because SOD is an extremely potent anti-inflammatory enzyme, the former promising concept was carried out when human recombinant Cu/Zn-SOD in a liposomal formulation (lrhSOD) was manufactured *(34–36)*. The main advantage of lrhSOD is its administrability as a topical gel, and adequate tissue penetration of the active ingredient as a consequence of liposomal encapsulation technology has been demonstrated *(37,38)*. In an uncontrolled pilot study, this human SOD proved to be beneficial in painful early-stage PD, with significant and fast resolution of pain symptoms, comparable to the results of the prior studies with injectable bovine SOD *(39)*. Subsequently, a prospective placebo-controlled, double-blind, multicenter clinical trial was performed to confirm these encouraging results *(40)*. During a 4-wk period, 39 patients with painful PD lesions were treated either with lrhSOD gel (2 mg SOD per gram gel) or placebo twice daily. After evaluation at this primary study end point, patients were treated for another 8 wk in a crossover design to ensure SOD therapy for all study participants for 8 wk.

Significant pain reduction (>50% from baseline as evaluated by a 10-point visual ana-
logue scale) after 4 wk of treatment was achieved by 10 of 19 (52.6%) patients in the active
drug group and 4 of 20 (20%) of the placebo group. This difference was statistically
significant ($p = 0.017$). After 8 wk of lrhSOD therapy, 89% of patients showed significant reduction of pain, 47% had a reduction of plaque size, and 23% had an improvement
of deviation, whereas 10% of patients reported an increase of deviation. Except for mild
skin reactions in 2 patients, no side effects were observed from local lrhSOD administration. In summary, lrhSOD therapy was rated successful by 71% of patients (40).

CONCLUSION

Despite the existence of a multitude of logical arguments and concepts for local drug
and physical therapies, none of the methods presented in this chapter have made their
way to become standard treatment. Similar to all conservative therapies, these procedures seem to be beneficial in resolving pain in the initial stage of PD (and maybe prevent
disease progression, which is reported to be as high as 40% in untreated cases), reduce
plaque size, and restore sexual function (41). The effect on penile deviation is unsubstan-
tial, but straightening of the penis is undoubtedly in the surgical domain (42). The results
of ultrasound and laser therapy do not seem any better, but are not much worse than those
reported for extracorporeal shockwave therapy, with costs not taken into consideration.
The ideal drug for local application is still to be defined. The lrhSOD may be a candidate,
but the advantage of enhanced transdermal penetration by liposomal drug encapsulation
may also be extended to other drugs with proven or suspected efficacy in PD. The aim
of having a gel for local self-administration as an ideal therapy should not be disregarded
and represents one of the future goals in urology. The availability of an easily admin-
istrable therapy will open the door to early treatment in the painful early stages of disease
and it is hoped will prevent development of distressing penile deformities that require
surgical correction.

REFERENCES

1. De la Peyronie F. Sur quelques obstacles qui sópposent à l'éjaculation naturelle de la semence. Mém
   Acad R Chir 1743; 1: 318–333.
2. El-Sakka AJ, Lue TF. Peyronie's disease. Curr Opin Urol 1999; 8: 203–209.
3. Levine LA. Review of current nonsurgical management of Peyronie's disease. Int J Impot Res 2003;
   15(suppl 5): S113–S120.
4. Wesson MB. Peyronie's disease (plastic induration), cause and treatment. J Urol 1943; 49: 350.
5. Tunuguntla HSGR. Management of Peyronie's disease—a review. World J Urol 2001; 19: 244–250.
6. First Latin American Erectile Dysfunction Consensus Meeting: Peyronie's disease. Int J Impot Res
   2003; 15(suppl 7): S36–S40.
7. Felipetto R, Vigano L, Pagni GL, Minervini R. Laser and ultrasonic therapy in simultaneous emission
   for the treatment of plastic penile induration. Minerva Urol Nefrol 1995; 47: 25–29.
8. Mazo VE. A new method for treating Peyronie's disease. Khirurgiia 1989; 42: 30–31.
9. Dugois P. The action of ultrasonics on Peyronie's disease, accelerated by α-chymotrypsin. Lyon Med
   1961; 93: 238.
10. Liakhovitskii NS. Experience in the use of ultrasonics in the therapy of plastic induration of the penis.
    Urologiia 1960; 25: 64.
11. Heslop RW, Oakland DJ, Maddox BT. Ultrasonic therapy in Peyronie's disease. Br J Urol 1967; 39:
    415–419.
12. Frank IN, Scott WW. The ultrasonic treatment of Peyronie's disease. J Urol 1971; 106: 883–887.

13. Miller HC, Ardizzone J. Peyronie's disease treated with ultrasound and hydrocortisone. Urology 1983; 21: 584–585.
14. Levine LA, Merrick PF, Lee RC. Intralesional verapamil injection for the treatment of Peyronie's disease. J Urol 1994; 151: 1522–1524.
15. Gärtner R, Heise H. Induratio penis plastica—Lokalbehandlung mit einer Prednisolon-Dimethylsulfoxid (DMSO)—Zubereitung. Derm Mschr 1977; 168: 48–52.
16. Gelbard M, Lindner A, Chvapil M, Kaufman J. Topical β-aminopropionitrile in the treatment of Peyronie's disease. J Urol 1988; 129: 746–748.
17. Kelly RB. Pathways of protein secretion in eukariots. Science 1985; 230: 25.
18. Aggler J, Frisch SM, Werb Z. Changes in cell shape correlate with collagenase gene expression in rabbit synovial fibroblasts. J Cell Biol 1984; 98: 1662.
19. Lee RC, Ping JA. Calcium antagonists retard extracellular matrix production in connective tissue equivalent. J Surg Res 1990; 49: 463.
20. Lee RC, Doong H, Jellama AF. The response of burn scars to intralesional verapamil. Report of five cases. Arch Surg 1990; 129: 107–109.
21. Roth M, Eickelberg O, Kohler E, Erne P, Block LH. Ca2+ channel blockers modulate metabolism of collagens with the extra cellular matrix. Proc Natl Acad Sci USA 1996; 93: 5478–5483.
22. Rehman I, Benet A, Melman A. Use of intralesional verapamil to dissolve Peyronie's disease plaque: a long-term single-blind study. Urology 1998; 51: 620–626.
23. Fitch WP, Easterling WJ. Topical verapamil, trifluoperazine and magnesium sulfate for Peyronie's disease. Int J Impot Res 2001; 13: S62.
24. Fitch WP, Easterling WJ. Topical verapamil for the treatment of Peyronie's disease. Available at: http://www.topicalverapamil.com/studyPDTv.asp.
25. Martin DJ, Badwan K, Parker M, Mulhall JP. Transdermal application of verapamil gel to the penile shaft fails to infiltrate the tunica albuginea. J Urol 2002; 168: 2483–2485.
26. Levine LA, Estrada CR, Shou W, Cole A. Tunica albuginea tissue analysis after electromotive drug administration. J Urol 2003; 169: 1775–1778.
27. DeVries JDM, Leenarts JAF, Nieuleman EJH, Debruyne FMJ. Die Behandlung der Peyronie's Disease mit SOD-Injektion. Attraktive Alternative zu den bisherigen Therapieverfahren? Akt Urol 1988; 6: 321.
28. Bartsch G, Menander-Huber KB, Huber W, Marberger H. Orgotein, a new drug for the treatment of Peyronie's disease. Eur J Rheumatol Inflamm 1981; 4: 250.
29. DeGrande G, Riso O, Rizza G. Nostra Esperienza con l'orgoteina nella induratio penis plastica [Our experience with orgothein in induratio penis plastica]. Urologia 1985; 52: 547–553.
30. Pisani E, Mantovani F, Patelli E, Austoni E. Orgothein by infiltration and iontophoresis in the treatment of induration penis plastica. In: Proceedings of the 56th Congress of Italian Society of Urology; 1983; Verona.
31. Gustafson H, Johansson B, Edsmyr F. Peyronie's disease: experience of local treatment with orgotein. Eur J Urol 1981; 7: 346.
32. Primus G. Orgotein in the treatment of plastic induration of the penis (Peyronie's disease). Int Urol Nephr 1993; 25: 169.
33. Berlin T. Orgotein vs hydrocortisone in the treatment of Peyronie's disease. A randomized study. J Urol 1986; 135(suppl): 103A–392A.
34. Bayer K, Jungbauer A, Uhl K. Humane rekombinante Superoxiddismutase. Bioengineering 1990; 6: 24–30.
35. Vorauer K, Skias M, Jungbauer A. Scale-up of recombinant protein purification by hydrophobic interaction chromatography. J Chromatogr 1992; 625: 217–226.
36. Vorauer-Uhl K, Wagner A, Katinger H. Long term stability of rh-Cu/Zn-superoxide dismutase (SOD)-liposomes prepared by the cross-flow injection technique following International Conference on Harmonisation (ICH)-guidelines. Eur J Pharm Biopharm 2002; 54: 83–87.
37. Schriebl K, Wagner A, Fürnschlief E, Katinger H, Vorauer-Uhl K. Aspects and limitations of in-vivo penetration studies of liposomal formulations—case study of liposomal human Cu/Zn-superoxide dismutase. Submitted to Int J Pharm.
38. Jadot G, Vaille A, Maldonado J, Vanelle P. Clinical pharmacokinetics and delivery of bovine superoxide dismutase. Clin Pharmacokinet 1995; 28: 17–25.

39. Riedl CR, Plas E, Vorauer K, Vcelar B, Wagner A, Pflüger H. Pilot study on liposomal recombinant human superoxide dismutase for the treatment of Peyronie's disease. Eur Urol 2001; 40: 343–348; editorial comment 348–349.

40. Riedl CR, Sternig P, Galle G, et al. Liposomal recombinant human superoxide dismutase for the treatment of Peyronie's disease: a randomized placebo-controlled double-blind prospective clinical study. Eur Urol 2005; 48: 656–661.

41. Maan Z, Arya M, Shergill I, Joseph JV, Patel HRH. Peyronie's disease: an update of the medical management. Expert Opin Pharmacother 2004; 5: 799–805.

42. Briganti A, Salonia A, Deho F, et al. Peyronie's disease: a review. Curr Opin Urol 2003; 13: 417–422.

10 Combination Nonsurgical Therapy

Vincenzo Mirone, MD

SUMMARY

Over the years, physicians have been searching for an effective way to treat Peyronie's disease (PD). This disorder remains poorly understood. As a result, there is no straightforward reliable therapy. When it is felt that medical therapy is in order, it is best started at the early stages of acute inflammation, when the therapy can potentially prevent the evolution of fibrosis. A variety of combined treatments have been tried in the past appearing to give better results than monotherapy. Various types of energy transfer, including shockwave therapy, orthovoltage radiation, ultrasound, laser therapy, and shortwave diathermy, have been used for PD. The best reported clinical results have been obtained by combining laser therapy with shockwave therapy, especially for pain resolution. Treatment outcomes concerning reducing penile curvature and plaque resorption have been disappointing. Published reports have demonstrated the best results of combination therapy with shockwave therapy and intralesional injection of verapamil as this approach appears not only to reduce pain but also to improve penile deformity. This chapter reviews the results of nonsurgical combination therapy in the treatment of PD.

Key Words: Extracorporeal shockwave therapy (ESWT); intralesional injection therapy; laser therapy; nonoperative therapy; Peyronie's disease (PD).

INTRODUCTION

The history of medical progress has always been accomplished by seeking new methods of treatment based on experience, observation, and experiments. Over the years, physicians have been searching for the right way to deal with Peyronie's disease (PD). It has always been poorly understood.

There are many kinds of etiopathogenic hypotheses (traumatic, infective, immune, autoimmune), and the disease's natural history can develop in variable ways, ranging from slow or fast evolution. Because of the disease's numerous characteristics, following a common standard for an effective therapy is very difficult. There are no clear reasons for the disease and no straightforward treatment.

As early as 1652, Tulp suggested the application of oil poultices, and in 1743 la Peyronie tried a therapy using douches with local Barèges spa water. Other methods, such as iodine, mercury, camphor, and iodoform were applied but without success.

From: *Current Clinical Urology:*
Peyronie's Disease: A Guide to Clinical Management
Edited by: L. A. Levine © Humana Press Inc., Totowa, NJ

Table 1
Combination Therapy

ESWT	Laser
ESWT	Verapamil
Radiotherapy	Vitamin E
Iontophoresis	(Lidocaine, verapamil)

ESWT, extracorporeal shockwave therapy.

At the beginning of 1950, Teasley introduced a valid therapy by injecting cortisone directly into the plaque of the penis. A few years later, Bodner created one of the first therapy combinations by adding hyaluronidase to Teasley's treatment.

The etiology and natural history of PD still remain unknown, but different drug types have been used, such as immunosuppressors, anti-inflammatories, cortisones, and antioxidants. Furthermore, because of the various phases of development in PD, an accurate assessment of staging the lesion is of great importance for the definition of an appropriate therapy.

Most authors agree that, when possible, the treatment of PD should be observation, especially in patients with a slight curvature and no erectile dysfunction. When a medical therapy is thought to be suitable, it should be started at the early stages of an acute inflammation, when the therapy can still prevent or at least stop the evolution in fibrosis. Different kinds of combination therapy have been tried, and it seems that a combination therapeutic approach produces better results than monotherapy.

TREATMENTS

Different types of energy transfer, such as shockwave lithotripsy, orthovoltage radiation, ultrasound, laser therapy, and shortwave diathermy, have been used as a treatment for PD (Table 1).

Extracorporeal shockwave therapy (ESWT) for the treatment of calcified orthopedic diseases has been on the increase because of its positive results when treating PD (1).

Laser therapy is one of the latest procedures in the treatment of PD. High- and low-level laser therapy are used locally, and the laser's biological action is based on local vasodilatation of arterioles and capillaries. This allows tissues to use more oxygen and correct metabolic imbalance.

In the use of laser therapy in combination with ESWT, results were strongly variable depending on patients' parameters, such as degree of penile curvature, patients' age, disease duration, and plaque's ecographic appearance.

The best clinical results have been obtained by combining these two procedures (laser therapy and ESWT), especially for pain resolution. Results concerning penile curvature and plaque resorption have been deeply inferior.

A combined therapy (association of ESWT and an injection of calcium channel blockers [CCBs]) seems to obtain the best results (2). This combined therapy not only reduces pain but also improves penile curvature (3). The intralesional therapy includes injection of a CCB, purified clostridial collagenase, steroids, and interferons.

The treatment with injection of a CCB such as verapamil is the preferred intralesional therapy used today. It is based on its effectiveness on cytokine expression in the early phases of inflammation and wound healing and increasing effect on the proteolytic activity of collagenase. With this kind of therapy, curvature improves, half of the patients report better sexual performance, and almost 80% note an arrest in disease progression, but it does not decrease penile shaft narrowing. The only side effects are pain and ecchymosis.

Clostridial collagenase is usually used only for moderate degrees of PD because it alters the collagen content of penile plaque, but severe curvature does not respond significantly to this therapy.

Treatment with steroids has been used mainly for recalcitrant painful plaque, but this treatment does not really treat curvature. Steroids decrease collagen synthesis because of their anti-inflammatory properties, but they also have many local side effects, such as local tissue atrophy and skin thinning.

Interferons, as well as clostridial collagenase, seem to be more useful only in patients with small plaques, but the only side effects in this treatment are influenza symptoms.

Medical therapy includes colchicine, acetyl-L-carnitine, potassium aminobenzoate, and vitamin E. All are used as oral systemic agents. Colchicine induces collagenase activity and decreases collagen synthesis, which are both ideal effects because plaques are a localized fibrosis caused by increased collagen (4,5). The side effects are mainly diarrhea, nausea, or liver disorders (6). Colchicine works in the inflammatory phase as well as in the fibrotic phase of this disease. The decrease or disappearance of plaque, the improvement of the curvature, and relief of pain during erection along with minimal side effects make colchicine considered a very potential treatment of men with PD (6).

Acetyl-L-carnitine also seems to bring a significant decrease in penile pain and plaque size. The mechanism of action of potassium aminobenzoate is based on the increased activity of monoamine oxidase, which decreases serotonin, and this effect decreases fibrogenesis. Gastrointestinal upset seems to be the most frequent side effect. Vitamin E is normally used in the treatment of PD for its antioxidant properties.

Iontophoresis is a painless treatment based on transdermal drug mixture (dexamethasone, lidocaine, and verapamil) transported into the diseased tissues. It is especially effective in the early stages of PD and for deviation less than 60°. The combination of dexamethasone and verapamil, both effective in this disease, brings better results than drug monotherapy, and lidocaine is used in this drug mixture, not to cure the lesion, but to reduce pain and increase dexamethasone transport (7).

In contrast with multiple injections that are difficult to perform and do not distribute the drug to the entire lesion, iontophoresis in a homogenous way delivers drugs to the entire lesion without any pain for the patient. The main and most important effects of iontophoresis are relevant pain reduction in almost all patients, and better erectile function and sexual activity and reduced penile curvature in almost half of the patients. What seems to be important is also the disease duration; the longer the disease lasts, the less successful are the results of iontophoresis. Usually, the patient needs about 2 wk of therapy to reach a painless state.

The greatest advantages of this procedure are that it strongly slows and prevents deterioration of the plaque's lesions, especially in the early stages (less than 12 mo) of PD. It is completely painless and almost without side effects for the patient.

Radiotherapy is also used as a treatment in plastic induration of the penis. Its strength is based on noninvasiveness; most patients note less penile pain after this treatment, and almost half of the patients describe improved sex life, regression of the plaque, and less penile curvature (8).

What is important in this kind of therapy is the dose–response relation because more benefit seems to be derived from low-dose radiotherapy than from high-dose therapy. Also, in this case the earlier the treatment is started, the more satisfying the results will be *(8)*.

The literature often states that plastic induration of the penis improves frequently in a spontaneous way in untreated patients within 12–18 mo. Almost all of the patients respond to radiotherapy within 2 mo. It is then reasonable to underline that, with this noninvasive treatment, patients will suffer less and are going to benefit earlier.

OUR EXPERIENCE

We used the association of ESWT and verapamil as a combination therapy to treat PD. ESWT seems to improve vascularization, and this mechanism is likely to bring metabolic activation of connective tissue and consecutively to absorb the calcification *(9)*. ESWT causes positive results mainly in the improvement of sexual function and reduction of pain during erection, even though the effect on penile deviation and on plaque size seems not to be relevant *(1)*. Verapamil is the preferred calcium channel blocker used in the intralesional therapy. Because of their singular characteristics, we chose to combine these two procedures.

Reports asserted that the inflammation is the result, rather than the cause, of the process in the tunica *(10)*. Devine et al. *(11)* associated minimal trauma, possibly during sexual intercourse in susceptible men, with the occurrence of PD. Their data strengthen the hypothesis that PD is initiated and sustained by tissue trauma and identified fibrin as a critical determinant in the pathogenesis of this condition.

Previous studies have shown the importance of calcium in the metabolism of fibroblasts and in the neosynthesis of collagen. Therefore, calcium antagonists such as verapamil were studied particularly for their antifibroblastic effect. It has been demonstrated that ESWT, successfully used in orthopedic or salivary stones because of its lithotriptic power, can also be useful to break Peyronie's plaques *(9)*. Furthermore, the suggestion of a synergy between mechanical and biochemical plaque-disintegrating actions has been supported by our results *(2)*.

To confirm or refute our previous therapeutic model for PD, a well-standardized method is strongly needed to evaluate better the histology and the evolution of the plaque in consecutive pathogenetic steps.

In our experience, 130 patients mean age 49 yr (range 28–61 yr) were divided into three treatment groups: (1) shockwaves alone in 21 patients; (2) a combination of shockwaves and verapamil (perilesional injection) in 36 patients; and (3) verapamil alone in 73 patients *(2)* (Table 2).

The shockwaves are produced by a therapeutic source and focused by a paraboloid reflector. The focal point is 40 mm from the edge of the therapeutic source (Fig. 1). The aperture is 85.5°, and its focus expands, changing the energy level; the ranges are $25 \times 2.4 \times 2.4$ mm. The waves are therefore extracorporeal, and they hit the patient's body, passing throughout an interface and some superficial gelatin. The patients were quiet in the supine position with flexed legs. The penis was placed on a support that could be vertically adjusted (Fig. 2).

After our standardized procedure *(10)*, we decided to verify its effectiveness by performing a new technique of penile biopsy, suitable for Peyronie's plaque as well as any other pathology of the penis requiring a biopsy (Fig. 3) *(12)*. We performed local anesthesia with 5 mL of 10% noropine on the site of the disease and with the patient in the supine

Table 2
Our Results

	Group A: ESWT alone		Group B: Verapamil + ESWT		Group C: Verapamil alone	
	N	%	N	%	N	%
Ultrasound plaque volume reduction	11/21	52.3	22/36	61.1	31/73	42.4
Pain alleviation	16/21	76.1	19/23	82.6	36/61	59
Improvement in penile narrowing	3/5	60	3/4	75	3/12	25
Curvature reduction	11/14	78.5	16/21	76.2	33/51	64.7
Subjective improvement in intercourse	9/12	74.9	7/9	77.7	31/56	55.3

ESWT, electrohydraulic shockwave therapy.

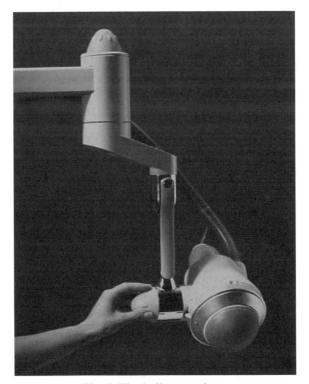

Fig. 1. The balloon probe.

position. The skin and the superficial fascia of the penis were incised for 2–3 mm, and the "tube shape" cutting edge of the punch was applied on the plaque, keeping the device normal to the main axis of the penis. The blade was then slowly advanced, turning the opposite edge of the tool (Fig. 4), giving rise to rotational progression of the cylinder into the plaque and obtaining a cylindrical core of tissue. The wound was then sutured with 4-0 plain catgut stitches. The core obtained was up to 3–4 mm long and 2 mm in diameter and was immediately washed of blood and any residual tissue (Fig. 5), placed in Bouin's solution, and submitted for histological analysis.

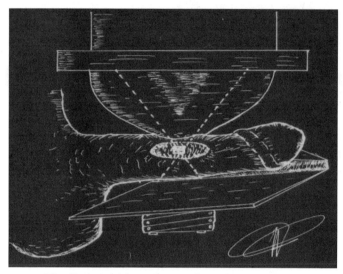

Fig. 2. A graphic representation of the treatment.

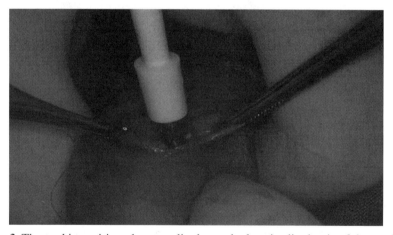

Fig. 3. The tool is positioned perpendicular to the longitudinal axis of the penis.

A few weeks later, mean 58 d (range 16–86 d), different surgical treatments for PD were performed: Nesbit operation (29 patients), plaque excision with auto-/heterologous graft (16 patients), or penile prosthesis implant (7 patients). During open surgery, a second tissue specimen for each patient was obtained and processed exactly as the Acu-Punch (Acuderm Inc.) cores. The Acu-Punch and the surgical biopsies were all performed by the same operator; the Acu-Punch cores and surgical biopsies were analyzed by the same pathologist with light, scanning, and transmission electron microscopy (Figs. 6 and 7).

Our goal was to evaluate the efficacy of the treatment in improving plaque volume, pain, and penile deformity. A reduction of plaque was found in 260 of 380 patients (68.4%) treated with ESWT and verapamil and in 2 of /92 patients (30.4%) treated with verapamil injections alone. The suggestion of a synergism between mechanical and biochemical plaque-disintegrating actions of ESWT and verapamil, respectively, was supported by our results *(2,12)*.

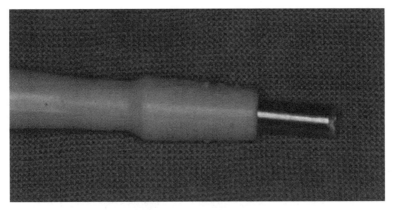

Fig. 4. Acu-Punch (Acuderm Inc.).

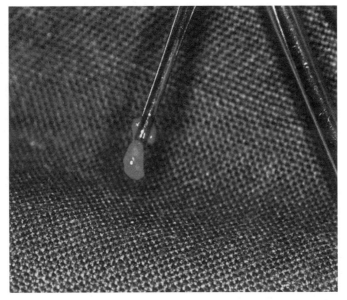

Fig. 5. The core obtained is 3–4 mm long and 2 mm in diameter and consists of both tunica albugineal and cavernosal tissue.

In conclusion, we can say that the therapeutic association could be an effective nonoperative treatment to stabilize the progression of PD.

CONCLUSION

Every therapeutic agent demonstrates a valid scientific basis that is connected to the physiopathology of the illness, even though it may be unknown. Because singularly prescribed treatment did not give the foreseen results, the proposal for a combined therapy was adopted.

Advances in basic research of wound healing and scarring have aided our understanding of PD. With continued discovery, treatment of PD will move toward halting and reversing the fibrosis and scarring responsible for this disease. Initial management of PD should be conservative with expectant therapy and medical management.

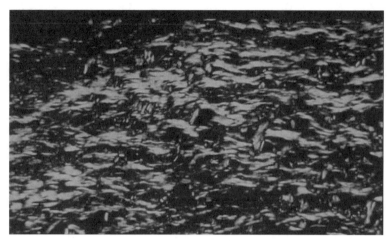

Fig. 6. Histological analysis of Acu-Punch core obtained from Peyronie's plaque pre-extracorporeal shockwave therapy.

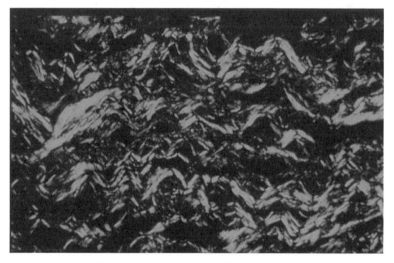

Fig. 7. Histological analysis of Acu-Punch core obtained from Peyronie's plaque post-extracorporeal shockwave therapy.

While waiting to discover a standard method of treatment that is followed under rigid observation, a physiopharmacological therapy has also been utilized in our institution for the last 8 yr, producing better results than any other so far. Further progress for treatment could derive from histomorphometric studies creating a valid understanding of the induratio penis plastica diagnosis and presenting a useful knowledge of illnesses associated with penile tissues.

These methods could demonstrate their utility in the selection of patients for the various types of combined therapy and to understand the prognosis.

REFERENCES

1. Hauck W, Mueller UO, Bschleipfer T, Schmelz HU, Diemer T, Weidner W. Extracorporeal shock wave therapy for Peyronie's disease: exploratory meta-analysis of clinical trials. J Urol 2004; 171: 740–745.

2. Mirone C, Imbimbo A, Palmieri F. Fusco: our experience on the association of a new physical and medical therapy in patients suffering from induratio penis plastica. Eur Urol 1999; 36: 327–330.
3. Levine LA. Review of current nonsurgical management of Peyronie's disease. Int J Impot Res 2003; 15(suppl 5): S113–S120.
4. Kerrshenobich D, Vargas F, Garcia-Tsao G, Perez Tamayo R, Gent M, Rojkind M. Colchicine in the treatment of cirrhosis of the liver. N Engl J Med 1988; 318: 1709–1713.
5. Harris D Jr, Krame SM. Effects of colchicine on collagenase in cultures of rheumatoid synovium. Arthritis Rheum 1971; 14: 669–684.
6. Akkus J, Breza S, Carrier A, Kadioglu J, Rehman T, Lue F. Is colchicine effective on Peyronie's disease? A pilot study. Urology 1994; 44: 291–295.
7. Riedl R, Plas E, Engelhardt P, Daha K, Pflueger H. Iontophoresis for treatment of Peyronie's disease. J Urol 2000; 163: 95–99.
8. Rodrigues I, Hian Njo K, Karim AB. Results of radiotherapy and vitamin E in the treatment of Peyronie's disease. Int J Radiat Oncl Biol Phys 1995; 31(3): 571–576.
9. Hauck W, Attinkilic BM, Ludwig M, et al. Extracorporeal shock wave therapy in the treatment of Peyronie's disease. First results of a case controlled approach. Eur Urol 2000; 38(6): 663–670.
10. Digelmann RF. Cellular and biochemical aspects of normal and abnormal wound healing: an overview. J Urol 1997; 157:298–302.
11. Devine CJ Jr, Somers KD, Jordan GH, Schlossberg SM. Proposal: trauma as the cause of the Peyronie's lesion. J Urol 1997; 157: 285–290.
12. Mirone C, Imbimbo A, Palmieri N, Longo F, Fusco G. Tajana: a new biopsy technique to investigate Peyronie's disease associated histologic alterations: results with two different forms of therapy. Eur Urol 2002; 42: 239–244.

11

Extracorporeal Shockwave Therapy in Peyronie's Disease

Ekkehard W. Hauck, MD and Wolfgang Weidner, MD

SUMMARY

Extracorporeal shockwave therapy (ESWT) has been on the rise for the treatment of Peyronie's disease. There have been 21 original papers, 1 meta-analysis, and 2 review articles published. Analyzing these studies systematically, ESWT seems to have an effect on penile pain during erection and on the improvement of sexual function. It seems that pain resolves faster after ESWT treatment than during the course of natural history. The effect on plaque size and penile curvature is less impressive. The most recent studies do not provide evidence that ESWT has an effect on curvature and plaque size. Despite the lack of severe side effects, the data concerning efficacy published to date do not justify recognizing ESWT as an evidence-based, standard procedure for the treatment of Peyronie's disease.

Key Words: Extracorporeal shockwave therapy; ESWT; Peyronie's disease; analysis.

INTRODUCTION

During the initial progressive stage of Peyronie's disease (PD), therapy should be conservative. However, most concepts of oral and intralesional drug treatment are not effective *(1,2)*. No substance is available that can cure all symptoms of PD in all patients. However, surgery is only indicated in the stable, nonprogressive stage of the disorder *(3)*. Moreover, not all patients who are candidates for surgical procedures are willing to undergo them. Deducing from these aspects, a high number of patients affected by PD ask for an alternative treatment, especially after unsuccessful drug therapy. It is their intention to avoid a surgical correction or to regard it as the last alternative. Extracorporeal shockwave therapy (ESWT) has been emphasized as a semi-invasive procedure to fill this therapeutic gap.

HISTORY

The use of ESWT for treatment of PD was first described by Bellorofonte et al. in 1989 *(4)*. This Italian paper reported more or less anecdotally on a series of a 16 patients who had undergone ESWT for penile fibrosis as a result of different causes, such as after priapism, removal of a penile implant, after cavernosography, or, in 9 cases, PD. After a decade

From: *Current Clinical Urology:*
Peyronie's Disease: A Guide to Clinical Management
Edited by: L. A. Levine © Humana Press Inc., Totowa, NJ

of silence concerning this alternative approach, a larger series of 52 patients treated by ESWT was presented by Butz and Teichert at the annual meeting of the American Urological Association in 1998 *(5)*. ESWT has been on the rise, mainly in Europe. This has resulted in an increasing amount of articles, with 21 original papers *(5–25)*, 1 meta-analysis *(26)* and 2 review articles *(27,28)* published. At major international and many local meetings, there has been an incredible flood of abstracts of limited scientific value presented during the last several years.

MODE OF ACTION

Despite the wide distribution of ESWT, not much is known about its mode of action in PD. The rationale for use in this fibrotic disorder has still not been clarified. Extracorporeal shockwave lithotripsy is well known to urologists as first-line therapy for the treatment of nephrolithiasis. The shockwaves crush the stone into small pieces that can leave the urinary tract spontaneously or can be extracted by endourological maneuvers. Shockwaves are also applied successfully for the treatment of salivary stones *(29)*.

Special lithotripters have been constructed for the superficial administration of shock waves in orthopedic diseases. Since the early 1990s, ESWT has been widely used to treat various calcified and noncalcified orthopedic disorders *(30)*. Four indications seem to be accepted: tendinosis calcarea of the shoulder, also called periarthritis humeroscapularis; the tennis or golfer elbow, epicondylopathia humeri radialis; calcaneal spur; and in some respects, pseudarthrosis *(30,31)*.

However, a definite mode of action for the treatment of nephrolithiasis has not been described thus far. An improvement of vascularization with consecutive resorption of calcification or dissolution has been discussed as one possible mechanism of ESWT *(30, 31)*. Concerning the noncalcified diseases, a change in the milieu of the free radicals or a direct disturbance of pain receptors could be the reason for the pain-relieving effect *(31)*. Another possible effect could be analgesia after hyperstimulation of the pain receptors by shockwaves.

Because PD is also an inflammatory disease at the initial stage with fibrosis of the tunica albuginea or calcified plaques during its course, ESWT was introduced in the treatment of this disorder. However, the definite modes of action remain unclear.

Basic research on animal models and histological clinical investigations that can definitely explain the effect of ESWT in PD is not available. Only one study has been performed that investigated the effect of ESWT on the penis of the rat *(32)*. This controlled approach in an animal model resulted in no different effects concerning hemodynamic and histopathology parameters comparing the group treated by ESWT with the control group *(32)*.

Only one study investigated histological effects on specimens of penile punch biopsy in patients who received ESWT *(23)*. A reduction in packing and clumping of the collagen fibers has been observed by histological examination in the plaques after ESWT *(23)*. Such findings were not observed in patients after clinically unsuccessful treatment.

CLINICAL STUDIES

Problems of Interpretation and Comparison

For further evaluation, only the results from the studies that have been published in peer-reviewed journals as original articles have been considered. There have been 21 articles published from 15 groups of authors. From five study groups with increasing series, only the most recent article was included *(8,13,17,20,23)*. However, as described in the methodology of our explorative meta-analysis, there are several reasons why a direct comparison of these studies is very difficult and should be carefully assessed *(26)*:

1. The study groups differed considerably in the medical history of the subjects and severity of symptoms.
2. Selection of outcome measures was inconsistent, and measurement itself was not standardized.
3. Effect-size categorization was poorly documented and inconsistent. What constitutes a clear success, a modest success, or no success at all varied from study to study. Thus, success frequencies between studies may be caused by real differences or differences in success category definitions.
4. In orthopedics, even if confined on a well-defined anatomical region, little topological differences may come with sizable differences in ESWT outcome *(30,33)*. Exact information on plaque size, location, and consistency may be critical, but typically it is not available.
5. Treatment protocols vary widely, and some of them may be more effective than others.
6. Only 5 of the 21 studies represent prospective controlled approaches according to their own definitions *(12–14,17,23,25)*, and none is single blinded—real vs simulated ESWT —as described in orthopedic studies *(33)*. A case-controlled design was only performed by 1 study group *(12)*.
7. PD is known to show quite divergent natural outcomes *(34,35)*. Therefore, the effect size of ESWT in all studies without a proper control group cannot be estimated.

Technical Parameters

In the 15 studies, ESWT was performed by seven different types of lithotripters. The most common type was the Storz Minilith SL1 lithotripter, which was used in 9 studies. Shockwaves were applied by Wolf Piezolith 2300 *(4)*, Wolf Piezolith 2500 *(8)*, EDAP LT-02 *(15)*, Siemens Lithostar *(6)*, Siemens Multiline *(17)*, and ReflecTron *(24)* lithotripters. As Table 1 shows, the technical parameters of the settings had a wide, range from one to five settings between 2 and 90 d. Only in the series using the Storz Minilith SL1 did the amount of applied energy seem to be more or less uniform, with an energy flow density of 0.11–0.17 mJ/mm^2 per shockwave.

Patient Populations

The study groups differed considerably in the medical history of the subjects and severity of symptoms. Treatment of PD before ESWT varied from none *(17)*, to different conservative approaches, to a series that also included patients with previous surgery *(18)*. The clinical data of the patients are summarized in Table 2.

Results

No severe complications were reported. Only penile pain during administration of ESWT, frequently skin hematoma, and rarely hematuria relating to urethral bleeding were observed after the intervention. Table 3 provides an overview of the results of treatment. Success rates varied widely for all outcomes: reduction of plaque size in 0–68% of the patients, reduction of penile curvature in 0–64%, reduction of penile pain in 56–100%, and improvement of sexual function in 12–80% *(26)*.

Table 1
Technical Parameters

Studygroup	ESWT technique	Number of settings (n)	Time between settings (d)	Shock waves per setting (n)	Energy per shockwave
Abdel-Salam et al. (6)	Siemens Lithostar	5 (4–10)	?	4000	15–21 kV
Baumann et al. (8)	Wolf Piezolith 2500	6	14–28	2500	3
Bellorofonte et al. (4)	Wolf Piezolith 2300	6	7	800	40–100 MPa
Butz (9)	Storz Minilith SL1	3–5	1–7	3000	?
Colombo et al. (10)	Storz Minilith SL1	4	2	3000	0.09–0.14 mJ/mm^2 4
Hamm et al. (11)	Storz Minilith SL1	3.9 (3.5)	?	3000	0.11 mJ/mm^2 2–5
Hauck et al. (13)	Storz Minilith SL1	1–4	≥90	4000	0.04–0.17 mJ/mm^2 4–5
Husain et al. (14)	Storz Minilith SL1	3	?	3000	0.11–0.17mJ/mm^2 4–5
Kiyota et al. (15)	EDAP LT-02	3–5	?	?	0.11–0.17 mJ/mm^2
Lebret et al. (17)	Siemens Multiline	1.6 (1–3)	90	3000	450–960 bar
Manikandan et al. (18)	Storz Minilith SL1	3–6	2 groups: 1 vs 3C	3000	0.3 mmJ/mm^2 4–5
Michel et al. (20)	Storz Minilith SL1	5	7	1000	0.11–0.17 mJ/mm^2 3–5
Mirone et al. (23)	Storz Minilith SL1	3	2	?	0.07–0.17 mJ/mm^2 ?
Oeynhausen et al. (24)	ReflecTron	4.5 (3–6)	30	2000–4000	0.13–0.15 mJ/mm^2 4–5
Strebel et al. (25)	Storz Minilith SL1	5	7	3000	0.11–0.17mJ/mm^2

Table 2

Baseline Data of the Patients in 17 Studies on ESWT in Peyronie's Disease

Study group	Number of patients (n)[a]	Age (yr, mean, range)	History (mo, mean, range)	Plaque calcification (n, %)	Penile curvature (°, mean, range)	Stable disease	Treatment before ESWT
Abdel-Salam et al. (6)	24	55 (36–67)	26 (6–240)	?	?	+	?
Baumann et al. (8)	74	54 (29–70)	19 (12–72)	?	?	(+)	+
Bellorofonte et al. (4)	9	41 (32–65)	?	?	?	?	?
Butz (9)	72	55 (26–74)	17 (3–96)	?	?	?	?
Colombo et al. (10)	82	54 (44–74)	23 (3–120)	36/82 (44%)	?	?	?
Hamm et al. (11)	28	57 (34–72)	>12	?	?	+	?
Hauck et al. (13)	96	53 (24–69)	27 (3–52)	42/96 (44%)	48 (15–90)	–	+
Husain et al. (14)	34	56 (24–69)	19 (4–60)	?	51 (20–90)	?	?
Kiyota et al. (15)	4	52 (35–65)	?	?	20–40	?	+
Lebret et al. (17)	54	56 (29–76)	16 (3–60)	?	48 (20–110)	?	–
Manikandan et al. (18)	42	55 (32–72)	17 (3–60)	?	20–75	?	+
Michel et al. (20)	35	58	34	?	50	+	?
Mirone et al. (23)	380	47 (32–71)	>6	?	?	?	+
Oeynhausen et al. (24)	30	55 (28–72)	25 (4–96)	19/30 (63%)	>30->60	?	+
Strebel et al. (25)	52	55 (29–77)	19 (4–168)	30/52 (57%)	40 (0–80)	?	?

[a]The number of patients included in the follow-up is provided.

Table 3
Results of Treatment by ESWT

Study group	Follow-up (mo, mean, range)	Mode of evaluation	Reduction of plaque size (n, %)	Reduction of penile curvature (n, %)	Reduction of pain during erection (n, %)	Improvement of sexual function (n, %)
Abdel-Salam et al. (6)	3–9	Photo Ultrasound Interview Examination	14/24 (58%)	14/24 (58%)	17/24 (72%)	14/24 (58%)
Baumann et al. (8)	24 (4–69)	Telephone Interview Examination	?	37/74 (50%)	42/47 (89%)	41/74 (55%)
Bellorofonte et al. (4)	12	Ultrasound Artificial erection Rigiscan	?	3/9 (33%)	?	5/9 (55%)
Butz (9)	12	Photo/drawing Ultrasound Interview	?	36%	66%	50%
Colombo et al. (10)	<1	Photo Questionnaire Ultrasound Examination	34/82 (41%)	24/78 (31%)	31/44 (70%)	?
Hamm et al. (11)	?	Artificial erection Photo Questionnaire IIEF Ultrasound Examination	?	18/28 (64%)	13/16 (81%)	20/28 (71%)
Hauck et al. (13)	9 (3–53)	Artificial erection Photo Ultrasound Interview Examination	41/96 (43%)	28/96 (29%)	26/37 (76%)	25/96 (26%)

126

Study	Age	Methods				
Husain et al. (14)	8 (5–11)	Artificial erection / Questionnaire / Ultrasound / Examination	?	15/32 (47%)	12/20 (60%)	?
Kiyota et al. (15)	<1	?	1/4 (25%)	0/4 (0%)	4/4 (100%)	?
Lebret et al. (17)	13 (3–?)	Photo / Questionnaire IIEF / Examination	23/54 (43%)	29/51 (54%)	31/34 (91%)	6/24 (25%)
Manikandan (18)	6 (2–18)	Artificial erection / Photo / Interview / Examination	?	22/38 (58%)	21/25 (84%)	5/42 (12%)
Michel et al. (20)	18	Artificial Erection / Pain Scale / Interview / Examination	0	5/24 (21%)	16/17 (94%)	9/35 (26%)
Mirone et al. (23)	?	Ultrasound / Interview / Examination	260/380 (68%)	?	312/340 (92%)	303/380 (80%)
Oeynhausen et al. (24)	4	Photo / Interview	20/30 (67%)	17/29 (58%)	13/16 (81%)	17/30 (56%)
Strebel et al. (25)	11 (4–17)	Ultrasound Examination / Photo/Drawing / Examination / Ultrasound / Questionnaire	?	16/52 (31%)	28/30 (93%)	11/40 (28%)

Despite the varied percentage change of the symptoms in the different studies, the quantity of improvement of each symptom should be regarded. Exact data on quantification of changes in plaque size were not provided in most studies. Only the two most recent studies *(13,25)* provided exact data on the change of plaque size. In these two studies, no significant changes of plaque size were observed in comparing the total number of patients before and after the intervention *(13,25)*. In the study by Hauck et al. *(13)*, the mean plaque size remained stable, with 509 mm^2 (range 25–1600) before ESWT and 499 mm^2 (0–1600) after ESWT. Exactly the same course was reported by Strebel et al. *(25)*. In this series, the mean plaque size was 246 mm^2 (21–875) before and 242 mm^2 (9–900) after therapy. This tendency was confirmed by another study that reported no significant differences concerning plaque size before and after ESWT *(20)*.

Concerning the changes of penile curvature, the situation is similar. An early study described a significant ($p < 0.001$) decrease of mean curvature of 12.8°, from 50.5° (20–90°) to 37.7° (10–80°) *(14)*. This tendency of statistically significant improvements of curvature could not be confirmed by three further studies that provided information concerning quantity of changes for the total population of patients. Michel et al. *(20)* observed a decrease of mean curvature from 59.3° to 49.3° without reaching significance *(20)*. In the series from Hauck et al. *(13)*, the mean curvature decreased without significance from 48.3° (15–90°) to 42.5° (0–90°). The subanalyses, depending on the degree of curvature before the intervention (0–30°, 31–60°, 61–90°), revealed a statistically significant decrease of curvature of 7.2° only for the subset between 31 and 60°. In this group, curvature decreased by 7.2°, from 47.7° (35–60°) to 38.5° (0–80°). In the study from Strebel et al. *(25)*, no significant changes of curvature for the total group of patients were observed *(25)*. The mean curvature was 40° (0–80°) before treatment and 37° (0–80°) after the intervention.

The more subjective symptoms of penile pain and the changes in sexual function are more difficult to quantify as no standardized instruments were used in most studies. Thus, most results defining a positive response after ESWT relied on the more or less subjective assessment of the patient or the clinician.

EXPLORATIVE META-ANALYSIS OF THE CLINICAL STUDIES

Only one early study was performed in a case-controlled approach *(12)*; it compared the effect of ESWT, with untreated patients representing the natural course of the disease. In this series, only a borderline significant effect on the decrease of penile curvature was observed. There were no significant differences concerning changes of plaque size, penile pain, or the subjective assessment of sexual function compared with the controls *(12)*. In the remaining, often retrospective, studies, no controls were available. During the natural course, improvement of symptoms, especially the spontaneous resolution of pain with time, has been described in the majority of patients *(34,35)*. Also, placebo-controlled studies of drug therapy revealed remarkable "response rates" for placebo *(36,37)*. Thus, the effect concerning the different parameters cannot really be assessed objectively without appropriate controls.

An exploratory meta-analysis of the studies published as peer-reviewed articles or abstracts at the annual meetings of the American Urological Association and the European Association of Urology was performed *(26)*. As mentioned in the section on problems in interpretation and comparison, an exploratory meta-analysis was carried out because a methodologically sound meta-analysis *lege artis* did not appear appropriate as treated groups differed considerably in structure; the selection of outcome measures was inconsistent, and the measurement was not standardized. Thus, this study has an exploratory character *(26)*. Four control groups taken from the literature were included, two from reports on the natural history *(34,35)* and two comparison groups from series on ESWT *(12,23)*.

The results of this exploratory meta-analysis can be summarized as follows *(26)*: ESWT seems to have an effect on penile pain during erection and on the improvement of sexual function. It seems that pain resolves faster after ESWT treatment than during the natural course. The effect on plaque size and penile curvature is less impressive. Deducing from the data of this exploratory meta-analysis, the effect on plaque size and curvature remains questionable. ESWT is not an evidence-based therapy at the present time.

DISCUSSION

The different studies had a wide range of treatment outcome. There are many reasons why it is problematic to compare the results of the different studies. However, some questions should be discussed.

ESWT seems to have a good effect on penile pain during erection. Evidently, pain seems to resolve faster after ESWT treatment than during the natural course. However, the question remains whether it is really valuable to treat the symptom pain that usually resolves spontaneously with time.

It is very difficult to assess the ability to perform sexual intercourse. The International Index of Erectile Function has been validated for administration in patients with PD *(38)*, but this instrument is not an ideal tool to measure the changes in problems resulting from penile deformity. Moreover, in most studies no standardized or validated instrument for the assessment of sexual function was used. Hypothetically, it is the relief of pain that improves the performance of sexual intercourse. It is more than questionable that the rather limited success rates concerning the decrease of penile curvature are really the reason for improvements of sexual function.

It seems remarkable that, in the most recent well-designed studies *(13,20,25)*, no statistically significant effect on decrease of penile curvature was evident regarding the total populations. The question still remains whether a statistically significant decrease of penile pain is really of clinical value for the patient. One study described a significant ($p < 0.001$) decrease of mean curvature by 12.8°, from 50.5° to 37.7° *(14)*. Another study revealed a statistically significant decrease of curvature only for the subset of patients with curvatures between 31 and 60°. In this group, mean curvature decreased by 7.2°, from 47.7 to 38.5°. Despite the statistically significant findings, it seems doubtful that a decrease of mean curvature of 12.8 or 7.2° is a real benefit for the patient *(13)*.

Exact data on changes of plaque size were only reported in the most recent two studies *(13,20)*. In these studies, no change of mean plaque size was evident, in contrast to other studies that reported a decrease of plaque size in a certain percentage of patients. However, the question is whether a softening or decrease of plaque size as described in some studies is of real clinical value for the patient.

Several studies concluded that a controlled, single-blinded, multicenter study with a careful, detailed documentation of the disease symptoms before the intervention and of the outcomes is required to investigate the real effect of ESWT. However, deducing from the data of the available clinical studies and the exploratory meta-analysis, doubts arise whether such a design could reveal statistically and clinically significant effects of ESWT.

Summarizing, to date ESWT has not been an evidence-based therapy for PD. If the uncontrolled studies are analyzed carefully, the efficacy concerning the objective symptoms of penile curvature and plaque size remain more than questionable. It seems that pain is relieved faster after ESWT than during the natural course of the disease. However, the question remains whether a symptom that usually disappears during the natural course is worth treating by an expensive, time-consuming method like ESWT.

Considering these vague facts concerning the efficacy of ESWT, the official statement of the German Urological Society stated that ESWT should not be recommend as first-line or standard therapy for PD *(39)*. This statement is also supported by the National Institute of Clinical Excellence in the United Kingdom. The guidelines recommend that, in the scope of the evidence on efficacy, the use of ESWT does not appear adequate without special arrangements for consent and for audit or research. The National Institute of Clinical Excellence is not undertaking further investigation at present *(40)*.

CONCLUSIONS

ESWT seems to be a safe procedure without severe side effects. However, the data published so far do not provide evidence to employ ESWT as a standard procedure for the treatment of PD.

REFERENCES

1. Levine LA. Review of current nonsurgical management of Peyronie's disease. Int J Impot Res 2003; 15(suppl 5): S113–S120.
2. Mynderse LA, Monga M. Oral therapy for Peyronie's disease. Int J Impot Res 2002; 14: 340–344.
3. Levine LA, Lenting EL. A surgical algorithm for the treatment of Peyronie's disease. J Urol 1997; 158: 2149–2152.
4. Bellorofonte C, Ruoppolo M, Tura M, et al. Possibility of using the piezoelectric lithotriptor in the treatment of severe cavernoufibrosis [in Italian]. Arch Ital Urol Nephrol 1989; 61: 417–422.
5. Butz M, Teichert HM. Treatment of Peyronie's disease (PD) by extracorporeal shock waves (ESW). J Urol 1998; 159(suppl 5): 118. Abstract 457.
6. Abdel-Salam Y, Budair Z, Renner C, et al. Treatment of Peyronie's disease by extracorporeal shock wave therapy: evaluation of our preliminary results. J Endourol 1999; 13: 549–552.
7. Baumann M, Tauber R. Peyronie's disease: Extracorporeal shock wave therapy (EPT) as a new treatment [in German]. Akt Urol 1998; 29: 1–5.
8. Baumann M, Böhme H, Tauber R. Extracorporeal shock wave therapy (ESWT) in combination with local verapamil injections in the treatment of IPP (induratio penis plastica) [in German]. Akt Urol 2001; 32(suppl 1): 61–64.
9. Butz M. Extracorporeal shock wave therapy (ESWT) in induratio penis plastica—development and topical ranking [in German]. Akt Urol 2001; 32(suppl 1): 55–57.
10. Colombo F, Massimiliano N. Shock waves in the treatment of La Peyronie's disease. Outcomes evaluation by ultrasonography. La Peyronie's disease [in Italian]. Arch Ital Urol Androl 2000; 72; 388–391.
11. Hamm R, Mclarty E, Ashdown J, Natale S, Dickinson A. Peyronie's disease—the Plymouth experience of extracorporeal shock wave treatment. BJU Int 2001; 87: 849–852.
12. Hauck EW, Altinkilic BM, Ludwig M, et al. Extracorporeal shock-wave therapy (ESWT) in the treatment of Peyronie's disease—first results of a case-controlled approach. Eur Urol 2000; 38: 663–670.
13. Hauck EW, Hauptmann A, Bschleipfer T, Schmelz HU, Altinkilic BM, Weidner W. Questionable efficacy of extracorporeal shock wave therapy in Peyronie's disease: results of a prospective approach. J Urol 2004; 171: 269–299.
14. Husain J, Lynn NNK, Jones DK, Collins GN, O'Reilly PH. Extracorporeal shock wave therapy in the management of Peyronie's disease: initial experience. BJU Int 2000; 86: 466–468.
15. Kiyota H, Ohishi Y, Asano K, et al. Extracorporeal shock wave treatment for Peyronie's disease using EDAP LT-02: preliminary results. Int J Urol 2002; 9: 110–113.

16. Lebret T, Herve JM, Lugane PM, et al. Extracorporeal shock wave lithotripsy (ESWL) in the treatment of la Peyronie disease. Use of a standardized lithotriptor (Siemens multilinie) on "young" plaques (less than 6 mo) [in French]. Prog Urol 2000; 10: 65–70.

17. Lebret T, Loison G, Hervé JM, et al. Extracorporeal shock wave therapy in the treatment of Peyronie's disease: experience with standard lithotriptor (Siemens-multiline). Urology 2002; 59: 657–661.

18. Manikandan R, Islam W, Srinivasan V, Evans CM. Evaluation of extracorporeal shock wave therapy in Peyronie's disease. Urology 2002; 60: 795–800.

19. Michel MS, Ptaschynk T, Musial A, et al. Shock wave therapy of Peyronie's disease: 18 mo follow-up of a prospective study for standardized and objective evaluation of symptom changes under artificial erection [in German]. Akt Urol 2001; 32(suppl 1): 68–71.

20. Michel MS, Ptaschnyk T, Musial A, et al. Objective and subjective changes in patients with Peyronie's disease after management with shock wave therapy. J Endourol 2003; 17: 41–44.

21. Mirone V, Imbimbo C, Palmieri A, Fusco F. Our experience on the association of a new physical and medical therapy in patients suffering from induratio penis plastica. Eur Urol 1999; 36: 327–330.

22. Mirone V, Palmieri A, Granata AM, Piscopo A, Verze P, Ranavolo R. Ultrasound guided extra shock wave treatment of la Peyronie's disease [in Italian]. Arch Ital Urol Androl 2000; 72: 384–387.

23. Mirone V, Imbimbo C, Palmieri A, Longo N, Fusco F, Tajana G. A new biopsy technique to investigate Peyronie's disease associated histologic alterations: results with two different forms of therapy. Eur Urol 2002; 42: 239–244.

24. Oeynhausen D, Oelbracht K, Zumbé J. Extracorporeal shock wave therapy (ESWT) in the treatment of Peyronie's disease [in German]. Akt Urol 2001; 32(suppl 1): 58–60.

25. Strebel RT, Suter S, Sautter T, Hauri D. Extracorporeal shock wave therapy for Peyronie's disease does not correct penile deformity. Int J Impot Res 2004; 16: 448–451.

26. Hauck EW, Mueller UO, Bschleipfer T, Schmelz HU, Diemer T, Weidner W. Extracorporeal shock wave therapy for Peyronie's disease: exploratory meta-analysis of clinical trials. J Urol 2004; 171: 740–745.

27. Michel MS, Köhrmann KU, Alken P. Treatment of Peyronie's disease by shock waves: a critical review [in German]. Aktuel Urol 2001; 32(suppl 1): 65–67.

28. Groth T, Monga M. Extracorporeal shock wave therapy for Peyronie's disease. Arch Androl 2003; 49: 205–213.

29. Iro H, Schneider H, Födra C, et al. Shock wave lithotripsy of salivary duct stones. Lancet 1992; 339: 1333–1336.

30. Wild C, Khene M, Wanke S. Extracorporeal shock wave therapy in orthopedics. Assessment of an emerging health technology. Int J Technol Assess Health Care 2000; 16: 199–209.

31. Haupt G. Use of extracorporeal shock waves in the treatment of the pseudarthrosis, tendinopathy and other orthopedic diseases. J Urol 1997; 158: 4–22.

32. Kadioglu A, Tefekli A, Erol B, et al. Hemodynamic and histopathologic effects of extra-corporeal shock waves (ESW) on rat penis: preliminary results. Int J Impot Res 2001; 13(suppl 1): S59. Abstract M80.

33. Rompe JD, Hopf C, Nafe B, Burger R. Low-energy extracorporeal shock wave therapy for painful heel: a prospective controlled single-blind study. Arch Orthop Trauma Surg 1996; 115: 75–79.

34. Gelbard MK, Dorey F, James K. The natural history of Peyronie's disease. J Urol 1990; 144: 1376–1379.

35. Kadioglu A, Tefekli A, Erol B, Oktar T, Tunc M, Tellaloglu S. A retrospective review of 307 men with Peyronie's disease. J Urol 2002; 168: 1075–1079.

36. Safarinejad MR. Therapeutic effects of colchicine in the management of Peyronie's disease: a randomized double-blind, placebo-controlled study. Int J Impot Res 2004; 16: 238–243.

37. Teloken C, Rhoden EL, Grazziotin TM, Da Ros CT, Sogari PR, Souto CAV. Tamoxifen vs placebo in the treatment of Peyronie's disease. J Urol 1999; 162: 2003–2005.

38. Wiltink J, Hauck EW, Phädayanon M, Weidner W, Beutel ME. Validation of the German version of the International Index of Erectile Function (IIEF) in patients with erectile dysfunction, Peyronie's disease and controls. Int J Impot Res 2003; 15: 192–197.

39. Weidner W, Hauck EW. Significance of extracorporeal shock-wave therapy (ESWT) in plastic penile induration. Statement of the DGU [in German]. Urologe A 2004; 43: 597–598.

40. Dillon A. Extracorporeal shockwave therapy for Peyronie's disease. National Institute of Clinical Excellence. 2003. Available at: www.nice.org.uk/IP182overview.

12 The Nesbit and Plication Procedures for Peyronie's Disease

David J. Ralph, MS, FRCS(Urol)

SUMMARY

The Nesbit operation, first used for Peyronie's disease in 1977, is still the most common operation performed to correct a penile curvature. Whereas there have been various modifications of the original technique over the years, the basic principle of shortening the tunica on the contralateral side to the plaque is applied. The operations are simple to perform, and the results are consistently excellent. This chapter describes the original technique and offers a comparison both with the modifications and with the alternative of grafting.

Key Words: Curvature; Nesbit; Peyronie's; plication; surgery.

INTRODUCTION

The first surgical removal of a Peyronie's plaque was performed by George McClellan in 1827, and by 1926 success with 32 cases had been reported *(1)*. With the advance in surgical techniques, plaque excision only was subsequently replaced by excision with dermal grafting to the defect, popularized by Devine and Horton in 1974 *(2)*. Other grafts used included vein *(3)*, lyophilized dura *(4)*, rectus aponeurosis *(5)*, tunica vaginalis *(6)*, and Dacron *(7)*. Concerns over the high incidence of erectile dysfunction with plaque excision were confirmed by Austoni et al. in 1995, when 20% of 418 patients developed postoperative erectile dysfunction *(8)*.

Since then, plaque excision has been replaced by plaque incision and grafting with either saphenous vein *(9)* or autologous materials *(10)*. In 1965, Reed Nesbit *(11)* described the correction of erectile deformities caused by congenital abnormalities by shortening the opposite side of the penis using plication or the excision of an ellipse of tunica albuginea. This principle was first applied to Peyronie's disease (PD) in 1977 by Pryor and Fitzpatrick *(12)* using the classical elliptical excision of the tunica opposite the plaque. Modifications of the Nesbit operation are commonly used (tunical incision with plication, plication alone or combinations with elliptical excision), but all with the same principle of shortening the contralateral side of the penis *(13–16)*. Penile prostheses are reserved for patients who also have an impaired erection or extensive disease *(17)*.

From: *Current Clinical Urology:*
Peyronie's Disease: A Guide to Clinical Management
Edited by: L. A. Levine © Humana Press Inc., Totowa, NJ

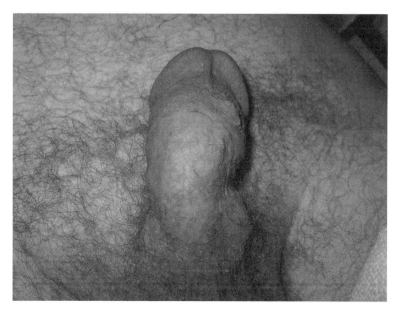

Fig. 1. A complex waisting deformity—a contraindication to the Nesbit operation.

This chapter assesses the operations utilizing the Nesbit principle, when and to whom it should it be offered, and the expected results and complications.

INDICATIONS AND ASSESSMENT FOR SURGERY

Surgery should be performed only when the disease is stable to ensure good long-term results. It is often difficult to decipher the end of the active phase, but in general disease duration for 1 yr and stability for a minimum of 3 mo is a good guide *(18)*.

Patients with dorsal deformities less than 45° may be able to manage without surgery. Younger patients, or those with ventral or lateral curvatures where penetration would be more difficult, tend to have lesser degrees of curvature corrected *(18)*. It is meddlesome to operate just because there is a lump or a minor erectile deformity. Also, some patients may have severe emotional distress, usually regarding the deformity and penile shortening, and would benefit from psychosexual counseling preoperatively.

In general terms, the choice of procedure to correct the deformity rests between a Nesbit-type operation or a grafting technique, and patients should be offered a choice between the two types of procedures *(19)*. In general, a Nesbit-type operation is a simple technique that gives excellent results but will result in a variable degree of penile shortening directly proportional to the severity of the original deformity but without impairment of erectile function *(18)*. A grafting technique is a more complex procedure but also gives excellent results with less penile shortening although with a higher risk of postoperative erectile dysfunction (ED *[20,21]*).

Clearly, those patients with minor deformities or already on treatment for ED would be better suited to a Nesbit operation. Those patients who have severe or complex wasting deformities (Fig. 1) but otherwise normal erectile function would be best suited to a grafting technique *(20,21)*. It must be remembered that patients with PD are at a risk of ED *de novo* as they commonly have arterial disease elsewhere in their body, and up to 67% will have arterial risk factors *(22)*. Then, one would expect erectile function to

Table 1
Suggested Surgical Options in Peyronie's Disease

Erection	Deformity	Suggested operation
Normal	<60°	Nesbit
	>60°	Graft
	Complex	Graft ± plication
Impaired	<60°	Nesbit + medication
	>60°	Penile prosthesis
	Complex	Penile prosthesis

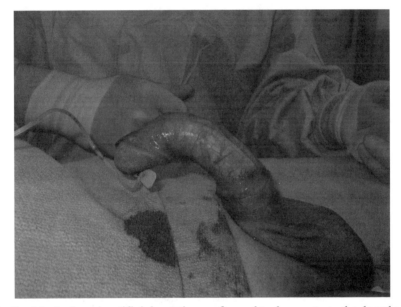

Fig. 2. Penile skin degloved; artificial erection performed to demonstrate the dorsal curvature.

deteriorate over time irrespective of surgery, and this must be taken into consideration when choosing the type of operation. Patients with extensive disease, ED risk factors, and particularly those with a distal flaccidity may be better suited to a penile prosthesis insertion to maintain length and function. A summary of the surgical options is shown in Table 1.

SURGICAL TECHNIQUES

As for all surgery in PD, the stretched penile length needs to be recorded pre- and post-operatively. The classical Nesbit operation is performed through a circumglandular incision—circumcising the man if necessary to prevent a secondary paraphimosis. The penile skin is then degloved, and an artificial erection is induced by injecting saline from a rapid transfusion apparatus without the use of a tourniquet as it sometimes makes for an inaccurate assessment of the bend (Fig. 2). It is also essential to observe the bend at the time of full erection; otherwise, the deformity may be underestimated. The site of maximum bend is marked with a stay suture.

Buck's fascia is incised longitudinally and dissected medially to bare the tunica albuginea (Fig. 3). This technique permits elevation of the corpus spongiosum ventrally or

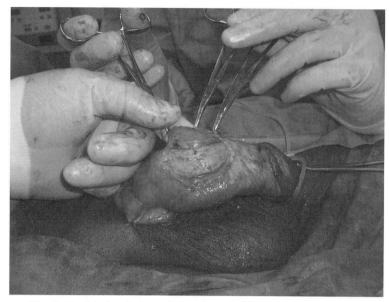

Fig. 3. Buck's fascia is mobilized medially to expose the tunica.

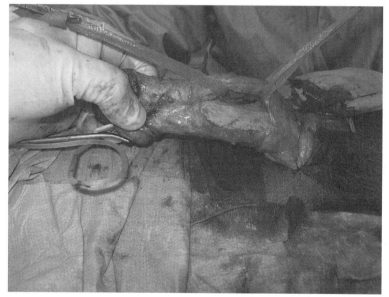

Fig. 4. Urethra mobilized to allow the excision of a single ellipse.

the dorsal neurovascular bundle without appreciable damage (Fig. 4). Alternatively, the dorsal tunica can be exposed by excising the deep dorsal vein and dissecting Buck's fascia laterally (Fig. 5).This type of mobilization typically allows for a single midline ellipse to be excised, and the suture line is covered by the urethra ventrally and therefore not palpable by the patient.

Alternative procedures excising two ellipses on either side of the urethra often result in more tissue excision with possible formation of a waist. The Nesbit ellipse is marked out opposite the site of maximum deformity, and for every 10° of bend, the ellipse is 1-mm

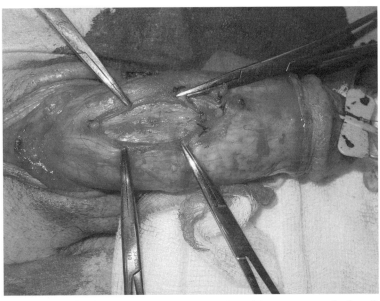

Fig. 5. Excision of the deep dorsal vein and lateral dissection of the neurovascular bundle gives good exposure to allow for a dorsal elliptical excision of the tunica to correct a ventral curvature.

wide. In a retrospective study, it was found that the mean width of the ellipse was 7 mm, and the angle of deformity was 68° *(18)*. When in doubt, it is possible to apply two Alliss forceps to the tunica albuginea (when the penis is flaccid) and then inflate the penis to check the correction (Fig. 6). On removal of the Alliss forceps, the remaining impression of the jaws that is left on the tunica also acts as a guide.

The ellipse is excised with minimum disturbance to the underlying muscle of the corpus cavernosum and the defect closed with 0-PDS sutures with the knots on the inside (Fig. 7). It is important to take good bites of tunica with the sutures to prevent "cutting out" and subsequent recurrent deformity. Finally, an artificial erection is induced to check that the penis has been straightened, and any minor residual deformity can be corrected by additional plication sutures. During closure, it is important to incorporate the dissected Dartos layer to prevent some penile shortening (Fig. 8). To prevent excessive penile shortening, a light compression dressing is applied for 2 d, and the penis is kept elevated to prevent swelling. The patient is then commenced on a phosphesterase type 5 inhibitor to promote nocturnal erections at 1 wk postoperatively for 3 wk or until he recommences sexual activity *(19)*.

The same principles apply for the alternative techniques of corporoplasty and plication that involve shortening the longer side of the penis, and the specific details are described in the following text.

In 1984, instead of excising an ellipse of tunica, Lemberger et al. described making a longitudinal incision in the tunica that when closed transversely shortened the longer side *(14)*. Based on the Heineke-Mikulicz principle, the technique was popularized by Yachia in 1990 when he reported a series of 10 cases *(13)*. It is important that the length of the longitudinal incision is not too long; otherwise, a dog-ear phenomenon is created when sutured transversely. Therefore, patients with a severe curvature may need more than one incision, each sutured to achieve straightening.

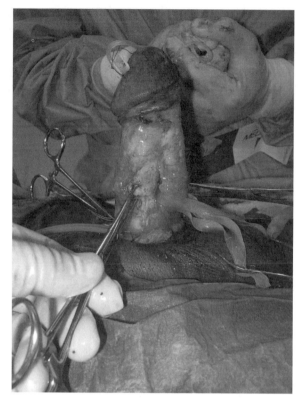

Fig. 6. Alliss forceps help mark out the site of the ellipse to be excised.

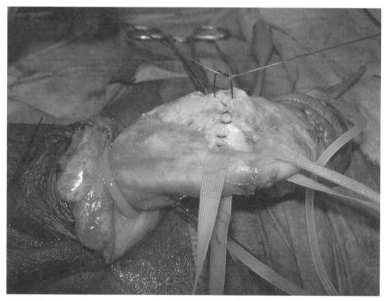

Fig. 7. Inverting sutures are used to ensure that the knots are buried.

The techniques of penile plication were introduced in 1985 by Essed and Schroeder in five patients using nonabsorbable sutures inserted in a figure-eight fashion to enable the suture knots to be buried *(15)*. At the same time, Ebbehoj and Metz also described

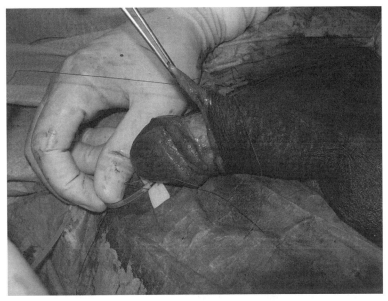

Fig. 8. Reattachment of the subcutaneous tissues to prevent some penile shortening.

Table 2
Results of the Nesbit Operation for Peyronie's Disease

Study group	Year	Number	Satisfaction (%)
Sulaiman and Gingell *(24)*	1994	78	79
Poulsen and Kirkeby *(25)*	1995	48	91
Ralph et al. *(18)*	1995	359	82
Porst *(26)*	1997	118	86
Savoca et al. *(27)*	2000	157	88
Syed et al. *(28)*	2003	42	79

the technique of using multiple rows of sutures to shorten the longer side for congenital curvature *(23)*. Minor variations in plication techniques have been made since then, most recently by Gholami and Lue *(16)*, who marked out 16 points to enable accurate placement of the sutures.

The advantages of penile plication are that there is minimal tissue dissection, and overcorrection can be rectified easily by removal of the suture. The problem with this procedure is that the correction depends on the strength of the suture material and not on wound healing. It is important, therefore, that a suture of high tensile strength is used, but if nonabsorbable, then the patient may complain of the knots causing pain.

RESULTS

Nesbit Operation

The results of the Nesbit technique are very satisfactory, and the largest series are shown in Table 2. Satisfaction is usually defined as the ability to have sexual intercourse without erectile dysfunction or a significant residual curvature.

Table 3
Relationship of Penile Shortening
to Coital Function Following the Nesbit Operation in 359 Patients

| Shortening (cm) | | Coitus | | |
	n	Normal	Possible	Impossible
Less than 1	311	—	—	
1 to 2	31	22	8	1
More than 2	17	11	4	2

From ref. *18*.

Table 4
Cause of Failure
of the Nesbit Procedure for Peyronie's Disease

Deformity (greater than 30°)	31
Surgical error	3
Suture failure	8
Progression of disease	20
Impaired erection	9
Penile shortening (greater than 2 cm)	19
Previous Nesbit	3
Progression of disease	3
Postoperative infection	3

From ref. *29*.

One of the reasons for failure is postoperative ED, and this is more likely in patients with poor-quality erections preoperatively. This was shown in two studies in which satisfaction rates increased from 74 to 90% *(18)* and 77 to 94% *(26)* in selected patients who had normal erectile function. Many patients with PD have either vascular disease or vascular risk factors that are likely to progress with time, and therefore any ED may worsen also *(22)*. To achieve good results, it is imperative to have an assessment of erectile function prior to surgery and to counsel those who are receiving treatment that progression and possible prosthesis implantation may be needed at a later date.

Penile shortening is inevitable with a Nesbit operation but only rarely is it significant enough to prevent sexual intercourse (Table 3). Measurement of the penile length at the time of surgery may help the patient appreciate that most of the shortening that occurs is caused by the fibrosis of their PD and not the surgery. Shortening of the penis by more than 2 cm was reported in 4.7% of 359 men in one series *(18)* and more than 1.5 cm in 14% of men in another series *(27)*. Severe shortening is more likely in patients who have a very severe curvature or those who have a significant complication of hematoma and infection. In an attempt to minimize shortening, patients are often given oral, injection, or vacuum therapy immediately postoperatively to encourage erections, although no scientific data have proven the benefit of such therapy.

The causes of failure of the Nesbit operation were assessed by Andrews et al. *(29)* in 2001 (Table 4). An immediate recurrence of the deformity is usually caused by sutures cutting out. Recurrences at 2–3 mo are the result of suture failure, hence the importance of taking good bites of tunica with a reliable suture of high tensile strength. Recurrence after 1 yr is usually caused by progression of the disease *(29)*.

Table 5
Results of Penile Plication for Peyronie's Disease

Study group	Year	Number	Satisfaction (%)	Recurrent deformity (%)
Nooter et al. *(33)*	1994	33	64	5
Klevmark et al. *(34)*	1994	51	82	5
Klummerling and Schubert *(35)*	1995	54	89	10
Thiounn et al. *(30)*	1998	29	62	20
Schulteiss et al. *(31)*	2000	21	67	43
Chahal et al. *(32)*	2001	69	52	14
Gholami and Lue *(16)*	2002	116	93	15
Cormio et al. *(37)*	2002	30	92	—
Van der Drift et al. *(36)*	2002	31	58	47
Van der Horst et al. *(38)*	2004	28	57	18
Greenfield et al. *(39)*	2005	68	98	1.5

Other possible postoperative complications that may occur include a urethral injury, glans numbness, and suture granuloma *(18)*.

Penile Plication

The results of penile plication are also generally good although possibly inferior to the standard Nesbit procedure *(30–32)*. The operation is, however, simpler and is ideal for the correction of minor deformities or in combination with a Nesbit or grafting operation to ensure absolute straightness. Most reports use the Essed technique, although variations are common, and the results are often reported for both congenital and acquired deformities. The results of plication for PD alone are shown in Table 5.

There is no standardization of reporting regarding outcome measures (what is deemed a success, unvalidated questionnaires, assessment of deformity, etc.), so comparisons are difficult to make. Overall, however, recurrent deformity appears to be higher with plication than with a standard Nesbit operation—as high as 57% in one series *(32)*. It is my opinion that this is because the whole operation depends on the strength of the suture and not on wound healing. This was also found in the new 16-dot plication technique by which multiple small rows of parallel sutures are placed with the penis erect. The recurrent deformity in this series was 15%, and suture failure would be the expected cause *(16)*. Penile shortening is also a concern, with 41–90% of patients complaining *(30–38)*, although the degree is likely to be similar to the standard Nesbit operation. In recent single center series of 102 men undergoing tunica plication, pre- and postoperative penile stretched length was measured. The mean length loss was 0.36 cm, with a range of 0–2.5 cm. Further analysis demonstrated that penile shortening was proportional to the original deformity angle and the original length, and more so in patients with a ventral curvature *(39)*. Palpable suture knots are common in one-third of patients *(31)*, and this is particularly so if nonabsorbable sutures are used.

Modified Nesbit Corporoplasty

There are many variations of the classical Nesbit operation that may include excision of multiple ellipses without urethral mobilization or additional plication sutures (Table 6).

Table 6
Results of the Modified Nesbit Operation for Peyronie's Disease

Study group	Year	Number (%)	Satisfaction (%)
Lemberger et al. *(14)*	1985	26	73
Sassine et al. *(40)*	1994	30	95
Licht and Lewis *(41)*	1997	30	83
Rehman et al. *(42)*	1997	26	78

Table 7
Results of the Nesbit Operation for Congenital Curvature

Study group	Year	Number	Satisfaction (%)	Recurrent deformity (%)
Poulson and Kirkeby *(25)*	1995	95	91	9
Porst *(26)*	1997	110	99	5
Kelami *(43)*	1987	100	96	4
Popken et al. *(44)*	1999	55	95	9
Andrews et al. *(45)*	1999	106	96	4

Table 8
Results of Penile Plication for Congenital Curvature

Study group	Year	Number	Satisfaction (%)	Recurrent deformity (%)
Ebbehoj and Metz *(46)*	1987	140	94	4
Erpenbach et al. *(47)*	1991	39	95	5
Klevmark et al. *(34)*	1994	48	81	5
Manning et al. *(48)*	1999	30	77	23
Schultheis et al. *(31)*	2000	40	77	23
Greenfield et al. *(39)*	2005	34	100	0

These combinations are standard practice, and each series usually contains modified cases. A defined modification described by Lemberger et al. and named the Yachia technique uses a unique principle of a longitudinal incision sutured transversely to shorten the longer side of the penis *(14,15)*. The results of this operation seem to be favorable, but all of the series had small numbers.

Comparison With Congenital Curvature

The Nesbit operation for congenital curvature of the penis gives excellent results (Table 7). The results are better than for PD, and this can be accounted for by the lack of postoperative erectile dysfunction in this group of young healthy men and the fact that penile shortening is less prevalent. Shortening has not occurred because of the original disease as in PD, and patients with congenital curvatures often have a large penis. With this comparison, patients with PD can be reassured that the Nesbit operation itself is unlikely to affect erectile function and is not responsible for the majority of shortening that occurs.

The results of penile plication for congenital curvature are shown in Table 8. The satisfaction rate is less than the Nesbit operation, and the recurrent deformity rate is higher.

This represents the fact that the whole operation depends on the strength of the sutures used rather than wound healing as for a Nesbit operation.

With these comparisons, it would seem that, for better patient results and satisfaction, the Nesbit operation is superior to plication in the treatment of the curvature caused by Peyronie's disease.

REFERENCES

1. Polkey HJ. Induratio penis plastica. Urol Cut Rev 1928; 32: 287–308.
2. Devine CJ, Horton CE. Surgical treatment of Peyronie's disease with a dermal graft. J Urol 1974; 111: 44.
3. Sachse H. Venenwandplastik bei Induratio penis plastica. Urolooge 1976; 15: 131–132.
4. Kelami A. Surgical treatment of Peyronie's disease using human dura. Eur Urol 1977; 3: 191–192.
5. Bruschini H, Mitre AI. Peyronie's disease: surgical treatment with muscularis aponeurosis. Urology 1979; 13: 505–506.
6. Das S. Peyronie's disease: excision and autografting with tunica vaginalis. J Urol 1980; 124: 818–819.
7. Lowe DH, Parsons CL, Ho PC. Surgical treatment of Peyronie's disease with Dacron graft. Urology 1982; 19: 609–610.
8. Austoni E, Colombo F, Mantovani F, Patelli E, Fenice O. Chirurgia radicale e conservazione dell' erezione nella malattia di La Peyronie. Arch It Urol 1995; 67: 359–364.
9. Brock G, Kadioglu A, Lue TF. Peyronie's disease: a modified treatment. Urol 1993; 42: 300–304.
10. Carson CC, Chun JL. Peyronie's disease: surgical management with autologous materials. Int J Impot Res 2002; 14: 329–335.
11. Nesbit RH. Congenital curvature of the phallus: report of three cases with description of corrective operation. J Urol 1965; 93: 230.
12. Pryor JP, Fitzpatrick JM. A new approach to the correction of the penile deformity in Peyronie's disease. J Urol 1979; 122: 622–623.
13. Yachia D. Modified corporoplasty for the treatment of penile curvature. J Urol 1990; 143: 80–82.
14. Lemberger RJ, Bishop MC, Bates CP. Nesbits operation for Peyronie's disease. Br J Urol 1984; 56: 721–723.
15. Essed E, Schroder FH. New surgical treatment for Peyronie's disease. Urology 1985; 25: 582–587.
16. Gholami SS, Lue TF. Correction of penile curvature using 16 dot plication technique: a review of 132 patients. J Urol 2002; 167: 2066–2069.
17. Carson CC, Hodge GB, Anderson EE. Penile prosthesis in Peyronie's disease. Br J Urol 1983; 55: 417–421.
18. Ralph DJ, Al-Akraa M, Pryor JP. The Nesbit operation for Peyronie's disease: 16-yr experience, J Urol 1995; 154: 1362–1363.
19. Levine LA, Lenting EL. Experience with a surgical algorithm for Peyronie's disease. J Urol 1997; 158: 2149–2152.
20. Montorsi F, Salonia A, Maga T, et al. Evidence based assessment of long-term results of plaque incision and vein grafting for Peyronie's disease. J Urol 2000; 163: 1704–1708.
21. El-Sakka AI, Rashwan HM, Lue TF. Venous patch graft for Peyronie's disease. Part II: outcome analysis. J Urol 1998; 160: 2050–2053.
22. Kadioglu A, Tefekli A, Erol B, Oktar T, Tunc M, Tellaloglu S. A retrospective review of 307 men with Peyronie's disease. J Urol 2002; 68: 1075–1079.
23. Ebbehoj J, Metz P. New operation for "krummerik" (penile curvature). Urology 1985; 25: 582–587.
24. Sulaiman MN, Gingell JC. Nesbit's procedure for penile curvature. J Androl 1994; 15: 545–565.
25. Poulsen J, Kirkeby HJ. Treatment of penile curvature—a retrospective study of 175 patients operated upon with plication of the tunica albuginea or with the Nesbit procedure. Br J Urol 1995; 75: 370–374.
26. Porst H. Congenital and acquired penile deviations and penile fractures. In: Penile Disorders (Porst H, ed.). Springer-Verlag, Berlin, 1997, pp. 37–56.
27. Savocca G, Trombetta C, Campalini S, De Stefani S, Buttazi L, Belgrano E. Long term results with Nesbit's procedure as treatment of Peyronie's Disease. Int J Impot Res 2000; 12: 289–294.
28. Syed AH, Abbasi Z, Hargreave TB. Nesbit procedure for disabling Peyronie's curvature: a median follow-up of 84 mo. Urology 2003; 61: 999–1003.

29. Andrews HO, Al-Akraa M, Pryor JP, Ralph DJ. The Nesbit operation for Peyronie's disease: an analysis of failures. BJU Int 2001; 87: 658–660.
30. Thiounn N, Missirliu A, Zerbib M, et al. Corporeal plication for surgical correction of penile curvature. Experience with 60 patients. Eur Urol 1998; 33: 401–404.
31. Schultheiss D, Meschi MR, Hagemann J, Truss MC, Stief CG, Jonas U. Congenital and acquired penile deviation treated with the Essed plication method. Eur Urol 2000; 38: 167–171.
32. Chahal R, Gogoi NK, Sundaram SK, Weston PM. Corporal plication for penile curvature caused by Peyronie's disease: the patients' perspective. BJU Int 2001; 87: 352–356.
33. Nooter RI, Bosch JLHR, Schrder FH. Peyronie's disease and penile curvature: long-term results of operative treatment with the plication procedure. Br J Urol 1994; 74: 497–500.
34. Klevmark B, Andersen M, Schultz A, Talseth T. Congenital and acquired curvature of the penis treated surgically by the plication of tunica albuginea. Br J Urol 1994; 74: 501–506.
35. Klummerling S, Schubert J. Peyronie's disease. Investigation of staging, erectile failure and operative management. Int Urol Nephrol 1995; 27: 629–637.
36. van der Drift DG, Vroege JA, Groenendijk PM, Slob AK, Schroder FH, Mickisch GH. The plication procedure for penile curvature: surgical outcome and postoperative sexual functioning. Urol Int 2002; 69: 120–124.
37. Cormio L, Zizzi V, Bettocchi C, et al. Tunica albuginea plication for the correction of penile curvature. Scand J Urol Nephrol 2002; 36: 307–310.
38. van der Horst C, Martínez Portillo FJ, Seif C, Alken P, Juenemann KP. Treatment of penile curvature with Essed-Schröder tunical plication: aspects of quality of life from the patients' perspective. BJU Int 2004; 93: 105–108.
39. Greenfield JM, Lucas S, Pinchcofsky H, Levine LA. Factors affecting the loss of length associated with tunica albuginea plication for correction of penile curvature. J Urol 2006; 175: 238–241.
40. Saissine AM, Wespes E, Schulman CC. Modified corporoplasty for penile curvature: 10 years experience. Urology 1994; 44: 419–421.
41. Licht MR, Lewis RW. Modified Nesbit procedure for the treatment of Peyronie's disease: a comparative outcome analysis. J Urol 1997; 158: 460–463.
42. Rehman J, Benet A, Minsky LS, Melman A. Results of surgical treatment for abnormal penile curvature: Peyronie's disease and congenital deviation by a modified Nesbit plication (tunica shaving and plication). J Urol 1997; 157: 1288–1291.
43. Kelami A. Congenital penile deviation and its treatment with the Nesbit-Kelami technique. Br J Urol 1987; 60: 261–263.
44. Popken G, Wetterauer U, Schultze-Seemann W, Deckart AB, Sommerkamp H. A modified corporoplasty for treating congenital penile curvature and reducing the incidence of palpable induration. BJU Int 1999; 83: 71–75.
45. Andrews HO, Al-Akraa M, Pryor JP, Ralph DJ. The Nesbit operation for congenital curvature of the penis. Int J Impot Res 1999; 11: 119–122.
46. Ebbehoj J, Metz P. Congenital penile angulation. Br J Urol 1987; 60: 264–266.
47. Erpenbach K, Rothe H, Derschum W. The penile plication procedure: an alternative method for straightening the penis. J Urol 1991; 146: 1276–1278.
48. Manning M, Junemann KP, Spahn M, Alken P. Operative korrektur der penisverkrummung—indikationen und grenzen der Essed-Schroder technik. Akt Urol 1999; 30:163–169.

13 Penile Plication Using the 16-Dot Technique

Robert C. Dean, MD and Tom F. Lue, MD

SUMMARY

Peyronie's disease, characterized by the formation of a fibrous plaque within the tunica albuginea of the corpora cavernosa, has long caused sexual dysfunction. Plication surgery has allowed a simple technique to correct the penile curvature caused by Peyronie's disease. The 16-dot plication technique corrects the penile curvature with a high level of patient satisfaction and yet can be performed under local anesthesia. Slight adjustments can be made during the procedure, which allows greater precision toward penile strengthening. The 16-dot penile plication procedure has an 85% long-term success rate for achieving a straight erection by patient reporting. Minimal complications are reported, with penile shortening (0.5–1.5 cm) reported at 41%. With a mean operative time of 45 min and the ability to perform the procedure under local anesthesia, the 16-dot plication procedure is an important tool for the urologist for treatment of Peyronie's disease.

Key Words: Penile curvature; penile straightening; Peyronie's disease; plication; surgery.

Peyronie's disease (PD) is characterized by the formation of a fibrous plaque within the tunica albuginea of the corpora cavernosa, causing a curvature, narrowing, or shortening of the penis. This deformity can be so severe that vaginal intromission becomes very difficult or impossible. Several surgical techniques have been described to repair the deformity. In 1965, Nesbit described the surgical correction of curvature of the penis by one or multiple elliptoid resections of the tunica albuginea on the longer side of the penis (1). A variation of this procedure, described by Saalfeld et al. (2) and Yachia (3), involves making longitudinal incisions on the healthy convex aspect of the penis and closing them horizontally using the Heineke-Mikulietz method.

Corporeal plication was popularized by Essed and Schroeder (4) as well as Ebbehoj and Metz (5) as a valid treatment for PD. In 1992, Donatucci and Lue (6) described the plication of penile curvature simplified through the use of intracavernosal papaverine injection. We have since modified our previous technique (6,7) for congenital and acquired penile curvature with our 16- or 24-dot, minimal tension technique using multiple parallel plications after penile erection is achieved with intracavernosal papaverine (8).

From: *Current Clinical Urology:*
Peyronie's Disease: A Guide to Clinical Management
Edited by: L. A. Levine © Humana Press Inc., Totowa, NJ

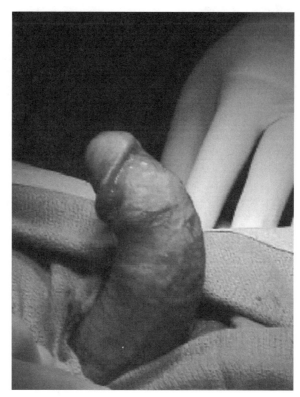

Fig. 1. Dorsal curvature of penis after papaverine injection.

The 16- or 24-dot, minimal tension plication technique is usually performed under local anesthesia with intravenous sedation. After the patient is comfortably positioned on the operating table, 2 mL (60 mg) papaverine are injected into the corpus cavernosum using a 25-gage needle. While the surgeons are scrubbing, the genital area is prepped and painted with the antiseptic of choice. A full erection should result. The degree and position of the curvature are assessed. The incision is then planned accordingly.

For dorsal curvature of the penis (Fig. 1), either a circumcising or a ventral longitudinal incision can be used, depending on patient preference. If preservation of uncircumcised foreskin is desired, a longitudinal incision should be used. We should bear in mind that a circumcising incision often requires more extensive degloving dissection. More edema and pain can be expected postoperatively after such degloving. If a ventral penile scar is acceptable to the patient, the longitudinal incision is better tolerated. Bupivicaine at a 0.25% concentration is given along the planned longitudinal incision or around the base of the penis for a circumcising incision. Buck's fascia is then incised longitudinally adjacent to the corpus spongiosum. Extending just lateral to the corpus spongiosum, the ventral tunica albuginea is exposed along the length of the curvature.

The center of the curvature is then marked. The entry and exit points of the sutures are marked, measuring approx 0.5–1 cm apart. The points are placed 2–3 mm lateral to the corpus spongiosum. Every four dots correspond to one suture; most curvatures require two or three sutures on each side of the corpus spongiosum to straighten the deformity (total 16 or 24 dots) (Fig. 2). In rare cases with severe angle of deformity or an extremely long phallus, four pairs of sutures (32 dots) are used. The 2-0 braided polyester suture (e.g., Ticron) is placed through the full thickness of the tunica albuginea. With the erection

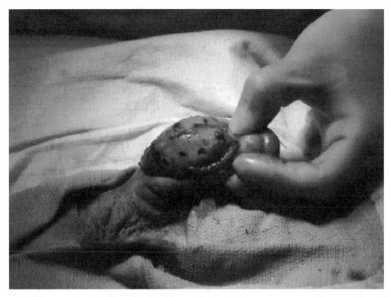

Fig. 2. Planned suture entry sites marked with pen lateral to corpus spongiosum. Erection attained throughout operation with papaverine.

still relatively full, the sutures are tied with a single throw of a square knot, and a rubber-shod clamp is placed just above each half-knot. With manual compression of the base of the penis, a rigid erection is created, and the straightness of the penis can be properly assessed. Any correction can be made by loosening or tightening the sutures; then, reevaluation is performed.

Only when there is a satisfactory consensus by the operating team are the knots permanently secured (Fig. 3). Smooth forceps are used to grasp the suture just beneath the first throw of the knot, the clamp is released, and four more throws are then placed. Because the sutures are tied while the penis is erect, there is minimal tension in the flaccid state. This prevents tissue strangulation, which may result in tunical damage during spontaneous rigid erection. Increasing the number of pairs of sutures ensures a minimal tension repair. At least two pairs of sutures (16 dots) should be used in any given repair to ensure minimal tension. The wound is closed after detumescence is assured.

For ventral curvatures, if a dorsal penile scar is acceptable to the patient, then a dorsal longitudinal incision is made. Buck's fascia is then incised longitudinally in the midline so the neurovascular bundle is not damaged. A space between the dorsal vein and the paired dorsal arteries is developed by careful blunt dissection using a fine hemostat. This is an extremely safe area for placement of sutures because nearly all of the dorsal nerve fibers are lateral to the dorsal arteries. The curvature center is marked, as are the entry and exit points.

For lateral curvatures, either a circumcising or a lateral longitudinal incision is used. Because of the presence of a more extensive neurovascular network, dissection under optical magnification is paramount. If the nerve bundles cross the path of the sutures, then the sutures need to be passed under the nerves to prevent injury and subsequent pain or paresthesia.

For combined curvatures (dorsal lateral or ventral lateral), the same technique as for the pure dorsal or ventral curvature can be used except for the placement of the dots. To correct the lateral component as well as the dorsal or ventral curvature, the space between

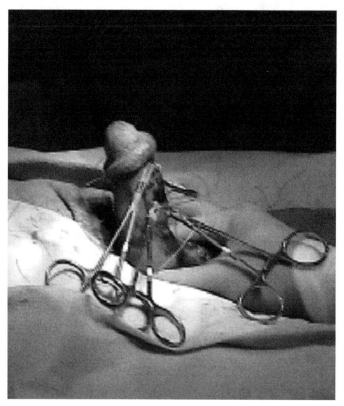

Fig. 3. Straightened penis following placement of suture with tension after placing first throw of knot. Clamps hold the tension of suture in place to allow for evaluation of the straightened penis.

the middle dots (of each four-dot set) on the long side of the lateral curvature is lengthened. This produces more shortening on the long side and therefore results in correction of these combined curvatures.

If an erection is still present at the completion of the case, then 10–20 mL of blood is aspirated from the corpora cavernosa with a 21-gage scalp vein needle. Every 3–5 min, 500 µg diluted phenylephrine are injected until the penis is flaccid. Careful monitoring of heart rate and blood pressure is important at this time. The injection site is then closed with a 5-0 polyglyconate suture ligature. Antibiotic solution is used to irrigate the wound thoroughly before the Dartos fascia is reapproximated over the Ticron sutures. The skin is closed with several vertical mattress sutures of 5–0 Dexon™ (Tyco Healthcare) interspersed with simple interrupted sutures. The incision is covered with Xeroform® (Sherwood) gauze, and finally a Coban™ (3M) dressing applied snugly around the penis. Most important, ice is applied for at least 12 h postoperatively. This ensures minimal edema. The dressing is checked within an hour postoperatively to ensure it is not too tight, and the patient is discharged home within 2 h.

RESULTS

A review of 132 patients who underwent the dot plication technique at University of California at San Francisco from 1995 to 2000 revealed the following statistics: The overwhelming presenting preoperative complaint (Table 1) was difficulty with intercourse or partner discomfort (81%). This was followed by penile pain (11%) and poor

Table 1
Presenting Complaints

Difficulty with intercourse or partner discomfort	81%
Penile pain	11%
Poor self-image	8%

Table 2
Postoperative Complaints

Shortening of penis (0.5–1.5 cm)	41%
Bother from suture	12%
Pain with erection	11%
Narrowing of penis	9%
Decreased penile sensation	6%
Hematoma	4%
Pain when flaccid	1%

Table 3
Recurrence Rate

	6 mo	Long term (mean 2.6 yr)
Straight erections	93%	85%
Slight curvature	7%	12%
Severe curvature		3%

self-image (8%). The most common postoperative complaint was shortening of the penis (41%). Loss of penile length ranged from 0.5 to 1.5 cm. Other complaints included bother from suture in 12%, pain with erection in 11%, narrowing of the penis in 9%, decreased penile sensation in 6%, hematoma formation in 4%, and pain when flaccid in 1% (Table 2). The preoperative angle of penile curvature ranged from 30 to 120°, with the average 64°. More than one direction of penile curvature was noted in 34% of patients.

Preoperative erectile function was good in 63%, moderate (requiring sildenafil) in 25%, and poor (requiring injection with or without a vacuum constriction device) in 12%. Erectile function was self-reported and confirmed by duplex color ultrasound after intracavernous injection and self-stimulation preoperatively. At 6 mo, 93% reported straight erections, 7% reported a slight curvature, and 3% complained of worse erectile function. Long-term follow-up (7 mo to 6 yr) showed 85% with straight erections and 15% with recurrence of curvature, which was severe only in 3% (Table 3). All 12 patients who had undergone failed Nesbit procedures were satisfied with the plication procedure and had straight erections postoperatively. Of all the patients with congenital curvature (16 patients), one man with a left lateral curvature had it recur after 1 yr. Four patients underwent secondary procedures: penile-lengthening procedure for recurrence of curvature with venous grafting in one patient, penile prosthesis surgery for erectile dysfunction (ED) not responsive to medical therapy in two, and penile-lengthening procedure with cadaveric pericardium as well as prosthesis surgery for medically refractory ED in one patient.

Mean operative time was 45 min. Local anesthesia only was used in 85% of the cases. Local anesthesia and intravenous sedation with midazolam and fentanyl was used in the remainder. One patient fainted during office injection, and the procedure was performed using laryngeal mask anesthesia.

SUMMARY

PD may be treated with a lengthening or shortening procedure. In the appropriate patient population, a lengthening approach is obviously desired. However, given that most patients present with comorbidities, including arteriogenic ED, lengthy anesthesia is less appropriate. Despite the fact that this is a type of shortening procedure, only 41% of patients noted or complained of postoperative shortening.

Several important points about this technique set it aside from prior methods and ensure a high success rate. The skin incision is chosen to minimize the need for degloving whenever possible. By incising Buck's fascia, the neurovascular bundles can be visualized, and an intervascular space devoid of nerves can be created. This minimizes the risk of opening healthy tunica albuginea and damaging the underlying erectile tissue in a population of patients with less-than-rigid erection. Failure of the Nesbit procedure *(1)* does not preclude plication surgery. Some of the patients evaluated long term (mean 2.6 yr) may have had *de novo* erectile dysfunction or worsening penile curvature caused by the disease process not related to the plication surgery. In this technique, neither the urethra nor the neurovascular bundles is mobilized, decreasing the chances of injury as compared to the technique of Essed and Schroeder *(4)*. An erection is maintained throughout the procedure, allowing real-time evaluation and adjustment of the repair and preventing over- or undercorrection. Paired multiple nonabsorbable multifilament sutures are used to distribute the total force required to straighten the curvature. This allows the sutures to be tied with minimal tension. This is the most crucial aspect of this plication technique. Minimal tension precludes the problems of suture breakage or cut-through reported in other series *(9–13)*.

This plication technique can be used to correct all types and degrees of penile curvature successfully except indentation or hourglass deformities. It has yielded satisfactory results with minimal morbidity. The great majority of patients with congenital curvature or acquired PD will have high success rates with this technique.

REFERENCES

1. Nesbit RH. Congenital curvature of the phallus: report of three cases with description of corrective operation. J Urol 1965: 93: 230–232.
2. Saalfeld J, Ehrlich RM, Gross JM, Kaufman JJ. Congenital curvature of the penis. Successful results with variations in corporoplasty. J Urol 1973; 109: 64–65.
3. Yachia D. Modified corporoplasty for the treatment of penile curvature. J Urol 1990; 143: 80–82.
4. Essed E, Schroeder FH. New surgical treatment for Peyronie disease. Urology 1985; 25: 582–587.
5. Ebbehoj J, Metz P. New operation for "krummerik" (penile curvature). Urology 1985; 26: 76–78.
6. Donatucci CF, Lue TF. Correction of penile deformity assisted by intracavernous injection of papaverine. J Urol 1992; 147: 1108–1110.
7. Baskin LS, Lue TF. The correction of congenital penile curvature in young men. Br J Urol 1998; 81: 895–899.
8. Gholami SS, Lue TF. Correction of penile curvature using the 16-dot plication technique: a review of 132 patients. J Urol 2002; 167: 2066–2069.
9. Andrews HO, Al-Akraa M, Pryor JP, Ralph DJ. The Nesbit operation for Peyronie's disease: an analysis of the failures. BJU Int 2001; 87: 658–660.
10. Poulsen J, Kirkeby HJ. Treatment of penile curvature—a retrospective study of 175 patients operated with plication of the tunica albuginea or with the Nesbit procedure. Br J Urol 1995; 75: 370–374.
11. Thiounn N, Missirliu A, Zerbib M, et al. Corporeal plication for surgical correction of penile curvature. Experience with 60 patients. Eur Urol 1998; 33: 401–404.
12. Nooter RI, Bosch JL, Schroder FH. Peyronie's disease and congenital penile curvature: long-term results of operative treatment with the plication procedure. Br J Urol 1994; 74: 497–500.
13. Klevmark B, Andersen M, Schultz A, Talseth T. Congenital and acquired curvature of the penis treated surgically by plication of the tunica albuginea. Br J Urol 1994; 74: 501–606.

14 Penile Straightening With Tunica Albuginea Plication Procedure

TAP Procedure

Laurence A. Levine, MD, FACS

SUMMARY

Penile straightening for Peyronie's disease may be accomplished through a variety of approaches. For the man with satisfactory rigidity for coitus but deformity that interferes with intromission, there are two main approaches: tunica plication and grafting techniques. According to previously published surgical algorithms, tunica plication appears to be the optimum technique for the man with curvature less than 60° without narrowing resulting in a hinge effect. This chapter describes the tunica albuginea plication procedure with which I have had excellent results with respect to correcting the deformity, preservation of sexual function, and predictable penile shortening depending on the direction and degree of curvature.

Key Words: Peyronie's disease; penile reconstruction; penile straightening; tunica plication.

INTRODUCTION

Surgery remains the gold standard of treatment for Peyronie's disease (PD) and is the most reliable way to correct the deformity associated with this disorder. The indications for surgical reconstruction include a stable, painless deformity with compromised ability or inability to engage in coitus as a result of deformity or diminished rigidity. In addition, men who have extensive plaque calcification are best considered for surgical correction as these patients tend to fail all medical therapy. Last, any man who desires the most rapid and reliable result should be offered surgery.

Because all patients with PD do not present alike, no single operation is likely to treat all patients successfully. Several factors should be evaluated that will assist the surgeon in determining the appropriate surgical approach. These include the nature of the deformity in terms of curvature, hinge effect, and hourglass deformity as well as erectile capacity. Erectile dysfunction (ED) is commonly associated with PD, and the man who has diminished preoperative rigidity needs to be counseled carefully about the surgical approach.

From: *Current Clinical Urology:*
Peyronie's Disease: A Guide to Clinical Management
Edited by: L. A. Levine © Humana Press Inc., Totowa, NJ

Men with significant preoperative ED who might be corrected surgically may still have significant ED postoperatively and therefore should be counseled to proceed to penile prosthesis. On the other hand, men who have satisfactory erections with or without pharmacotherapy may be offered surgical straightening without penile prosthesis.

Several surgical algorithms for PD have been presented; the first published algorithm in 1997 suggested that when rigidity was adequate regardless of the deformity a tunica albuginea plication (TAP) procedure was the preferred approach when the curvature was without significant hourglass or hinge effect or less than or equal to 60°. For the more complex, multidimensional curves of greater than 60° with or without a destabilizing hourglass or hinge effect, then plaque incision or partial excision with grafting was recommended (1).

All patients should undergo a detailed preoperative discussion as the goals for surgical reconstruction are to enhance or preserve preoperative rigidity, to straighten the penis, and to reestablish a shaft with normal caliber. We know that not all men who have undergone these procedures have been satisfied with the outcome; therefore, a detailed preoperative discussion of outcome expectations and informed consent should be obtained with every patient. The surgeon should discuss the possible side effects of surgery, including potential reduction of rigidity; diminished penile sensation; delayed ejaculation, which may take up to 6 mo to resolve; or shortening of the penis (regardless of the surgical approach). There is also a potential risk of persistent or recurrent curvature, which is unusual if disease has been stable for at least 6 mo. I counsel my patients to understand that sexual activity may not resume immediately after surgery and may take 2–6 mo to recover fully. Those patients who are not willing to accept these possible compromises should consider evaluation by a sex therapist prior to surgery.

Prior to beginning any reconstruction, penile stretched length should be measured. This is performed by measuring the dorsal shaft length from the pubis (by pushing down on the pubic fat pad) to the corona. This length uses two fixed points; measurement should be repeated pre-, intra-, and postoperatively (2).

For the patient who is a candidate for tunica plication, a variety of corporal plication procedures have been reported since the original description by Nesbit in 1965 (3). This procedure was used initially for boys with congenital chordee. A more detailed review of tunica plication options is found in Chapter 12.

This chapter focuses on a modification of the TAP procedure first reported by Duckett and Baskin in 1994 to correct congenital chordee with or without hypospadius (4). This procedure offers the benefit of other plication approaches as it is relatively simple to perform, corrects mild-to-moderate curvature (≤60°) in any direction with a very low rate of compromise to postoperative erectile capacity. All plication procedures are designed to be less invasive than the incision/partial excision and grafting operations, which are reserved for the more complex severe deformities in men without preoperative ED. Plication procedures are designed to be simple and relatively minimally invasive but have been noted to result in penile shortening; therefore, they are best used only for mild-to-moderate curvature (<60°) and for those without significant narrowing deformity.

SURGICAL APPROACH

An artificial erection is first created in the operating room with the aid of an injection of papaverine (60 mg) or alprostadil (20 µg) and infusion of saline using an infusion pump (Fig. 1). A circumcising incision is made approx 1.5 to 2 cm proximal to the corona. Tom

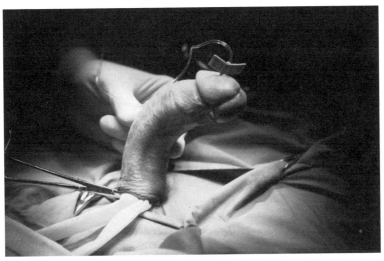

Fig. 1. Penile deformity defined intraoperatively with aid of vasoactive intracorporeal injection and saline infusion via butterfly needle through glans.

Lue has recommended a vertical ventral or dorsal skin incision for the man who refuses circumcision (see Chapter 13). The penis is degloved exposing Buck's fascia to the base of the penis. Hemostasis throughout the procedure is best accomplished with bipolar electrocautery. Loupe magnification is advised but not essential.

For Ventral Curvature

The surgical approach for ventral curvature is performed by elevating and resecting a segment of the deep dorsal vein dorsally contralateral to the area of maximum curvature. Circumflex and perforating veins are ligated and divided between 4-0 silk ties. Careful elevation of the neurovascular bundle lateral to the bed of the deep dorsal vein will expose the dorsal aspect of the tunica albuginea. At this point, a pair of transverse incisions approx 1.0–1.5 cm in length and separated by 0.7–1.5 cm is made directly over the septum (Fig. 2). The incision is carried down sharply with the scalpel through the longitudinal tunical fibers but not through the circular fibers. This will allow the erection to remain and reduce injury to the underlying cavernosal tissue. If the dorsal tunica between the two incisions is thick, as is frequently the case, this can be shaved down to reduce the bulk of the plicated tunica albuginea *(5)*.

The tunica is then plicated using 2-0 braided polyester suture (Tevdek, Teleflex Medical, Fall River, MA) in a vertical mattress fashion to bury the knot (Fig. 3). Typically, two or three of these Tevdek sutures are placed. The plication is then reinforced with several 3-0 PDS™ sutures (Ethicon, Somerville, NJ) placed in a Lembert fashion. Following each plication, penile straightness is checked by re-creating the erection by infusing saline (Fig. 4). Two or three plications usually are necessary to obtain full straightening. In our experience, straightening may take 1–6 plications. If one tries to plicate a much larger space between the two parallel incisions, this may result in "dog-ear" deformity, enhanced indentation, or general tunica irregularity. Therefore, it is recommended to keep the plications relatively short in transverse length and have no more than 0.7–1.5 cm between the two parallel transverse incisions.

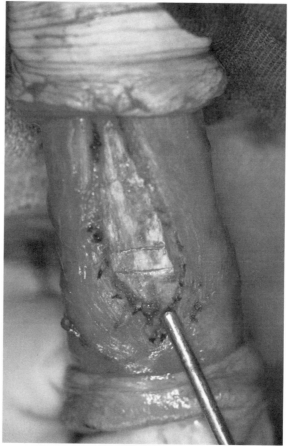

Fig. 2. Paired transverse parallel incisions through dorsal longitudinal fibers of tunica albuginea.

For Dorsal Curvature

When the curvature is dorsal, the plication incisions are made on the thicker ridge of tunica, adjacent to the urethra bilaterally (Fig. 5). Therefore, the mobilization of Buck's fascia should be made lateral to the urethral ridge and allow partial bilateral elevation of the urethra medially to expose the lateral aspect of the suburethral tunica (Figs. 6–8). The tunica ventrally is typically much thinner and therefore shaving is not indicated.

If the curvature has a substantial dorsal-lateral component, it may be that the plication on one side of the urethra will need to be broader than on the other to correct the lateral component. It may also be necessary to make the length of the transverse incisions longer on the contralateral side of the lateral curvature again to correct the lateral deformity.

One advantage of this approach is that, if overcorrection occurs, the sutures can simply be removed and repositioned to optimize the outcome without injuring or exposing the underlying cavernosal vascular tissue.

Once there is adequate straightening, Buck's fascia may be reapproximated with running 4-0 chromic suture. Any residual erection caused by the injected vasoactive agent should be reversed by either direct needle drainage or injection of dilute phenylephrine HCl solution (Baxter, Irvine, CA) at 100 µg/cc.

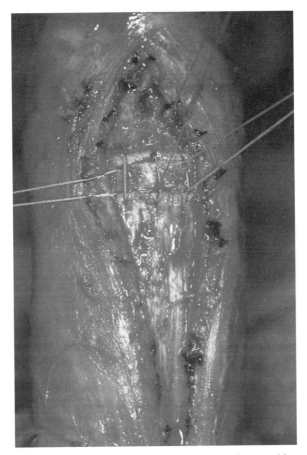

Fig. 3. Plication with 2-0 Tevdek suture with inverted knot.

The penile shaft skin is then reapproximated with horizontal mattress 4-0 chromic sutures on a cutting needle. The dressing for the TAP procedure is accomplished with application of a Xeroform® (Tyco Health Care, Mansfield, MA) dressing placed over the incision and covered by a dry sterile dressing. Finally a Coban™ dressing (3M, St. Paul, MN) is lightly wrapped from the glans to the base of the penis; the dressing is left on for 3 d. Although there is concern about applying a pressure dressing to the penis, the Coban should only be placed loosely to reduce postoperative swelling and bleeding. As long as this dressing is gently applied and then molded to the surface of the penis so it does not interfere with urination, it can be left in place for 3 d, which we have performed in well over 400 cases with no adverse events (Fig. 9).

At Rush University Medical Center, Chicago, we reviewed our experience with 154 consecutive TAPs performed on men with PD *(6)*. The highlights of our review focused on factors that contribute to loss of length following the TAP procedure. Although it is intuitive that the degree of curvature and the direction of curvature will have a bearing on the perceived and real length loss, this was demonstrated conclusively in this report.

Basically, given that the measurement of length in our institution is made on the dorsal aspect of the penis and represents the aspect of the penis, which is most readily appreciated

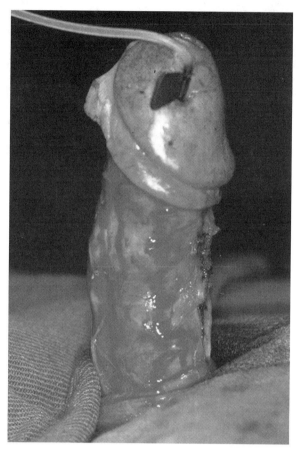

Fig. 4. Straightened penis.

by the patient during direct examination or indirectly in the mirror, our analysis demonstrated that patients with a dorsal curvature had the smallest mean percentage loss (0.5%) vs those with a ventral component, for whom a mean loss of length of up to 5% was measured. There also was a direct correlation between the degree of curvature and length lost; patients who had curvature less than 45° had a mean length loss of 1%, whereas those with over 60° curvature had a 4% mean length loss.

This study supported the empirical suggestion in the previously noted surgical algorithm that plication procedures should be reserved for curvatures of less than 60° to minimize length loss, particularly in men with PD (1). This study also demonstrated that the majority of patients who complained of loss of length postoperatively had also complained of loss of length preoperatively. This was also true for diminished erectile function and penile sexual sensitivity. In our experience with the TAP procedure, adequate straightening (defined as <20° residual curve) was accomplished in 99% of men. There was one man who had a 70° ventral curve and postoperatively had a 30° dorsal curve, which bothered the patient, but he declined surgical correction.

The TAP procedure appears to satisfy the goals of penile straightening for men with mild-to-moderate deformity with minimal risk of surgically induced ED and remains our procedure of choice except in those men with severe deformity or an unstable penis due to advanced indentation or hourglass deformity causing a hinge effect.

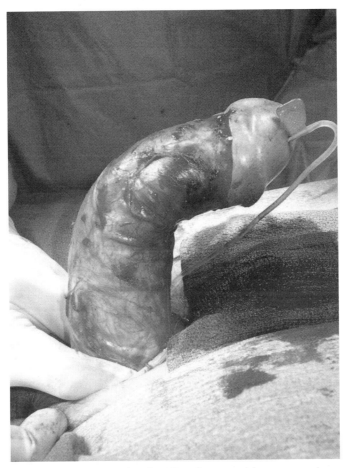

Fig. 5. Degloved erect penis demonstrating dorsal curve without narrowing or indentation.

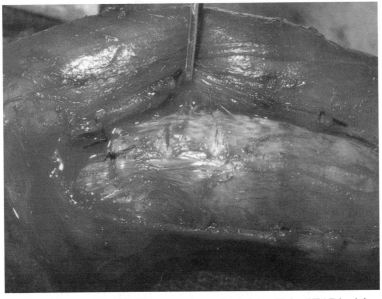

Fig. 6. Buck's fascia is elevated medially to expose urethral ridge. Paired TAP incisions made over thickened tunica on ridge.

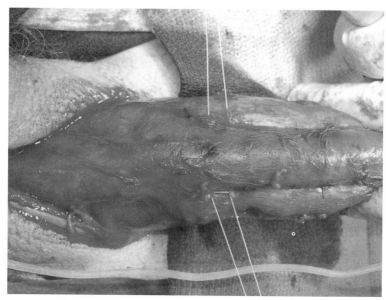

Fig. 7. The paired TAP incisions and plication are made bilaterally adjacent to urethra. Suture is placed to bury the knots.

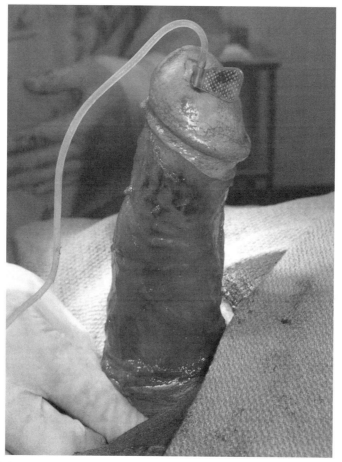

Fig. 8. Straightened erection, with three sets of paired plications employed in this case.

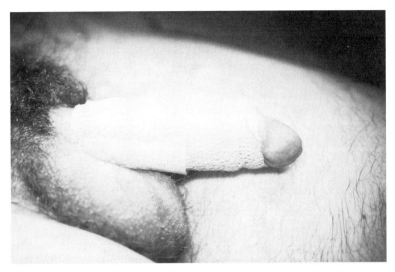

Fig. 9. Coban dressing in place, lightly applied from distal to proximal allowing exposure of glans.

REFERENCES

1. Levine LA, Lenting EL. Experience with a surgical algorithm for Peyronie's disease. J Urol 1997; 158: 2149–2152.
2. Levine LA, Greenfield JM. Establishing a standardized evaluation of the man with Peyronie's disease. Int J Impot Res 2003; 15(suppl 5): S103–S112.
3. Nesbit RM. Congenital curvature of the phallus: report of three cases with description of corrective operation. J Urol 1965; 93: 230.
4. Baskin LS, Duckett JW. Dorsal tunica albuginea plication for hypospadius curvature. J Urol 1994; 151: 1668–1671.
5. Rehman J, Benett A, Minsky LS, Melman A. Results of surgical treatment for abnormal curvature. Peyronie's disease and congenital deviation by modified Nesbit plication (tunical shaving plication). J Urol 1997; 157: 1288–1291.
6. Greenfield JM, Levine LA. Factors affecting the loss of length associated with tunica albuginea plications for correction of penile curvature. J Urol 2006; 175: 238–241.

15

Incisional Corporoplasty for the Correction of Peyronie's Disease Caused Penile Curvature

Daniel Yachia, MD

SUMMARY

Shortening the convex part of the corpora cavernosa for the treatment of penile curvatures was recommended more than 150 yr ago. Almost a century later, the surgical technique for straightening congenital penile curvatures by removing ellipsoid wedges from the convex side of the tunica albuginea, known as the *Nesbit corporoplasty*, was described. The modified corporoplasty described in this chapter was developed for achieving a straight and smooth penile shaft after the repair. This technique also is based on the principle of shortening the convex part of the corpora cavernosa, but without removing segments from the tunica albuginea and without dissection of the neurovascular bundle and its mobilization. In this technique, the longitudinal incisions done to the tunica albuginea of the corpora cavernosa are closed horizontally for shortening the convex part. Then, the bulges at the ends of the closure lines are buried with inverting sutures to smooth the penile shaft. This easily learned and performed technique can be used in most patients with Peyronie's disease who have a reasonable penile length for achieving excellent cosmetic and functional results.

Key Words: Incisional corporoplasty; Peyronie's disease; Yachia's corporoplasty.

INTRODUCTION

Peyronie's disease (PD) is a localized, sometimes disabling, condition mainly affecting the tunica albuginea of the corpora cavernosa. This is a condition of unknown etiology that results in fibrotic changes of the tunica albuginea, causing thickening and a loss of elasticity in this connective tissue. The deformity it may cause to the erect penis is sometimes so severe that penetration may become very difficult and even impossible. Like the congenital curvatures of the penis, the acquired curvatures are surgically curable deformations.

The aim of surgery is to make penetration comfortable by straightening the penis. Surgery is considered only in patients with stabilized disease and in whom the curvature affects their sexual performance. From all patients with PD, only about 10% may need surgical

From: *Current Clinical Urology:*
Peyronie's Disease: A Guide to Clinical Management
Edited by: L. A. Levine © Humana Press Inc., Totowa, NJ

correction *(1)*. This may be required when coital function becomes impaired or impossible. If a patient can penetrate without difficulty and both partners enjoy the sexual act, then there is no need to straighten the penis.

Surgical correction of the deformity should be considered in patients who did not respond to conservative treatments and who already have a stabilized disease. It is advisable to perform a surgical correction after an observation period of about 1 yr from the onset of the symptoms or after the stabilization of the curvature (followed up by 3 monthly autophotographies) and not before a 6-mo period after the disappearance of the painful erections.

Surgical procedures for correcting curvatures caused by PD are divided into three major groups:

1. Plaque surgery: excision of plaque and patching or incision through the plaque.
2. Corporoplasty: excisional, incisional, or plication procedures to the healthy part of the tunica albuginea.
3. Penile prosthesis implant.

Any of the corporoplasty techniques that straighten congenital penile curvatures can be used for straightening acquired penile curvatures. Corporoplasty was first used in PD patients by Pryor and Fitzpatrick in 1977 and published in 1979 *(2)*. They recommended this technique to patients with large plaques or diffuse fibrosis; with severe deformity, making penetration difficult or impossible; with established disease (at least 1 yr from the onset of the curvature). Pryor reported 77% satisfactory results with this technique *(3)*. Since then, similar results have also been reported by other authors using the original technique or its modifications *(4–9)*. The correction can be done using either the original technique as described by Nesbit *(10)* or by one of its modifications *(11,12)*.

An important point before performing a corporoplasty in these patients is to know the erectile ability status of the patient. The ideal patient for this surgery is the one having a rigid erection, with a minimum of 10-cm erect penile length from penile base to tip (the concave side length), but having severe penetration difficulties. A corporoplasty can be performed also in those patients who have an erectile dysfunction but respond to phosphodiesterase type 5 inhibitors or vasoactive injections and accept receiving such treatment after surgery.

NESBIT'S CORPOROPLASTY

Shortening the convex part of the corpora cavernosa for the treatment of ventral penile curvatures was recommended by Pancoast in 1844 *(13)*. More than a century later, the surgical technique for straightening congenital penile curvatures by removing ellipsoid wedges from the convex side of the tunica albuginea, known as *Nesbit corporoplasty*, was described by Nesbit in 1965 *(10)*. According to Nesbit, the first congenital penile deviation was treated by Young in 1932, but it was Nesbit himself who first described this entity in 1954 *(14)*.

Nesbit, with his publication in 1965, popularized the technique: In Nesbit's technique, after penile skin degloving for exposing the tunica albuginea, four to six symmetrically placed elliptical segments are outlined on the convex surface of the corpora, and these segments are excised. In those years, Nesbit recommended to close the defect with no. 2 silk *(10)*. In the same article, he also described his earlier experience using a plication technique to shorten the convex side of the penis to straighten the curvature by performing six vertical rows of plicating sutures using heavy silk. Despite the early satisfactory result, he noted that after 6 mo the patient reported complete recurrence of the erectile deformity, which had gradually developed. At operation, he found the plicating sutures pulled out of their attachments at the site of the repair.

CORPOROPLICATION

A nonexcisional method for shortening the convex side of the corpora was described by Ebbehøj and Metz in 1985. In this technique, 2-0 Prolene™ (Ethicon) sutures are placed using a double-crossover stitch, grasping deep into the tunica in four positions. Each of these sutures has four grasping points approximating the tunica to the center of the plication. The authors noted that application of one to four plications resulted in a straight erection in most cases. They also advised the patient that he would be able to palpate the small suture nodules under the penile skin (15).

KELÂMI'S CORPOROPLASTY MODIFICATION

Kelâmi described a refined modification of the Nesbit procedure by using Allis clamps to take as many "pinches" as necessary from the convex side until the penis straightens. According to this technique, the pinches of the tunica albuginea are excised in a diamond shape. Then, the diamond-shape defects are closed horizontally with a continuous U-shaped suture using 3-0 delayed absorption synthetic absorbable monofilament sutures. These sutures hold the edges of the diamond-shape corporeal windows closed until they disappear within 6–9 mo (11).

INCISIONAL CORPOROPLASTY

Alternative surgical techniques to excisional corporoplasty were proposed by Saalfield et al. (16) and Lemberger et al. (12). Both modifications were based on the Heineke-Mikulicz principle. Saalfeld's group tried to lengthen the shorter, concave side of the corpora cavernosa by making several transverse incisions that were closed longitudinally. This repair caused narrowing of the penile shaft at the repair site. Lemberger's group made longitudinal incisions at the convex part of the corpora and closed them horizontally. This repair caused several bulges at the repair site.

The corporoplasty described in this chapter is a refined modification of the incisional corporoplasty techniques. This modification was developed for achieving a straight and smooth penile shaft after the repair. Initially, I used this technique for straightening congenital penile curvatures in adults, then in congenital nonhypospadic and hypospadic pediatric penile curvatures and for straightening penile curvatures caused by PD (17).

Because of the relative potential risk of erectile dysfunction seen after plaque excision and patching for straightening the penis of patients with PD, I adapted the incisional corporoplasty technique for straightening also penile curvatures related to PD as well as other acquired penile curvatures of traumatic or iatrogenic origin.

The modification was developed to refine and simplify the existing corporoplasty techniques for obtaining a smooth penile shaft after repair, and to prevent accidental injuries to the corpus spongiosum or the neurovascular bundle. Because of the near vicinity of the neurovascular bundle or corpus spongiosum to the site where segments of the tunica are removed (in the excisional techniques), these structures are prone to injury. This is the reason why, during an excisional corporoplasty, before ellipsoidal or diamond-shaped wedges are removed from the tunica, the neurovascular structures should be mobilized.

Like all other corporoplasty techniques, this technique also is based on the principle of shortening the convex part of the corpora cavernosa. However, it differs from them because in this technique no tunica albuginea segments are removed and no neurovascular bundle or corpus spongiosum dissection and mobilization are performed.

All surgical manipulations done to the cavernous tissues produce some scar tissue at the site. The already impaired blood flow in older men can deteriorate further because of surgical manipulations, which cause development of local fibrosis in the cavernous tissues during the removal of the tunica albuginea segments. In the incisional corporoplasty technique described in this chapter, holding the scalpel blade in a certain way when making the longitudinal incision prevents cavernous tissue injury *(17,18)*.

This technique allows the surgeon to perform longitudinal incisions parallel to the neurovascular elements without mobilizing the bundle or corpus spongiosum. Even if the longitudinal incisions have to be done at the dorsal aspect of the penile shaft, they run parallel or between the neurovascular elements, abolishing the need to mobilize them.

PRESURGICAL EVALUATION

When evaluating a patient with PD for surgery, I recommend performing the following imaging procedures:

Autophotography. Because the curvature can barely be seen when the penis is flaccid, initial assessment of the deformation should be done by photographing the erect penis. Photographs taken from the sides, from above, and from the front, with a fully erect penis, document the deformation (Fig. 1). This allows documentation of the degree of deformation in a private setting. In case the patient cannot reach an erection, the procedure can be done in the office by using a vacuum erection device *(19)* or by intracorporal injection. Autophotography by showing the functional shape of the deformed erect penis allows the surgeon to choose the optimal technique for the surgical repair. Documenting the preoperative shape of the penis is important not only for allowing comparison of the surgical outcome but also for its medicolegal value.

Sonography of the penile shaft allows us to see the extent of the plaque.

Plain x-*ray of the penis* shows the presence of calcifications in the plaque.

STEPS FOR PERFORMING INCISIONAL CORPOROPLASTY

Step 1. Skin Incision and Penile Degloving

If the patient is circumcised, then a circumferential skin incision is done 5–10 mm below the corona. If not, then the patient is circumcised. Not performing a circumcision often results in severe postoperative preputial edema and sometimes in preputial necrosis or paraphimosis.

Penile skin degloving is done with sharp and blunt dissection until the whitish Buck's fascia is reached and is continued toward the penile base. Care should be taken not to injure the dorsal neurovascular bundle and the corpus spongiosum during this dissection.

Step 2. Artificial Erection

A tourniquet is applied at the base of the penis using the quarter-inch penrose drain held in place with a large hemostatic clamp. A large-gage butterfly needle is inserted directly

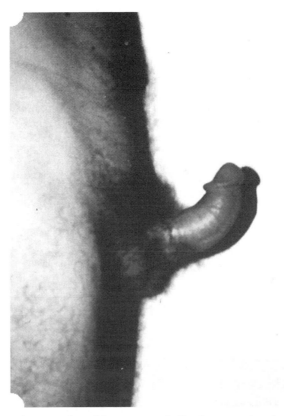

Fig. 1. Autophotography of the erect penis for documenting the deformity.

into one of the corpora or through the glans. Then, saline is injected to fill the corpora to create an artificial erection (Fig. 2). It is important to reach a maximal erection to demonstrate the entire deformation. The use of a tourniquet and saline injection for the artificial erection allows an almost-bloodless surgical field during the entire repair procedure. Although the artificial erection can be created by injecting vasoactive agents, I prefer not to do so because of the increased bloody surgical field after the corporotomy incisions.

Step 3. Artificial Straightening (Preview of Straightening)

Using Allis clamps with sharp teeth, pinches up to 1 cm are taken from the most convex side of the curvature (Fig. 3). To ease the pinching and prevent slippage of the clamps, it is advised to clean all the loose tissue over the Buck's fascia and reduce the tension of the erection by stopping the saline infusion for 1–2 min. Additional Allis clamps are applied until the curvature is completely straightened (Fig. 4). The number of pinches to be taken depends on the severity of the curvature.

Step 4. Albugineal Incisions

The Allis clamps are removed one at a time. The marks left by their teeth are the places and the length of each incision to be made (Fig. 5).

Holding the no. 11 scalpel blade horizontally, with its cutting edge upward, the blade is inserted into the tunica between the marks left by the clamp to perform the longitudinal

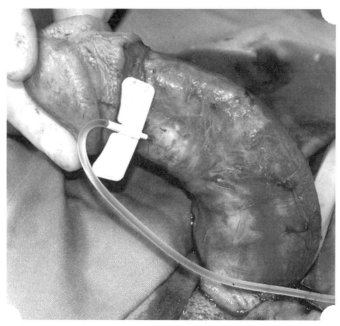

Fig. 2. Intraoperative artificial erection with saline injection into the (right) corpus cavernosum.

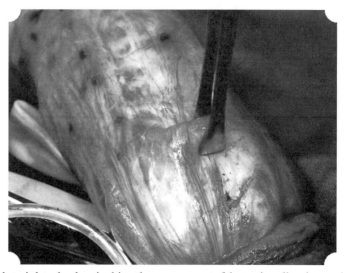

Fig. 3. Artificial straightening by pinching the convex part of the tunica albuginea using Allis clamps.

incision (Fig. 6). This maneuver allows incising the tunica only without damaging the cavernosal tissues (Fig. 7).

Step 5. Closure of Albugineal Incisions

The incision edges are held from their middle using small hooks to pull the edges horizontally. This maneuver turns the longitudinal incision to a transverse one (Fig. 8). The incisions are closed in a watertight manner using 3-0 delayed absorption suture material such as PDS™ (Ethicon) or Maxon™ (Davis & Geek) in a continuous-lock suture. I do not advise the use of either nonabsorbable material, which will remain permanently under

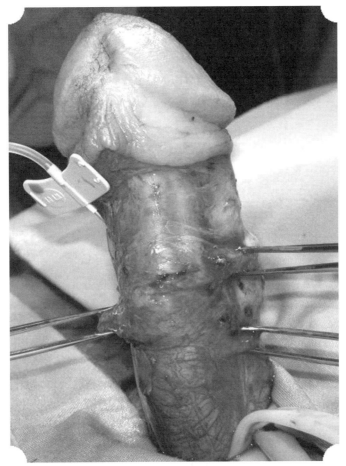

Fig. 4. Repair preview. Complete artificial straightening with several Allis clamps applied to the ventrolateral aspect of the penis to straighten the dorsal curvature.

the penile skin, or relatively rapid absorption suture material such as Vicryl™ (Ethicon), Dexon™ (Davis & Geck), or Monocryl™ (Ethicon) because these sutures lose their tension before the healing process is complete and can cause a recurrence of the curvature.

After closure of the incisions dog-ears form at the end of the suture line (Fig. 9). The dog-ears and the knots are buried by inverting sutures using the same suture material (Fig. 10). This maneuver smoothes the surface of the penile shaft (Fig. 11).

Step 6. Repeated Artificial Erection

After removing the tourniquet, the artificial erection is repeated to check the result of the correction (Fig. 12). In case of residual curvature, this is corrected by adding more incisions, repeating steps 4 and 5.

During the entire procedure, the surgical field is frequently irrigated with gentamicin solution.

Before reapproximating the shaft skin, hemostasis is obtained, especially to the inner surface of the skin, to prevent development of postoperative subcutaneous hematoma. The skin is sutured with fine, monofilament, absorbable suture material.

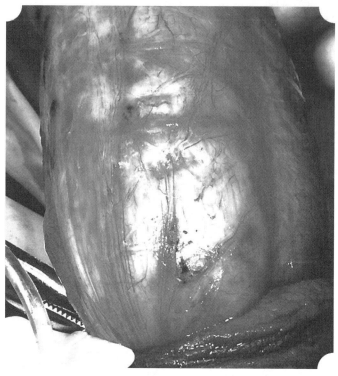

Fig. 5. Marks left on the tunica albuginea by the Allis clamps indicate the place and the length of the incisions.

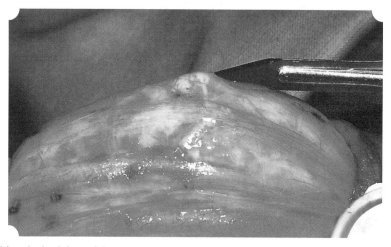

Fig. 6. Making the incision with the cutting edge of the no. 11 scalpel blade directed upward to prevent injury of the cavernous tissues.

To reduce the early postoperative pain, a penile block is performed by injecting 5 mL 0.5% bupivacaine to each side of the suspensory ligament.

POSTOPERATIVE CARE

At the end of the procedure, a slightly compressing elastic bandage is applied around the penis. An alternative to this elastic dressing is a silicone foam cast around the penis.

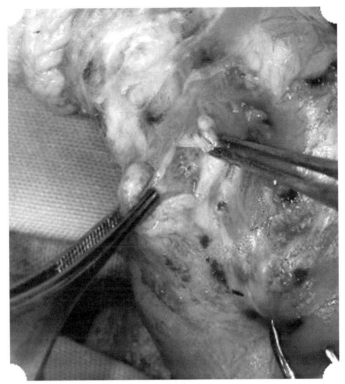

Fig. 7. Intact cavernosal tissue after performing the longitudinal tunical incision.

The dressing is kept for 48 hr to prevent edema or hematoma formation and to reduce the spontaneous postoperative erections, which are painful. Usually, there is no need to put a new dressing around the skin incision line.

In elderly patients with a history of obstructive voiding symptoms, a small-caliber indwelling catheter can be left at the end of the procedure for a few days. The catheter is inserted before the dressing is applied. If an indwelling catheter is not inserted, postoperative antibiotic prophylaxis is not mandatory.

If the procedure is done on an outpatient basis, then the patient can be discharged home 12 hr after surgery. If hospitalized, then he can be discharged the day after surgery.

Usually, when the penis is flaccid there is almost no pain after surgery. The patient should be informed that pain will appear during nocturnal spontaneous erections, but because of the pain, the duration of the erections are typically shorter than usual. Oral analgesics such as ibuprofen, dypirone, or paracetamol can be used for reducing the pain level during nocturnal or spontaneous erections.

The patient is advised to have no sexual activity for 45 d following surgery. At the end of this period, he is advised to return with new photographs of the erect penis taken a day before the visit for documenting and comparing the postoperative result with the preoperative deformation.

COMPLICATIONS, THEIR PREVENTION, AND THEIR TREATMENT

The risk of complications after the incisional corporoplasty is very low. The immediate complications can be hematoma formation and infection. A very important factor for

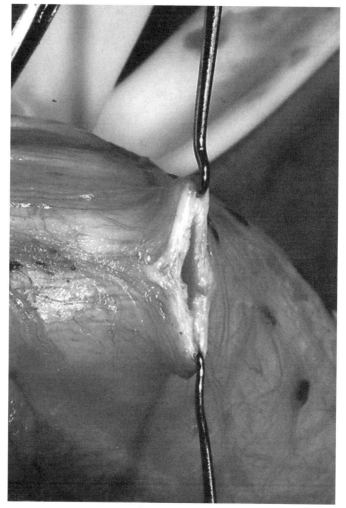

Fig. 8. Horizontalization of the longitudinal incision with a pair of small hooks applied to the middle of the incision edges, pulling them aside.

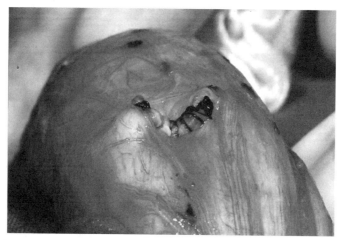

Fig. 9. Watertight transverse suture of the incision. Note the dog-ears at the ends of the suture line.

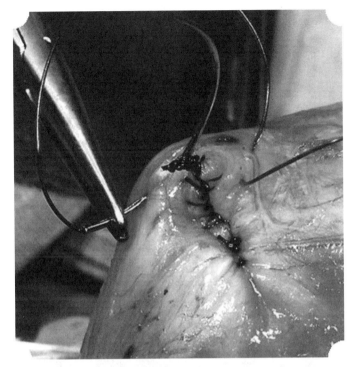

Fig. 10. Inverting sutures to bury the dog-ears and the knots.

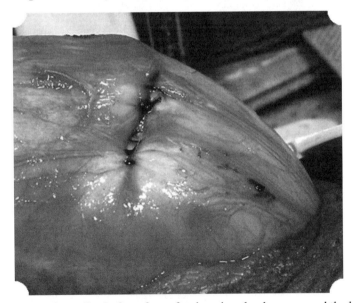

Fig. 11. Smooth penile shaft surface after burying the dog-ears and the knots.

hematoma formation is cavernosal blood leaking from the corporotomy incisions. It is important to make the closure of the incisions watertight and to check the incision after completion of the closure by a repeated artificial erection. It is also important to close with a small, absorbable, figure-eight suture the entrance hole of the large-caliber butterfly needle used for the artificial erection (if it was inserted directly into the corpus cavernosum and not through the glans).

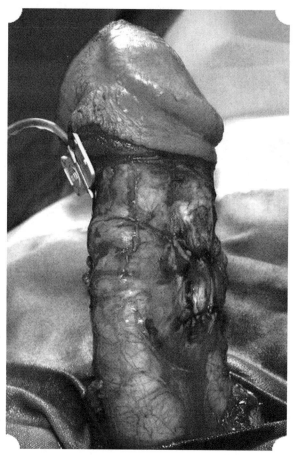

Fig. 12. Repeat intraoperative artificial erection to check the watertightness of the sutures and the straightening.

Another reason for postoperative hematoma formation is incomplete hemostasis of the penile shaft and the inner surface of the penile skin. Meticulous hemostasis is a must. If a postoperative hematoma develops because of large leaks from the corporotomy incision, the leak should be treated surgically. Large hematomas should be drained with antibiotic coverage. Smaller hematomas can be treated conservatively by applying a mildly compressive elastic bandage for a few days.

Wound infection is very rare. Performing repeated antibiotic solution irrigations during surgery reduces the risk of wound infection to a very low level. Advising the patients to use an antiseptic soap for washing the genitalia the night before and the morning of surgery as well as during the first week after surgery is recommended. Infection of the incision can result in skin wound dehiscence that may not need intervention if it is in a small area but may require excision and resuturing if a large area of the suture line opens.

Loss of penile skin or glans sensation has been infrequently reported. It is mainly caused by the circumferential skin incision. The sensation gradually returns within a few weeks. If during penile skin degloving damage is caused to the dorsal nerves, then the return of the sensation, especially the glans sensation, can take months. If the nerve damage is substantial, then the return of sensation can be patchy, with several areas of the glans remaining without sensation.

Late complications are very rare. The most important one is the recurrence of the curvature, developing within a few weeks after the repair. This is mainly caused when inadequate suture material is used. Use of suture material such as Dexon or Vicryl is not recommended because it becomes weak within a couple of weeks and cannot hold the incision edges closed during the healing period. I also do not recommend the use of non-absorbable suture material because they remain permanently under the skin and are felt by the patient or his partner. The use of delayed absorption material such as 3-0 PDS or Maxon is strongly advised. These sutures are strong enough and keep their tension long enough, until complete healing of the tunica albuginea occurs. Recurrence of the curvature can be caused by premature resumption of sexual activity. Rigid and prolonged erections before wound healing (during the 2–4 wk after surgery) can cause the suture material to cut through the tunica albuginea and may disrupt of the repair. This is rarely seen in patients with PD who have less-rigid erections than their younger counterparts undergoing a corporoplasty for congenital penile curvature. Late recurrence (over 6 mo) of the curvature is not considered a failure of the repair but indicates a new episode of the disease.

CONCLUSIONS

The simple technique and low complication rate of the incisional corporoplasty makes it our preferred technique to repair the penile curvature in patients with PD who have a reasonable penile length. This technique has been used on more than 300 patients with excellent cosmetic and functional results.

REFERENCES

1. Carson CC, Hodge GB, Anderson EE. Penile prosthesis in Peyronie's disease. Br J Urol 1983; 55: 417–421.
2. Pryor JP, Fitzpatrick JM. A new approach to the correction of the penile deformity in Peyronie's disease. J Urol 1979; 122: 622–623.
3. Pryor JP. Surgical treatment of Peyronie's disease using the Nesbit technique. Prog Reprod Biol Med 1983; 9: 98–103.
4. Goldstein M, Laungani G, Abrahams J, Waterhouse K. Correction of adult penile curvature with a Nesbit operation. J Urol 1984; 131: 56–58.
5. Coughlin PW, Carson CC, Paulson DF. Surgical correction of Peyronie's disease. The Nesbit procedure. J Urol 1984; 131: 282–285.
6. Daich JA, Angermeier KW, Montague DK. Modified corporoplasty for penile curvature: long-term results and patient satisfaction. J Urol 1999; 162: 2006–2009.
7. Savoca G, Scieri F, Pietropaolo F, et al. Straightening corporoplasty for Peyronie's disease: a review of 218 patients with median follow-up of 89 mo. Eur Urol 2004; 46: 610–614.
8. Giammusso B, Burrello M, Branchina A, et al. Modified corporoplasty for ventral penile curvature: description of the technique and initial results. J Urol 2004; 171: 1209–1211.
9. Rolle L, Tamagnone A, Timpano M, et al. The Nesbit operation for penile curvature: an easy and effective technical modification. J Urol 2005; 173: 171–173.
10. Nesbit RM. Congenital curvature of the phallus: report of three cases with description of corrective operation. J Urol 1965; 93: 230–232.
11. Kelâmi A. Congenital penile deviation and its treatment with the Nesbit-Kelâmi technique. Br J Urol 1987; 60: 261–263.
12. Lemberger RJ, Bishop MC, Bates CP. Nesbit's operation for Peyronie's disease. Br J Urol 1984; 56: 721–723.
13. Gross SD (citing Pancoast). The Diseases, Injuries and Malformations of the Urinary Bladder, Prostate Gland and the Urethra. 2nd ed. Blanchard and Lea, 1855.

14. Nesbit RM. The surgical treatment of congenital chordee without hypospadias. J Urol 1954; 72: 1178–1180.

15. Ebbehøj J, Metz P. New operation for "krummerik" (penile curvature). Urology 1985; 26: 76–78.

16. Saalfield J, Ehrlich RM, Grass JM, Kaugman JJ. Congenital curvature of the penis: successful results with variations in corporoplasty. J Urol 1973; 109: 64–68.

17. Yachia D. Modified corporoplasty for the treatment of penile curvature. J Urol 1990; 143: 80–82.

18. Yachia D. Our experience with penile deformations: incidence, operative techniques and results. J Androl 1994; 15(suppl): 63S–68S.

19. Yachia D. Negative-pressure induced erection for the assessment of impotent patients with Peyronie's disease. Br J Urol 1990; 66: 106–107.

16 Peyronie's Disease

Surgical Straightening With Tunica Plication and Tunica Transfer

Konstantinos Hatzimouratidis, MD, PhD
and Dimitrios G. Hatzichristou, MD, PhD

SUMMARY

The objective of surgical treatment for Peyronie's disease is to restore a painless, straight, and natural erection that is sufficient for intercourse. Plication procedures are associated with penile shortening, especially in cases of excessive curvature or rotation. Grafting procedures may prevent penile shortening, but they are often associated with poor postoperative anatomical and functional results caused by graft shrinkage and postoperative graft-associated corporeal veno-occlusive dysfunction. Surgical straightening of penile curvature with tunica plication and tunica albuginea free grafts is a simple and highly efficacious treatment modality with excellent functional results. It is associated with minimal postoperative shortening and eliminates major immediate and late complications, including recurrent curvature. It preserves erectile capacity in men with preoperative normal erectile function. Initial long-term patient satisfaction data, with lasting cosmetic and functional results, indicate that the proposed technique may be used as the indicated procedure for successful surgical treatment of excessive congenital or acquired penile curvature malformation.

Key Words: Grafts; penile induration; penis; Peyronie's disease; tunica albuginea.

INTRODUCTION

Peyronie's disease (PD) remains a pathophysiological and therapeutic dilemma because the cause and natural history of the disease are largely unknown *(1–3)*. Medical treatments are largely unsatisfactory in stabilized disease. The presence of calcified plaques and stable disease for at least 6 mo are well-accepted criteria for considering reconstructive surgery *(4)*. The objective of surgical treatment is to restore a painless, straight, and natural erection that is sufficient for intercourse *(5)*. Preoperative erectile dysfunction (ED) minimizes success because erectile inadequacy persists postoperatively *(6,7)*. Thus, the indication for surgical correction of angulation is limited to troublesome curvature but otherwise normal rigidity as the reason for sexual dysfunction *(8)*.

From: *Current Clinical Urology:*
Peyronie's Disease: A Guide to Clinical Management
Edited by: L. A. Levine © Humana Press Inc., Totowa, NJ

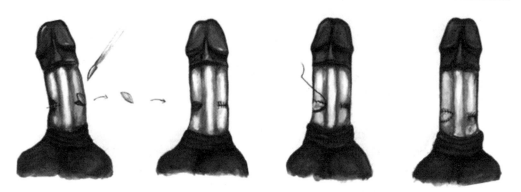

Fig. 1. Schematic drawing of the surgical procedure. At the point of maximal convexity, an elliptical segment of the tunica albuginea is excised and used as free graft. At the point of greatest concavity (site opposite the former incision), a symmetrical relaxing incision is made in the tunica albuginea, and the free graft is placed in the defect created.

The Nesbit procedure, which was initially applied for correcting congenital penile deviation, is considered the gold standard based on excellent results in terms of penile straightening and long-term durability. However, it is associated with penile shortening, especially in cases of excessive curvature or rotation *(9)*. Plication procedures are associated with the same drawbacks *(10)*. On the other hand, grafting procedures have been proposed in cases with significant penile curvature where Nesbit or plication procedures are expected to cause significant penile shortening or if shortening is unacceptable to patients.

These procedures can prevent penile shortening, but they are often associated with poor postoperative anatomical and functional results caused by graft shrinkage and postoperative graft-associated corporeal veno-occlusive dysfunction *(11,12)*. Several autologous tissue or even synthetic materials have been proposed, but only vein grafts—in conjunction with postoperative application of different graft shrinkage prevention techniques—gained certain acceptance *(13,14)*. In principle, tunica albuginea is considered the most appropriate grafting material because no other graft can share its unique properties. The surgical procedure, the results, and complications of tunica albuginea grafting are discussed in this chapter.

OPERATIVE TECHNIQUE

Indications

The patient indications for penile straightening with tunica plication and tunica transfer include significant penile deviation (usually greater than 45°) caused by congenital curvature or secondary to PD that has been stable for more than 6 mo after diagnosis. It is actually a combination of the typical Nesbit procedure with tunica albuginea free grafting (Fig. 1).

Anesthesia Requirements

The operation can be performed under general, regional, or local anesthesia (penile block). So, virtually every patient can be a candidate for this operation despite age or existing comorbidities as the operation can be managed as a day case.

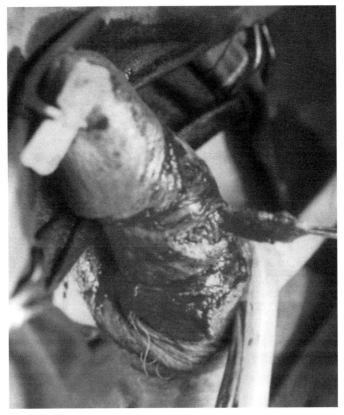

Fig. 2. Excision of the elliptical segment of the tunica albuginea at the point of greatest concavity.

Description of the Operative Technique

A circumcising incision is made and shaft dissection is done according to the typical degloving technique. The tunica albuginea is then exposed by incising Buck's fascia.

A 21-gage butterfly needle is then inserted into the glans penis, and artificial erection is induced by normal saline infusion after a tourniquet is applied to the base of the penis to minimize venous outflow. The aim of the artificial erection is to demonstrate the extent of the deformity and, using the knife, to identify the appropriate place and size of the elliptical segment necessary to be removed.

The elliptical segment of the tunica albuginea is then excised just opposite the point of maximal curvature (Fig. 2). In cases of dorsal or dorsolateral curvature, the elliptical segment must be excised from the ventral aspect of the penis, and mobilization of the corpus spongiosum is necessary. In cases with ventral or ventral-lateral curvature, the elliptical segment must be excised from the dorsal aspect of the penis after careful mobilization of the dorsal neurovascular bundle. Care is undertaken to avoid damage to the underlying tissue of the corpora cavernosa as much as possible.

After excision, the tunica albuginea segment is preserved in normal saline. The edges of the defects are approximated with interrupted or running 4-0 polydioxanone (PDS II™) sutures.

At the point of greatest concavity (site opposite the former incision), a symmetrical relaxing incision is made in the tunica albuginea, and two stay sutures of 4-0 polydioxanone

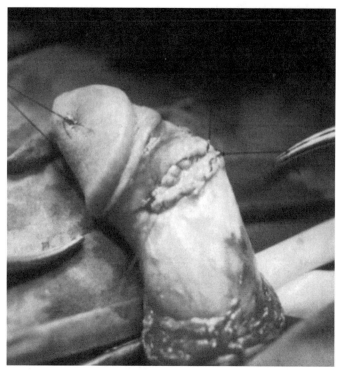

Fig. 3. The free graft is placed in the defect created at the point of greatest concavity.

(PDS II™, Ethicon, Somerville, NJ) are placed at the two ends of the incision, keeping their needles. The length of the relaxing incision is determined by the length of the elliptical tunica albuginea graft. The graft is placed in the defect, and its ends are sutured at the ends of the incisions using the two above-mentioned sutures (Fig. 3). The sutures run along the whole edge from each side, locking every other stitch to make the suture line watertight.

Artificial erection follows to assess the restoration of penile straightening and possible leakage (Fig. 4). When leakage is present, supplementary interrupted sutures of the same material can be placed. Further elliptical excisions and grafting should be done as needed to correct the deformity; for a curve up to 60°, one graft is usually sufficient; in cases of 90–120°, two grafts are necessary in most cases.

Before closing the Buck's fascia, confirmation of straightening is necessary by again producing artificial erection and removing the tourniquet from the base of the penis; despite the increased venous outflow, artificial erection is easy to achieve by increasing the infusion rate, especially in patients with normal corporeal veno-occlusive mechanism. Such erection not only demonstrates the final result of the operation, but also unmasks possible deviation at the base of the penis, which typically is "covered" by the tourniquet placement. Afterward, the penile skin is reapproximated at the coronal sulcus using 3-0 polyglactin (Vicryl Rapid™, Ethicon) sutures. A self-adhesive penile dressing with moderate compression using Coban™ (3M, St. Paul, Minnesota) dressing follows in the usual manner.

The patient is discharged either the same night of or the day after surgery. In the case of same-day discharge, the patient is instructed to visit the outpatient clinic the next day

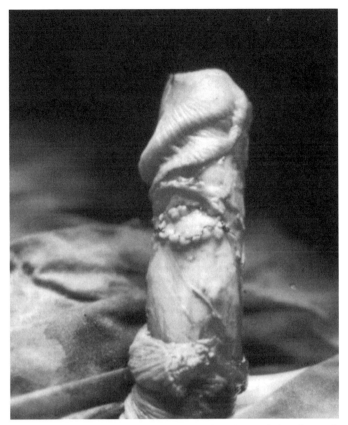

Fig. 4. Artificial erection is used to assess the restoration of penile straightening and possible leakage.

to remove the dressing and control for hematomas, mainly caused by nocturnal erections. Typically, a follow-up appointment at 1 mo postoperatively is scheduled, with instructions to avoid sexual activity during this period. In cases of hematoma formation, the dressing is replaced for a couple of days.

Follow-Up

Patients are followed at 1- and 6-mo intervals postoperatively. At the first follow-up visit, an intracavernosal injection of 10 μg alprostadil is given to identify the functional and aesthetic result of the operation. This step is important for both medical and legal purposes. Photographs of the penis in the erect state, taken by the patient or his partner, are a good alternative, avoiding the time-consuming process of pharmacological erection. At 6-mo follow-up visit, triplex ultrasonography of the corpora cavernosa before and after intracavernosal injection of 10 μg alprostadil is used to determine the absorption of the polydioxanone (PDS II) sutures as well as possible further progression of the primary pathological condition. At that time, questions regarding the postoperative sexual experience of the patient are mandatory.

CLINICAL TRIALS USING TUNICA ALBUGINEA GRAFTING

The first description of tunica albuginea grafting was by Goldstein and Blumberg *(15)*. The authors excised elliptical segments of the tunica albuginea that had been grafted to the contralateral corpus cavernosum as in the described technique. The indications included severe penile angulations in which penile shortening could be significant. They reported straightening of the penis with minimal shortening in three men.

Hatzichristou et al. treated 17 potent patients (4 with congenital penile curvature and 13 with stable PD) between 19 and 62 yr old (mean age plus or minus standard deviation 46.1 ± 14.5 yr) with the described surgical technique (16). Mean age of those with congenital deviation was 21.75 ± 2.2 yr (range 19–24 yr); patients with acquired penile deformities were considerably older (mean age 53.6 ± 4.7 yr, range 46–62 yr). The minimal disease duration before surgical treatment in the latter group was 1 yr (mean 25.8 ± 13.7 mo). During the operation, straightening was achieved in all patients, and the short-term results were considered excellent in all cases. Postoperatively, penile shortening was noticed by 8 patients (47%), of whom 2 (11.7%) considered it significant. Only 1 man considered decreased penile length emotionally bothersome. Erectile ability was preserved in all patients, and all reported functional erection within the initial 3 mo of follow-up. Immediate postoperative complications were minimal, including temporary penile edema in most patients and hematoma at the grafting site in only 1 patient. Hematoma was limited, and follow-up ultrasound 1 mo later showed normal findings.

During long-term follow-up (18–62 mo, mean ± SD 39.5 ± 13.7 mo), only 1 patient (5.9%) with the preoperative diagnosis of PD reported a minor relapse of about 10° of penile deviation, which had no functional effect on erectile capacity or the mechanical aspect of sexual intercourse. Curvature recurrence was attributed to progression of the underlying pathological condition, as determined by ultrasound 18 mo postoperatively. All patients reported that they were satisfied or very satisfied (on a 5-point satisfaction scale with 1 as very dissatisfied, 5 as very satisfied) with the postoperative straightening of the penis, the resumption of sexual intercourse, and the sustained preoperative level of erectile function. Furthermore, all patients would recommend the operation to others or undergo it again if necessary.

Teloken et al. also used tunica albuginea free grafts, but the surgical technique was different (17). The authors incised the plaque (horizontal, H-shaped, or cruciform incision was utilized) or removed it completely if it was relatively small. The graft was obtained from the crura through perineal access with the patient in the lithotomy position. Seven patients with stabilized PD for at least 2 mo were treated. In six cases, straightening was satisfactory. In one patient, the correction was not complete, but he could achieve vaginal penetration, and no further treatment was warranted. Concomitant technical plication was not necessary in any case, and none of the patients reported worse penile rigidity postoperatively. However, the follow-up was short (mean follow-up 6 mo, range 3–12 mo).

Schwarzer et al. (18) modified the technique described by Teloken et al. and published their preliminary results, also with a short follow-up, ranging from 1 to 17 mo. The plaque was incised, but the graft was obtained from the proximal corpus cavernosum (crura) through a separate horizontal infrapubic incision. Thus, there was no need for a second operative field, and the operative time was shorter. The authors treated 18 patients (48–69 yr old) with tunica albuginea free grafts. All patients had stabilized PD for at least 4 mo, and the curvature was between 40 and 90°. In 11 patients, two grafts were used; in the remaining 7 patients, only one graft was used. In 5 patients, a plication was also performed to correct minor residual curvature after grafting (deviation in these patients was over 70°). Complete correction of the curvature was seen in 12 patients, and mild residual curvature (<20°) was seen in 4 patients (2 patients lost in follow-up). Complications included mild penile hematoma in 2 patients. Two patients reported ED postoperatively caused by venous leak after penile irradiation in 1 patient and possible psychogenic causes in the other. Fourteen patients were very satisfied and would decide on the operation again; 2 patients were unsatisfied because of penile shortening.

IS TUNICA ALBUGINEA THE IDEAL GRAFT?

Grafting procedures have the advantage of straightening the penis, causing minimal or no shortening. Much debate exists in the literature about the ideal graft *(19)*. Numerous types of patch grafts, including vein *(20,21)*, Dacron *(12,22)*, full-thickness dermis *(23)*, temporalis fascia *(24)*, tunica vaginalis *(25)*, cadaveric dura mater *(26)*, cadaveric pericardial graft *(27)*, muscular aponeurosis *(28)*, and small intestinal submucosa *(29)* have been used as substitutes for the tunica albuginea in men who maintain their potency preoperatively. Although the ideal substitute has yet to be identified, characteristics would include easy procurement, low cost, and minimal inflammatory reaction with good tissue acceptance.

Dermal grafts were initially used, but delayed graft contraction with recurrent chordee, cysts, and swelling caused by retained hair follicles and sebaceous cysts under the graft have been late complications *(1,5,30)*. Most of the grafts are associated with inflammatory responses and fibrosis that could be detrimental to optimal healing in the setting of a Peyronie's plaque *(31)*.

The onset of ED after surgery is the major problem associated with patch grafts. Postoperative potency rates range from 12 to 100% *(11)*. The pathophysiology is currently attributed to the appearance of venous leakage at the site of the plaque and graft. With the exception of subjective preoperative erection grade, no single parameter predicted the occurrence of postoperative ED as described by Levine et al. *(32)*. The authors also suggested that the postoperative administration of sildenafil (sildenafil rehabilitation) may diminish ED. Vein grafts gained acceptance because of excellent potency-sparing results and long-term durability *(21)*. The success of the vein patch may be a result of limited dissection and the allowance for endothelial-to-endothelial surface healing to occur. They are associated with greater affinity to erectile tissue; endothelium-derived substances, such as nitric oxide, may have a possible beneficial effect on decreasing the risk of hematoma below the graft or fibrosis-associated corporeal veno-occlusive dysfunction.

Because tissue elasticity and compliance are essential for normal function of the corporeal veno-occlusive mechanism, using a natural autologous graft, such as the excised tunica albuginea with its unique structure and function, seems more appropriate for preserving normal veno-occlusive function and therefore potency *(33)*. Moreover, complications associated with grafting procedures, mainly graft scarring, are limited because no site-specific curvature relapse or erectile function deterioration was noted *(16)*. A wide range of recurrence rates has been recorded after the surgical correction of congenital or acquired penile curvature with a Nesbit or plication procedure. Except for the obvious argument of progression of the primary disease in patients with acquired deformities, in whom the risk of recurrence is higher, relapse even in those with congenital deviation may indicate possible weak points of the surgical technique *(34)*. Tunica albuginea is the "original" tissue with less tendency to shrink, cause inflammatory response, and bulge than other grafts.

The described technique is simple, short, and has a low learning curve. It shares essentially the same principles with the Nesbit technique and plication procedures with which most urologists are familiar. Furthermore, there is no need for a second incision to obtain the graft from the crura. These procedures require more operative time and access to the crura may be troublesome. Also, it may be difficult to obtain larger grafts. A possible disadvantage of the technique is the prolonged operative time, compared with the Nesbit procedure, although the time difference is hardly significant.

CONCLUSIONS

Surgical straightening of penile curvature with tunica plication and tunica albuginea free grafts is a simple and highly efficacious treatment modality with excellent functional results. It is associated with minimal postoperative shortening and eliminates major immediate and late complications, including recurrent curvature. It preserves erectile capacity in men with preoperative normal erectile function. Initial long-term patient satisfaction data, with lasting cosmetic and functional results, indicate that the proposed technique may be used as the indicated procedure for successful surgical treatment of excessive congenital or acquired penile curvature malformation. Larger patient series and comparative multicenter trials using a validated protocol are required in order to establish the "gold standard" technique for cases with significant curvature and normal erectile function.

REFERENCES

1. Gelbard MK, Dorey F, James K. The natural history of Peyronie's disease. J Urol 1990; 144: 1376–1379.
2. Devine CJ Jr, Somers KD, Jordan SG, Schlossberg SM. Proposal: trauma as the cause of the Peyronie's lesion. J Urol 1997; 157: 285–290.
3. El-Sakka AI, Hassoba HM, Pillarisetty RJ, Dahiya R, Lue TF. Peyronie's disease is associated with an increase in transforming growth factor-beta protein expression. J Urol 1997; 158: 1391–1394.
4. Pryor J, Akkus E, Alter G, et al. Peyronie's disease. J Sex Med 2004; 1: 110–115.
5. Rehman J, Benet A, Minsky LS, Melman A. Results of surgical treatment for abnormal penile curvature: Peyronie's disease and congenital deviation by modified Nesbit plication (tunical shaving and plication). J Urol 1997; 157: 1288–1291.
6. Bailey MJ, Yande S, Walmsley B, Pryor JP. Surgery for Peyronie's disease. A review of 200 patients. Br J Urol 1985; 57: 746–749.
7. Metz P, Ebbehoj J, Uhrenholdt A, Wagner G. Peyronie's disease and erectile failure. J Urol 1983; 130: 1103–1104.
8. Poulsen J, Kirkeby HJ. Treatment of penile curvature—a retrospective study of 175 patients operated with plication of the tunica albuginea or with the Nesbit procedure. Br J Urol 1995; 75: 370–374.
9. Ebbehoj J, Metz P. Congenital penile angulation. Br J Urol 1987; 60: 264–266.
10. Yachia D. Modified corporoplasty for the treatment of penile curvature. J Urol 1990; 143: 80–82.
11. Dalkin BL, Carter MF. Venogenic impotence following dermal graft repair for Peyronie's disease. J Urol 1991; 146: 849–851.
12. Faerber GJ, Konnak JW. Results of combined Nesbit penile plication with plaque incision and placement of Dacron patch in patients with severe Peyronie's disease. J Urol 1993; 149: 1319–1320.
13. Lue TF, El-Sakka AI. Venous patch graft for Peyronie's disease. Part I: technique. J Urol 1998; 160: 2047–2049.
14. El-Sakka AI, Rashwan HM, Lue TF. Venous patch graft for Peyronie's disease. Part II: outcome analysis. J Urol 1998; 160: 2050–2053.
15. Goldstein M, Blumberg N. Correction of severe penile curves with tunica albuginea autografts. J Urol 1988; 139: 1269–1270.
16. Hatzichristou DG, Hatzimouratidis K, Apostolidis A, Tzortzis V, Bekos A, Ioannidis E. Corporoplasty using tunica albuginea free grafts for penile curvature: surgical technique and long-term results. J Urol 2002; 167: 1367–1370.
17. Teloken C, Grazziotin T, Rhoden E, et al. Penile straightening with crural graft of the corpus cavernosum. J Urol 2000; 164: 107–108.

18. Schwarzer JU, Muhlen B, Schukai O. Penile corporoplasty using tunica albuginea free graft from proximal corpus cavernosum: a new technique for treatment of penile curvature in Peyronie's disease. Eur Urol 2003; 44: 720–723.
19. Hellstrom WJ, Usta MF. Surgical approaches for advanced Peyronie's disease patients. Int J Impot Res 2003; 15(suppl 5): S121–S124.
20. Fournier GR Jr, Lue TF, Tanagho EA. Peyronie's plaque: surgical treatment with the carbon dioxide laser and a deep dorsal vein patch graft. J Urol 1993; 149: 1321–1325.
21. Brock G, Nunes L, von Heyden B, Martinez-Pineiro L, Hsu GL, Lue TF. Can a venous patch graft be a substitute for the tunica albuginea of the penis? J Urol 1993; 150: 1306–1309.
22. Schiffman ZJ, Gursel EO, Laor E. Use of Dacron patch graft in Peyronie disease. Urology 1985; 25: 38–40.
23. Krishnamurti S. Penile dermal flap for defect reconstruction in Peyronie's disease: operative technique and four years' experience in 17 patients. Int J Impot Res 1995; 7: 195–208.
24. Gelbard MK, Hayden B. Expanding contractures of the tunica albuginea to Peyronie's disease with temporalis fascia free grafts. J Urol 1991; 145: 772–776.
25. Das S. Peyronie's disease: excision and autografting with tunica vaginalis. J Urol 1980; 124: 818–819.
26. Fallon B. Cadaveric dura mater graft for correction of penile curvature in Peyronie disease. Urology 1990; 35: 127–129.
27. Levine LA, Estrada CR. Human cadaveric pericardial graft for the surgical correction of Peyronie's disease. J Urol 2003; 170: 2359–2362.
28. Bruschini H, Mitre AI. Peyronie disease: surgical treatment with muscular aponeurosis. Urology 1979; 13: 505–506.
29. Soergel TM, Cain MP, Kaefer M, et al. Complications of small intestinal submucosa for corporal body grafting for proximal hypospadias. J Urol 2003; 170: 1577–1578, 1578–1579.
30. Devine CJ Jr, Horton CE. Surgical treatment of Peyronie's disease with a dermal graft. J Urol 1974; 111: 44–49.
31. Brannigan RE, Kim ED, Oyasu R, McVary KT. Comparison of tunica albuginea substitutes for the treatment of Peyronie's disease. J Urol 1998; 159: 1064–1068.
32. Levine L, Greenfield J, Estrada CR. Erectile dysfunction following surgical correction of Peyronie's disease and a pilot study of the use of sildenafil citrate rehabilitation for postoperative erectile dysfunction. J Sex Med 2005; 2: 241–247.
33. Schultheiss D, Lorenz RR, Meister R, et al. Functional tissue engineering of autologous tunica albuginea: a possible graft for Peyronie's disease surgery. Eur Urol 2004; 45: 781–786.
34. Schultheiss D, Meschi MR, Hagemann J, Truss MC, Stief CG, Jonas U. Congenital and acquired penile deviation treated with the essed plication method. Eur Urol 2000; 38: 167–171.

17 A Review of Plaque Incision With Focus on Temporalis Fascia Grafts

Martin Gelbard, MD

SUMMARY

This chapter reviews the history of plaque incision, the physical bases for expansion of cylindrical tissue, the numerical relationship between tunica extensibility and angular penile deformity, the effects of diameter loss on corporeal function, the design and placement of relaxing incisions, and operative technique based on 15 yr of experience with more than 130 cases. Special attention is given to the deployment and testing of relaxing incision and the use of autologous temporalis fascia as a free graft. Overall, without consideration of angle orientation or narrowing, results showed 75% of patients were corrected, 20% improved, and 7% were rendered dependent on medication for erectile rigidity.

Key Words: Axial deformation; cylindrical column strength; extensibility; graft darting; hourglass; indentation; plaque incision; stacked hoop model of corpora; temporalis fascia; tissue expansion; tunica preservation; wall tension.

CONNECTIVE TISSUE EXPANSION IN GENITAL RECONSTRUCTION

When we performed our first plaque incision and temporalis fascia graft in 1989, most urologists using grafts in the treatment of Peyronie's disease (PD) were doing so in conjunction with plaque excision *(1)*. A brief perusal of the table of contents for this book reveals a change in the pattern of practice with respect to this point: most reconstructive surgeons are now incising plaques rather than removing them. Why?

Earlier surgeons identified the loss of normal connective tissue mechanics in the scarred tunica albuginea of PD and attempted to increase focally the expansion of diseased regions of the corpora cavernosa by excising restrictive scarring. In 1950, Lowsley and Boyce described their 15-yr experience with plaque excision followed by free fat grafts *(2)*. Dissatisfied with the results of this technique, Horton and Devine went to the laboratory seeking a better, stronger graft material, combining the methods of urological surgery with those of plastic surgery to modernize the approach. Concluding that Peyronie's plaques were scars lacking elasticity, they pioneered the use of full-thickness dermal grafts

From: *Current Clinical Urology:*
Peyronie's Disease: A Guide to Clinical Management
Edited by: L. A. Levine © Humana Press Inc., Totowa, NJ

(3). Their concept was that complete removal of plaque and replacement with an elastic, readily available material (dermis) could restore the shape of the erect corpora.

Contemporary thinking has largely adopted Devine and Horton's hypothesis: plaque formation in PD represents locally inappropriate or abnormal wound healing, which results in areas of dense scar within the tunica albuginea. These contracted scars resist normal load-induced tissue elongation, creating regions with a deficit of functioning tunica albuginea. We sought to remedy this deficit by augmentation, rather than replacement, of the tunica.

Tissue expansion is a technique that has been in use for more than 40 yr for the correction of coverage deficits. It is primarily a method for the creation of additional skin by the use of implanted expanders. In urology, this technique has been adapted for vaginoplasty, urethral and penile reconstruction, scrotoplasty, epispadius/exstrophy, and traumatic skin loss *(4)*. Although relaxing incisions for the correction of PD were first described in conjunction with implantation of penile prostheses *(5)*, the dense contractures of PD are not amenable to staged expansion by inflatable, temporarily implanted expanders without irreversibly damaging the interior of the corpora cavernosa. But, diseased tunica albuginea can in fact be expanded, with preservation of corporeal function, by surgical section and inlay of autologous grafts.

Though clinical outcomes clearly support plaque incision, research into the fundamental pathobiology of this disorder raises new questions that bear on the issue. Mulhall et al. have shown that Peyronie's plaque-derived fibroblasts exhibit tumorigenicity when implanted into mice with severe combined immunodeficiency *(6)*. By showing that plaque-derived fibroblasts are biologically transformed compared to those derived from normal tunica or neonatal foreskin, this study posed an interesting question. Beyond the usual reconstructive goals, considerations about tissue geometry, and tunica albuginea veno-oclusive function, should other factors be taken into account when weighing plaque excision against incision? Mulhall et al.'s interesting look at the cellular biology of PD indicates that Peyronie's plaque is the source of fibroblasts with a pathological tendency to proliferate, although their study did not examine the behavior of fibroblasts harvested from unaffected regions of the tunica in men with this disorder. If the "normal" tunica in patients with PD does not harbor transformed fibroblasts, perhaps plaque removal would be beneficial.

Of course, this hypothetical conclusion has to be viewed against a body of clinical evidence that in my opinion still supports plaque incision over excision. Plaque (and the disease process itself) tends to stabilize over time as dense scar *(7)*, suggesting that, in vivo, fibroblast proliferation does not continue indefinitely. And, most important, the plaque in patients with long-term, stable PD behaves like mature scar—it can be expanded successfully by incision and graft inlay. That the contractures of this disorder do not usually recur postoperatively appears to be the strongest argument in favor of incision over excision, particularly because preservation of tunica seems to produce less postoperative veno-occlusive erectile dysfunction than its resection.

EXPANDING A CYLINDER: RELAXING INCISIONS, PEYRONIE'S DISEASE, AND THE IMPLICATIONS OF CORPOREAL GEOMETRY

Modeling the human corpora cavernosa as paired inflatable cylindrical pressure vessels is a bit of an oversimplification as the corpora appear uniquely specialized to function as they do. Although intraluminal pressures of 5–7 psi are required to produce rigidity in prosthesis cylinders, the corpora attain this state at only 1.5 psi *(8)*. Still, plaque incision and grafting involves restoration of cylindrical integrity and column strength, and surgeons undertaking these tasks need to be aware of the mechanical implications of their interventions.

First, I provide a few definitions to identify the goals sought in surgical reconstruction more precisely. Some authors have cited restoration of tunica elasticity as the objective in graft surgery for PD. Normal tunica albuginea does contain elastic fibers, and these have been observed to fragment in patients with PD. They are arrayed primarily in hoop orientation *(9)*, giving the tunica elastic behavior that is anisotropic. In other words, tunica elongates in all directions but "snaps back" forcefully only transversely—elasticity is the tendency of the material in question to generate an opposing restoring force that is proportional to its deformation. But, in surgical reconstruction, elasticity is not sought as much as tissue elongation or extensibility. Extensibility, an uncomplicated and clinically useful term, has been used to characterize overall connective tissue function of the penis *(10)*. It is simply the ratio of stretched to rest length and is based on the assumption that, within the range of forces occurring naturally, straightening of undulated collagen bundles establishes an upper limit to extension. As a result, the measurement is independent of the forces involved. Modification of tunica extensibility is at the heart of plaque incision and grafting. If diseased tunica can be induced to extend further under existing mechanical forces, angulation and diameter loss can be corrected—whether or not the graft material exhibits springlike elastic behavior.

Relationship Between Loss of Tunica Function and Angular Bending

Extensibility is a useful construct for exploring the behavior of tunica albuginea. Overall penile extensibility (penile length at maximal longitudinal traction divided by flaccid penile length) decreases significantly with age and reflects the mechanical behavior of tunica albuginea exclusive of skin and cavernous tissue. In one study, mean flaccid length of 13 cm was increased 4 cm on stretch, yielding an extensibility of about 1.35 *(10)*. Using a stacked-hoop model of the corpora, we have calculated that with an extensibility of 1.5, nearly 8 cm of dorsal plaque would be required to create a bend of 60° *(11)*. With all other factors constant, decreasing extensibility lessens bend, so this calculation actually underestimates how much plaque it would take to produce a 60° bend in someone with normal or reduced extensibility. The message here for plaque incision is that substantial angular deformity (as seen in surgical candidates) reflects the loss of tunica elongation over large segments (Fig. 1). With the exception of a young patient with high extensibility whose substantial bend may be the result of a more limited plaque, a single transverse relaxing incision is inadequate to correct angulation greater than 30°.

Diameter Loss: Effects and Correction

Many patients with PD exhibit hoop-oriented contractures in addition to the longitudinal scarring that produces angulation. As biomechanical analysis clarifies the placement of transverse relaxing incisions in the correction of curvature, it also calls attention to the effects of diameter restriction. Although severe indentation or hourglass deformity is only occasionally a patient's presenting complaint, some degree of girth restriction is present in most surgical candidates. Because resistance to axial deformation is related to corporeal cross-sectional area *(11)*, the management of narrowing is the key to restoration of column rigidity in patients with PD.

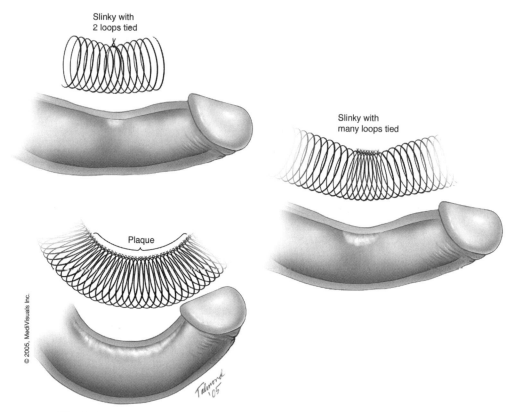

Fig. 1. Surgical candidates have lost tunica extensibility over large regions.

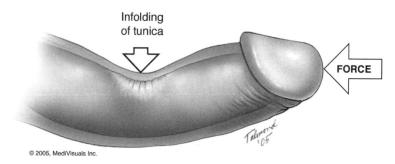

Fig. 2. Factors contributing to buckling.

Buckling of the erect curved penis during attempted intromission is a common functional disturbance in patients *(7)*. In mechanical terms, this problem, secondary to both longitudinal curvature and diameter loss, results from inward collapse of the concave segment of corpora during axial loading (Fig. 2). Curvature changes the axial compressive stress of intromission into transverse stress on the column of the pressurized corpora, which appears as tensile stress in the convex wall and compressive stress in the concave wall. Diameter loss defeats the ability of the concave wall to resist compression. Transverse loads in a pressurized cylindrical shell are ultimately borne by wall tension, making low-tension segments prone to structural failure.

The palpable hardness of a rigid erection can be thought of as if every point along the surface of the inflated tunica was responding to a force directed outward, perpendicular

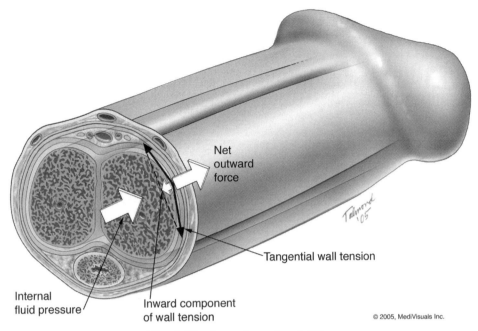

Fig. 3. Net forces in tunica rigidity.

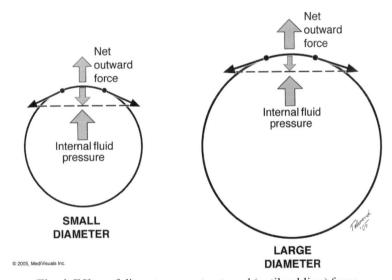

Fig. 4. Effect of diameter on net outward (antibuckling) force.

to each element of surface. This is actually a net force, the vector sum of the outward forces of interior sinusoidal fluid pressure and the inward forces generated by tunica albuginea wall tension. Transverse tangential wall tension can be resolved into an inward component that opposes the outward force of the pressurized interior. It is the net outward force, or the vector sum of these two opposing forces, that resists inward collapse associated with buckling (Fig. 3). In such a pressurized cylindrical shell, net outward force is highest in regions with the greatest radius of curvature; as the inward-directed component of wall tension decreases, the radius of curvature increases (Fig. 4). In other words, narrowed segments tend to fail because they exhibit reduced resistance to infolding.

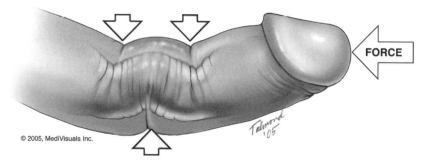

Fig. 5. Tendency of narrowed areas to collapse.

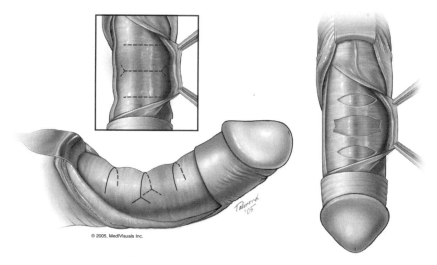

Fig. 6. Darting of relaxing incisions.

The physical principles here are similar to those underlying a standard undergraduate physics test problem: What happens if two balloons of unequal size are connected by a tube? Contrary to intuition, they will not equalize, but instead the small balloon will collapse, and the large one will expand. Similarly, there is a tendency for narrow regions to collapse when freely communicating corporeal segments of differing diameters co-exist (Fig. 5).

Proper placement of relaxing incisions can overcome diameter loss, but first it is instructive to look at the effect on diameter of the standard transverse relaxing incisions used to correct angulation. Transverse incisions of longitudinal plaque straighten the penis by gaping open in the direction of tunica deficit—along the long axis. As this relaxing incision opens, its perimeter remains relatively fixed owing to its location in a scarred region of tunica. The length generated because of distraction longitudinally is gained at the expense of its lateral corners, which are pulled inward, reducing width. This narrowing effect of transverse incisions can be overcome by darting the corners. Our experience is that darting a single transverse incision, usually the central one of three, is adequate to overcome the narrowing that results from multiple relaxing incisions in the patient with predominantly angular deformity *(12)* (Fig. 6).

In the patient with problematic diameter loss, some type of transverse expansion targeting specific areas of hourglass deformity is required. Girth can be locally expanded

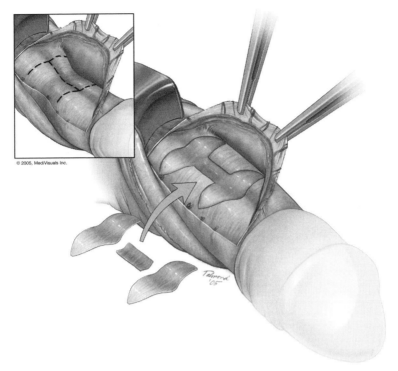

Fig. 7. H graft.

by interposing a longitudinal relaxing incision between transverse incisions in an H pattern. Usually, in the case of narrowing accompanying a region of angular deformity, the longitudinal incision is positioned in the midline (Fig. 7). In that case, the central portion is grafted first, prior to measuring and grafting the transverse incisions. Another technique is applicable to the correction of hourglass superimposed on an angulated segment. After two transverse relaxing incisions are cut for the correction of angulation, the intervening strip of tunica bounded by these incisions is divided obliquely. The two flaps thus formed are advanced laterally in opposite directions to widen the penis. Once these flaps have been sutured together in their new configuration, the resulting transverse defects are measured and grafted (Fig. 8).

Lateral indentation unassociated with angular deformity can be managed with a longitudinal relaxing incision deployed laterally through the indented area. It must be well darted, however, to prevent transverse expansion from pulling the proximal and distal extremities of the relaxing incision together, reducing length along the lateral meridian of the penis and creating lateral angulation.

Testing the Adequacy of Relaxing Incisions

Ultimately, the best test of graft inlay is the configuration of the resulting erection. For this reason, we have been liberal in our use of the saline insufflation artificial erection. Initially, we proceeded cautiously, making one relaxing incision at a time, grafting it with a watertight closure, then inducing saline erection. After 50 or 60 cases, certain patterns began to appear, which have since streamlined our approach. Currently, in a patient with more than 45° of dorsal curvature and no significant hourglass deformity, we space three transverse relaxing incisions across the area of maximal concavity, divide the temporalis fascia accordingly, and then graft all three areas before insufflating.

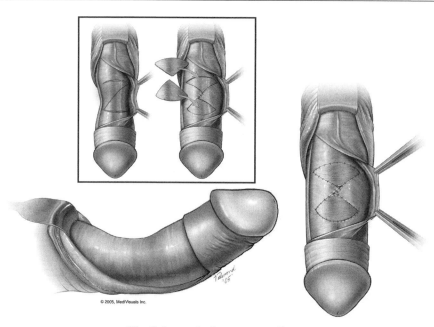

© 2005, MediVisuals Inc.

Fig. 8. Lateral advancement flaps.

However, because we generally will use all temporalis fascia harvested, it is useful to get some indication of the effect the relaxing incisions will have on the contracture before committing ourselves to a particular partitioning of the graft material. After marking and incising plaque, we assess whether the tension induced in the diseased tunica by stretch is relieved by these incisions. This is fairly straightforward with respect to longitudinal expansion in the correction of angular deformity: stretching the penis should cause the incisions to gape open evenly, and under these conditions there should be no tension transferred to the lateral corners of the incisions. If with stretch the tunica is palpably tense at the lateral extremities of the incisions, then the incisions need to be extended (Fig. 9). Testing the adequacy of longitudinal or compound relaxing incisions deployed for the expansion of diameter is slightly more difficult. Using holding sutures in the tunica to retract the neurovascular bundle away from the area of interest, elevation of the entire penile shaft over a finger placed behind the narrowed region will spread the tunica laterally and show if these relaxing incisions are sufficiently widening the area (Fig. 10).

OPERATIVE TECHNIQUE
Materials

Between 1987 and 2006, a total of 131 plaque incision and temporalis fascia graft procedures have been performed on 128 patients; 3 patients underwent a second procedure to correct persistent deformity. Patients ranged in age from 41 to 70 yr with deformities distributed as 78% dorsal bends, 10% dorsolateral bends, 7% true lateral bends, 4% ventral bends, and 1% indented without angulation. Of the patients with angulation, 30% were Kelami class II (30–60°), and 70% were class III (>60°). There were no patients with angulation less than 30°.

Temporalis fascia was harvested by a head-and-neck or plastic surgeon, usually via a retroauricular incision. The average specimen measured approx 4.5×5 cm, with a total surface area of approx 18 cm^2 *(13)* (Fig. 11). We have previously described the virtues of

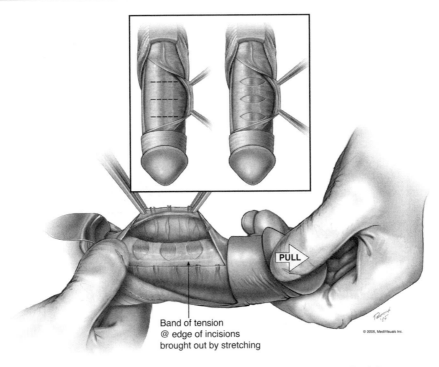

Fig. 9. Transfer of tension to edge of incomplete relaxing incision.

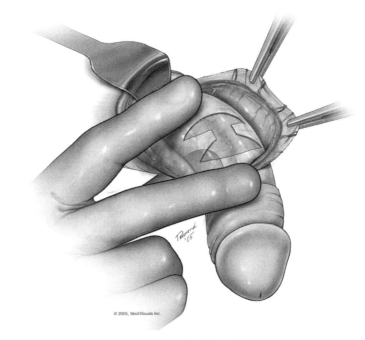

Fig. 10. Evaluating H-graft incision.

this material as flexible yet strong and having a lower metabolic requirement than highly vascularized dermis, a reduced tendency to contract as a free graft, and sufficient size to provide for the multiple grafts our technique employs.

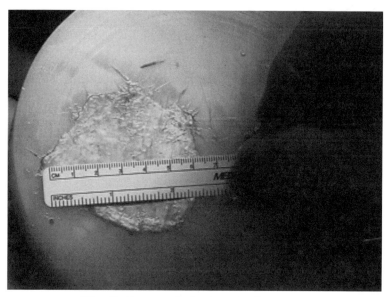

Fig. 11. Temporalis fascia on Teflon block.

Methods

EXPOSURE

In all cases except those with ventral curvature, a circumcising incision with proximal degloving seems to provide the best exposure. Attempting to preserve the prepuce in uncircumcised men frequently results in persistent distal edema, and therefore we usually recommend circumcision in these patients. In the case of ventral curvature, a ventral penoscrotal incision in the raphe works well.

To approach dorsal or dorsolateral plaque, Buck's fascia is opened longitudinally along the lateral meridians at 3 and 9 o'clock. The transverse-oriented circumflex veins that cross these incisions are elevated from the underlying tunica and divided with fine absorbable ties. Lifting the medially coursing side of these veins provides entry to the plane between the dorsal neurovascular bundle and the tunica albuginea, which is meticulously developed with sharp dissection using Joseph scissors. When one portion of the bundle has been elevated, a silastic vessel loop is passed to assist in mobilizing the remaining portion, which is handled with 4 × 4s and fingers only. To further limit the need for retractors or instruments on the bundle, 3-0 nylon holding sutures placed in the tunica are used to facilitate exposure during graft anastomosis (Fig. 12). In most cases of dorsal angulation, neurovascular bundle elevation is limited to expose just enough plaque at the concavity of the bend to permit placement of three transverse relaxing incisions spaced about 1 cm apart. Distal mobilization of the bundle is terminated at a point 1 cm proximal to the corona to avoid sensory loss in the glans. To expose ventral scarring in the paraurethral ridges, Buck's fascia is divided at 6 o'clock over the urethra and mobilized laterally.

INCISION

Prior to marking exposed plaque for incision, saline is insufflated until the artificial erection clearly shows the nature and location of curvature. When this has been done, a longitudinal line marking the intersection of the plane of curvature with the penile shaft is marked. In the case of dorsal angulation, this will be in the midline. Three transverse

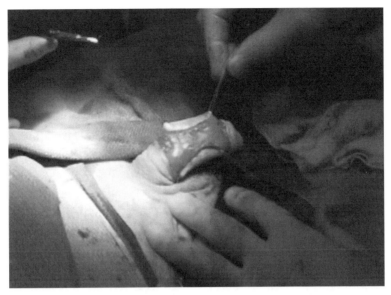

Fig. 12. Use of holding sutures.

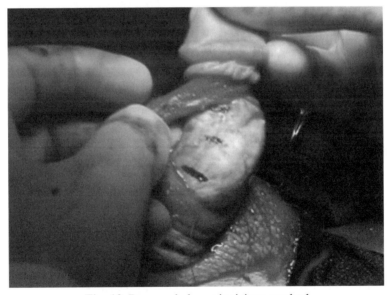

Fig. 13. Proposed plaque incisions marked.

relaxing incisions are then marked over the plaque, centering on this line, spaced approx 1 cm apart. If the zone of curvature in question is associated with substantial narrowing, then the incisions should be placed to allow one of the techniques for diameter expansion. In the absence of an identified hourglass segment, the middle relaxing incisions should be darted laterally to prevent longitudinal expansion from narrowing the penis.

Incisions are marked using a sharpened sterile cotton swab and methylene blue dye. We find it helpful to confirm that the transverse relaxing incisions are oriented properly, drawn without inadvertent obliquity, by bunching the dorsal neurovascular bundle together in the midline and viewing these incisions from the dorsal perspective (Fig. 13). Because of the distortion introduced by retracting the bundle to one side or another, the view afforded by this exposure can make it difficult to see if the lines are truly transverse. A no. 15 blade

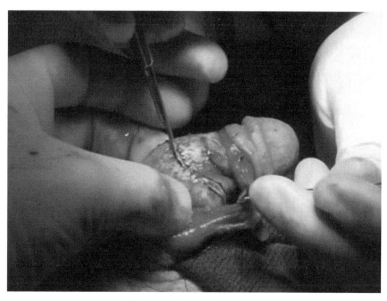

Fig. 14. Incision of plaque.

is then used to score the incisions, which are deepened with fine Joseph scissors, taking care to preserve all underlying sinusoidal tissue (Fig. 14).

A modification of technique is necessary when plaque calcification has been either identified preoperatively or encountered during surgery as a hard plaque that cannot be divided. In dealing with macroscopic calcification such as can be seen on low-kilovoltage x-rays (14), relaxing incisions should be planned to cross the calcified area in more than one place to allow maximal exposure. When the overlying tunica has been incised down to the calcification, usually located in the areolar tissue sleeve between the corpus cavernosum and the tunica albuginea, a sharp Freer ear, nose, and throat periosteal elevator is used in conjunction with fine scissor dissection to lift the tunica off the outer surface of the calcification (Fig. 15). It is then a fairly simple matter to push the sinusoidal tissue from the underside of this material and remove it completely. We have found in the majority of cases the overlying tunica thus preserved is quite satisfactory. Rarely, in the case of very large, irregular, or multifenestrated plaques, the overlying tunica is unintentionally thinned or divided, requiring use of a small portion of the temporalis fascia for midline repair.

Graft Harvest, Marking, Transfer, and Anastomosis

On obtaining the temporalis fascia, our ear, nose, and throat colleagues flatten it out onto a Teflon™ block. Once the relaxing incisions have been made and tested for adequacy as described, toothed Adson forceps are used to stretch each incision for measurement. When using temporalis fascia, grafts are cut to fit the relaxing incisions with no need to oversize them for shrinkage. It then remains only to divide the specimen in such a way that they provide proper size and shape to each graft. Although this occasionally presents a challenge requiring some imaginative space planning, we have found the average piece of temporalis fascia usually supplies three grafts without difficulty. In the most common instance of dorsal curvature, the proximal and distal grafts are cut elliptically to fit the gaps created by transverse incision; the central graft is left with squared-off ends for the darted middle incision. A heavy line of methylene blue is used to mark

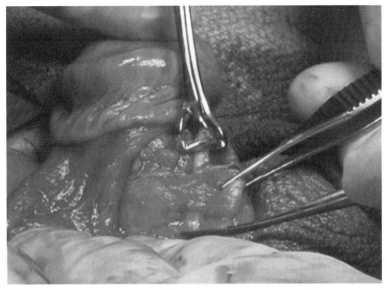

Fig. 15. Removal of dystrophic calcification, sparing tunica.

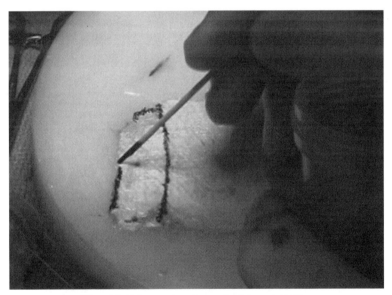

Fig. 16. Edges of graft marked for visibility.

the fascia for division into grafts, so that each graft keeps a painted blue edge (Fig. 16). This facilitates accurate suture anastomosis.

To provide exposure for the transfer and anastomosis of each graft, selected 3-0 nylon holding sutures in the tunica are passed under the neurovascular bundle to retract it safely out of the way. Then, 5-0 PDS™ sutures are passed through each lateral corner of the relaxing incision and through the corresponding corner of its graft, which allows the graft to be passed onto its corresponding defect without furling or distortion (Fig. 17). Proximal and distal midline sutures of the same material are then placed, maintaining graft position by four-point fixation and facilitating graft anastomosis using fine watertight running

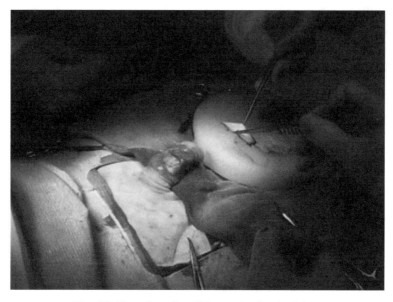

Fig. 17. Transfer of graft into relaxing incision.

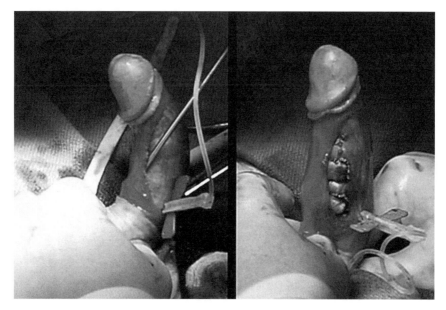

Fig. 18. Effect of free graft expansion with saline insufflation.

technique for each of the four quadrants. This allows the suture line to expand without purse-stringing.

TESTING AND FINE TUNING

When all relaxing incisions are grafted, saline insufflation artificial erection is induced using a no. 21 butterfly needle and pair of 20-cc syringes (Fig. 18). At this time any significant leaks can be closed with a figure-eight 5-0 PDS suture. Residual angulation can be addressed with either additional grafts (if material remains) or with small plications.

We have found Yacchia's technique for corporoplasty useful: After the application of Allis clamps, a no. 11 blade is used to open the tunica longitudinally between teeth marks, which is then closed transversely *(15)*. This is most commonly used to correct the slight dorsal glans tilt that remains in some cases of severe angulation owing to our unwillingness to place distal grafts under the coronal sulcus. Usually, a 1- or 2-mm plication is sufficient.

Results

Our original 1991 report of 12 cases treated by plaque incision and temporalis fascial grafts was updated at the National Institutes of Health International Conference on PD held in Bethesda, Maryland, in March 1993. At that time, among 40 patients, bending was corrected in 74%, significantly improved in 21%, and uncorrected in 5%. Bothersome erectile dysfunction was present in 12% of patients preoperatively. Postoperatively, 14% of patients required either vacuum erection devices or the use of intracavernous injections. In 1995, we reviewed experience with 69 cases, highlighting the difficulty encountered in patients with isolated lateral bends *(12)*. Among this group, 50% of patients had dorsal bends, 20% were lateral, 20% were dorsolateral, and 10% were ventral or ventrolateral. Of those patients afflicted with dorsal or ventral bending, surgery produced complete correction of deformity in 82% and improvement in 6%. Only 17% of patients with purely lateral bending were completely corrected by surgery, with 33% in this group demonstrating improvement. Currently, 131 surgeries have been done. Overall, without regard to orientation of bend or the presence/absence of hourglass deformity, we continue to see 75% of patients corrected and 20% improved by this technique. Approximately 7% of patients not using pharmacological therapy for erectile dysfunction preoperatively will require medication (usually phosphodiesterase inhibitors) postoperatively.

CONCLUSIONS

With careful selection of operative candidates and strict attention to technique, plaque incision and temporalis fascial graft inlay offers correction of deformity and improvement in sexual function in a high percentage of men with severe Peyronie's disease.

REFERENCES

1. Gelbard M, Hayden B. Expanding contractures of the tunica albuginea due to PD with temporalis fascia free grafts. J Urol 1991; 145: 722–725.
2. Lowsley O, Boyce W. Further experiences with an operation for the cure of certain cases of plastic induration (Peyronie's disease) of the penis. J Urol 1947; 57: 552–555.
3. Devine CJ, Horton CE. Surgical treatment of Peyronie's disease with a dermal graft. J Urol 1974; 111: 44–50.
4. Mathews R, Umesh P. Tissue expansion in urologic surgery. In: Reconstructive and Plastic Surgery of the External Genitalia (Ehrlich R, Alter G, eds.). Saunders, Philadelphia, 1999, pp. 153–158.
5. Raz S, deKernion J, Kaufman J. Surgical treatment of Peyronie's disease—a new approach. J Urol 1977; 117: 598–601.
6. Mulhall JP, Martin DJ, Lubrano T, et al. Peyronie's disease fibroblasts demonstrate tumorigenicity in the severe combined immunodeficient (SCID) mouse model. Int J Impot Res 2004; 16: 99–104.
7. Gelbard M, Dorey F, James K. The natural history of Peyronie's disease. J Urol 1990; 144: 1376–1381.
8. Pescatori ES, Goldstein I. Intraluminal device pressures in three-piece inflatable penile prostheses: the "pathophysiology" of mechanical malfunction. J Urol 1993; 149: 295–300.
9. Gelbard M. The disposition and function of elastic and collagenous fibers in the tunic of the corpus cavernosum. J Urol 1982; 128: 850–851.

10. Moreira de Gloes P, Wespes E, Schulman C. Penile extensibility: to what is it related? J Urol 1992; 148: 1432–1434.
11. Gelbard M. Peyronie's disease. In: The Penis (Hashmat AI, Das S, eds.). Lea and Febiger, Philadelphia, 1993, p. 244.
12. Gelbard M. Relaxing incisions in the correction of penile deformity due to Peyronie's disease. J Urol 1995; 154: 1457–1460.
13. Gelbard A, Aroesty D, Gelbard M. Harvesting large segments of temporalis fascia for penile reconstruction: the retroauricular approach. 2005; submitted.
14. Gelbard M. Dystrophic penile calcification in Peyronie's disease. J Urol 1988; 193: 738.
15. Yacchia D. Modified corporoplasty for the treatment of penile curvature. J Urol 1990; 143: 80.

18

Venous Patch Graft Surgery for Peyronie's Disease

Robert C. Dean, MD *and Tom F. Lue,* MD

SUMMARY

Multiple surgical procedures have been developed for the treatment of Peyronie's disease. With these penile-straightening surgeries, two broad surgical categories have emerged. These categories are penile-shortening procedures (plication) and penile-lengthening procedures (penile grafting). With the penile-grafting procedures, different grafting materials have been used. Presented here is the use of the autologous saphenous vein graft. The venous graft has many advantages, including (1) similar thickness of the replacing tunica albuginea, (2) an endothelial lining that prevents hematoma formation, (3) elasticity of the graft, and (4) the wall of the saphenous graft can establish a blood supply from the lumen of the corpus cavernosum, thus preventing graft ischemia and contracture. Also, there is decreased inflammation or reaction to the graft because it is autologous. With careful patient selection, the saphenous vein graft for Peyronie's disease is an excellent therapy for penile curvature.

Key Words: Graft; Peyronie's disease; penile straightening; saphenous vein; surgery.

INTRODUCTION

Surgical management of Peyronie's disease (PD) is quite varied. Modifications of procedures have been made to techniques that were first described almost 50 yr ago. The "perfect" surgery to correct penile curvature secondary to PD still eludes urologists. The urologist should embrace these various techniques and procedures for the patient with PD is better served when the urologist can customize a surgery to correct that patient's particular disease presentation. The varied anatomical, pathological, and physiological presentations of PDs are perhaps the reason for the wide array of surgical interventions necessary for a customized correction.

In certain indications, tunica-preserving procedures have had reasonable success. The most popular of these are tunical plication *(1,2)* and the Nesbit procedure *(3,4).* However, these procedures shorten the penis and do not correct the hourglass deformity or penile narrowing. Graft replacement surgery has gained wide popularity, with many autologous and synthetic materials reported with varying results, but notable shortcomings include graft contracture, curvature recurrence, neurovascular injury, and impotence. Ideally, a

From: *Current Clinical Urology:*
Peyronie's Disease: A Guide to Clinical Management
Edited by: L. A. Levine © Humana Press Inc., Totowa, NJ

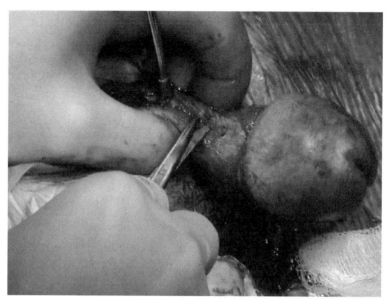

Fig. 1. Dissecting the neurovascular bundle laterally toward the corpus spongiosum.

grafting procedure should result in a straight penis without impairing erectile function. Also, the graft material should be accepted with minimal inflammatory response at the recipient's site. In this chapter, the technique and surgical outcome of plaque incision and saphenous venous patch grafting to correct the complex penile deformity associated with PD is discussed.

SURGICAL TECHNIQUE

For Penile Curvature

A circumcision incision is made proximal to the glans penis. If the patient is uncircumcised, then the foreskin can be preserved if a circumferential incision is made just proximal to the glans penis on the retracted skin of the penis. (Editor's note: There is risk of paraphimosis with this technique.) Next, dissect and reflect the skin and subcutaneous tissue in a degloving manner to the base of the penis. For a dorsally located plaque, identify and resect the deep dorsal vein after opening the Buck's fascia. Then, dissect Bucks' fascia, with the paired dorsal neurovascular bundles, off the tunica albuginea of the corpora cavernosa, leaving the fibrous tissue behind. This is performed from the 12 o'clock position (from the bed of resected deep dorsal vein) laterally.

The use of surgical loupes to dissect the bundles safely off the tunica is highly recommended. This is an extremely important step in this surgery for it restores the neurovascular bundle's length (Fig. 1). Also, despite great care to prevent stretch and injury to the paired neurovascular bundles, some patients will complain of glans sensitivity changes postoperatively. In addition, if an arterial communication between the dorsal and cavernous arteries is identified on preoperative duplex ultrasonography, great effort should be made to preserve these vessels. For the ventrally located plaque, one must dissect the corpus spongiosum off the corpora cavernosa.

To assess the patient's curvature, an artificial erection is created by inserting a 21-gage butterfly needle into the corpus cavernosum for injection of saline solution with manual

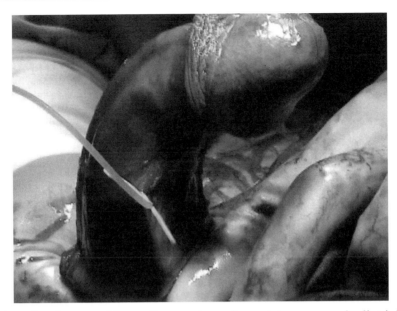

Fig. 2. Locating the apex of the penile curvature using an intracavernosal saline injection.

compression of the crura. The apex of the curvature is marked horizontally with a mark-ing pen. This mark will be the site of the relaxation incision, the middle bar of an H-shaped incision (Fig. 2). It should extend at least 1 cm beyond the plaque laterally. Often, the end point of this incision is near the corpus spongiosum. Once the H-shaped incision is made, the penis is stretched both longitudinally and transversely, and the tunical defect is mea-sured to determine the appropriate size of the vein graft. Occasionally, more than one incision may be necessary to correct a longer or complex deformity. One to two incisions are sufficient in all cases to correct deformity. An H-shaped incision generally suits most deformities (Fig. 3).

For graft harvest, either distal or proximal saphenous vein can be used. The femoral portion is preferred as this region of the saphenous vein provides a thicker graft and fewer separate segments are needed to form the final graft. An incision over the inner thigh is made and a segment of the saphenous vein is isolated. The length of the venous segment is determined by the size of tunical defect. The harvested vein is detubularized and divided into equal-length segments. Using small, nonpenetrating vascular clips on the adventi-tial surface, the segments are assembled (Fig. 4). The assembled saphenous patch graft is then sutured to the defect, endothelial side down facing the erectile tissue, with con-tinuous 4-0 polyglycolic acid suture. To prevent gathering of the tissue and graft, locking stitches are employed.

Intracavernosal saline injection is used again to induce an erection to check for any leakage and to assess the deformity (Fig. 5). If necessary, another patch graft or plication sutures are placed. Minor corrections are made by placing nonabsorbable plication sutures to compensate for over- or undercorrection or to correct for lateral curvature. Once there is no significant leakage and the penis is straight, Buck's fascia is closed using 4-0 poly-glycolic acid sutures. Closure of the penile wound is performed with absorbable 5-0 sutures. A urethral catheter is inserted. The leg wound is closed with 4-0 polyglycolic acid suture subcuticularly. The penis is wrapped with a circumferential, noncompression dress-ing. The patient's penis is checked 1–2 h later to ensure adequate blood supply to the glans.

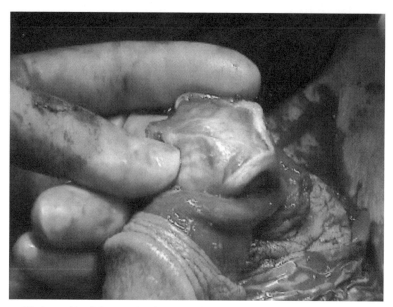

Fig. 3. After an H-shaped incision on the dorsum of the penis is made, the penis is stretched longitudinally and transversely so that the size of the tunical defect can be measured.

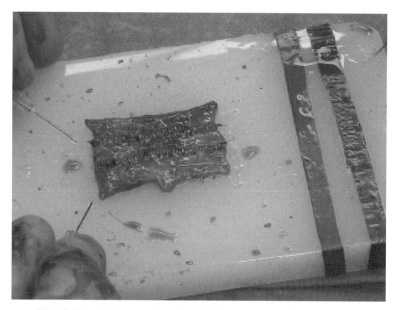

Fig. 4. Staple line on the adventitial surface of the vein graft.

On postoperative day 1, the penile dressing is changed, and the urethral catheter removed. The patient can then be discharged with instructions to change the dressing once a day for 10 d and to abstain from sexual intercourse for 6 wk *(5)*.

For Penile Indentation or Hourglass Deformity

The procedure is similar to the previous one described except for the following: (1) The neurovascular bundle is dissected from the paraurethral ridge toward the dorsal aspect; (2) a tunical incision is made on the lateral aspect of the penis with the middle bar of the

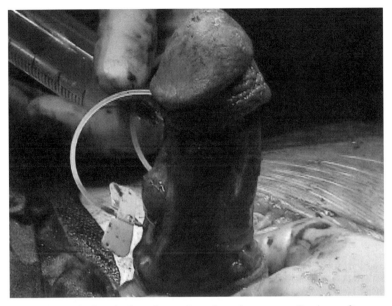

Fig. 5. Saline-induced erection after placement of vein graft.

H placed longitudinally; (3) a longitudinal graft is placed for unilateral indentations; and (4) two separate longitudinal grafts are needed for an hourglass deformity *(6)*.

For Penile Curvature With Hourglass Deformity

An H-type incision is made on the dorsum of the penis. Again, the middle bar of the H is made at the apex of the curve, but the lateral incisions are longer to correct the hourglass deformity. An H-shaped graft is constructed to expand the tunica albuginea both longitudinally and transversely.

For Severe Penile Shortening Caused by Peyronie's Disease

For patients with severe contracture of the penis, circumferential vein grafting is performed with the understanding that vacuum erection device or penile prosthesis will be necessary for sexual intercourse following the surgery. A similar approach is used to obtain exposure to the plaque of the penis as previously described. After a circumcising incision and a degloving dissection is performed to the base of the penis, the deep dorsal vein is resected. Under loupe magnification, the neurovascular bundles and the corpus spongiosum are carefully dissected off the corpus cavernosa. A relaxing horizontal incision is made through the center of the plaque and carried circumferentially around the tunica albuginea. The circumference and the longitudinal gap are measured to harvest an adequate length of the saphenous vein graft. A circular graft is created. The graft is sutured to the tunica albuginea to cover the defect. Following the recovery from this surgery, the patient is instructed to use a vacuum erection device to stretch the penis daily for 6 mo. This begins after the second postoperative month. Because of both the severity of the disease and the extent of the surgery, these patients are not likely to achieve full erection after the surgery. Therefore, again, the patient must be made aware of the need for the vacuum erection device for adequate erections for sexual intercourse *(7)*.

SURGICAL SELECTION AND OUTCOMES

In 1974, penile dermal grafting to cover the defect from Peyronie's plaque excision was first described by Horton and Devine (8). Because penile shortening with plication surgeries was unacceptable for many patients, especially those with severe curvature, Horton and Devine developed this technique. The success of this procedure has been widely reported; however, other reports have been less enthusiastic secondary to graft retraction and a substantial risk of erectile dysfunction postoperatively (9–11). The search for the ideal graft material began. Ideal graft material qualities include (1) pliability and compliance, (2) low antigenicity risk, (3) low infection risk, (4) minimal inflammation, and (5) high tensile strength (12). The search for the ideal graft material continues today.

The rationale for saphenous vein graft was born from the fact that the penis is essentially a blood vessel. The tunica albuginea is similar to a vessel wall. We believe the saphenous vein graft therefore has the following theoretical advantages for substitution of the diseased tunica albuginea: (1) The endothelium prevents hematoma formation under the graft by releasing nitric oxide; (2) the thickness of the venous wall is similar to the tunica albuginea; (3) there is excellent elasticity within the muscular coat of the venous graft; and (4) the wall of the saphenous graft can establish a blood supply from the lumen of the corpus cavernosum, thus preventing graft ischemia and contracture (13). The disadvantages include (1) the need for a second incision; (2) hematoma to the thigh or leg; (3) lymphocele formation; and (4) potentially limiting the supply of saphenous vein needed for grafting during coronary bypass surgery.

Patient selection is extremely important for individuals considering incision-and-grafting surgery with saphenous vein graft. Patients with minimal penile curvature or deformity secondary to PD should strongly consider plication surgery, especially if there is adequate penile length. Further investigations with intracavernousal injection and color duplex ultrasound are strongly recommended to aid in the evaluation of the penile curvature/deformity and the vascular anatomy. Injury to vascular communications of the dorsal and cavernosal arteries near the plaque could increase the risk of erectile dysfunction postoperatively. If these communications are present, then it is recommended that the patient have a plication surgery in lieu of a grafting procedure. Patients with erectile dysfunction, even responsive to medical therapy, should not undergo incision and grafting for these patients carry an almost 50% probability of worsening erectile dysfunction. All patients need to be counseled for the possibility of continued penile curvature, erectile dysfunction, penile ballooning, and penile shortening postoperatively.

Successful outcomes have been established in several reports for saphenous vein graft. The initial report from Lue et al. demonstrated complete penile straightening in 96% of patients, and 83% of patients had the same or improved penile length. Erectile dysfunction occurred in only 13% of the potent patients studied (14). Other authors have reported straightening rates from 75 to 96% and potency rates over 90%, with patient satisfaction rates approx 90% (15–17).

SUMMARY

Saphenous vein graft for penile curvature correction secondary to PD has become a standard procedure. The techniques required for this surgery are complex and delicate but are within reach of the practicing urologist. Careful patient selection is required, which is true in any surgical intervention for PD. The plaque incision and saphenous vein grafting procedure is a useful technique for correction of penile deformity secondary to PD.

REFERENCES

1. Mufti GR, Aitchison M, Bramwell SP, et al. Corporeal plication for surgical correction of Peyronie's disease. J Urol 1990; 144: 281–282.
2. Nooter RI, Bosch JL, Schroder FH. Peyronie's disease and congenital penile curvature: long-term results of operative treatment with the plication procedure. Br J Urol 1994; 74: 497–500.
3. Nesbit RM. Congenital curvature of the phallus: report of three cases with description of corrective operation. J Urol 1965; 93: 230–232.
4. Coughlin PW, Carson CC 3rd, Paulson DF. Surgical correction of Peyronie's disease: the Nesbit procedure. J Urol 1984; 131: 282–285.
5. Lue TF, El-Sakka AI. Venous patch graft for Peyronie's disease. Part I: technique. J Urol 1998; 160: 2047–2049.
6. Gholami SS, Lue TF. Peyronie's disease. Urol Clin North Am 2001; 28: 377–390.
7. Lue TF, El-Sakka AI. Lengthening shortened penis caused by Peyronie's disease using circular venous grafting and daily stretching with a vacuum erection device. J Urol 1999; 161: 1141–1144.
8. Devine CJ Jr, Horton CE. Surgical treatment of Peyronie's disease with a dermal graft. J Urol 1974; 111: 44–49.
9. Wild RM, Devine CJ Jr, Horton CE. Dermal graft repair of Peyronie's disease: survey of 50 patients. J Urol 1979; 121: 47–50.
10. Hicks CC, O'Brien DP 3rd, Bostwick J 3rd, et al. Experience with the Horton-Devine dermal graft in the treatment of Peyronie's disease. J Urol 1978; 119: 504–506.
11. Palomar JM, Halikiopoulos H, Thomas R. Evaluation of the surgical management of Peyronie's disease. J Urol 1980; 123: 680–682.
12. Carson CC, Chun JL. Peyronie's disease: surgical management: autologous materials. Int J Impot Res 2002; 14: 329–335.
13. Chang JA, Gholami SS, Lue TF. Surgical management: saphenous vein grafts. Int J Impot Res 2002; 14: 375–378.
14. El-Sakka AI, Rashwan HM, Lue TF. Venous patch graft for Peyronie's disease. Part II: outcome analysis. J Urol 1998; 160: 2050–2053.
15. Kadioglu A, Tefekli A, Usta M, et al. Surgical treatment of Peyronie's disease with incision and venous patch technique. Int J Impot Res 1999; 11: 75–81.
16. Akkus E, Ozkara H, Alici B, et al. Incision and venous patch graft in the surgical treatment of penile curvature in Peyronie's disease. Eur Urol 2001; 40: 531–536.
17. Metin A, Kayigil O, Ahmed SI. Plaque incision and venous patch grafting for Peyronie's disease. Int Urol Nephrol 2002; 34: 223–227.

19

Use of Porcine Small Intestinal Submucosal Graft in the Surgical Management of Peyronie's Disease

L. Dean Knoll, MD

SUMMARY

This chapter reports long-term outcomes and the incidence of postoperative erectile dysfunction with the use of a xenographic porcine jejunal submucosal graft as a closure material for the tunica albuginea after Peyronie's plaque incision. There were 122 patients with penile curvature of 60° or greater who underwent plaque incision with closure of the tunical defect with this material. Surgical correction of the penile curvature was achieved in 90% of the patients. At a mean follow-up of 36 mo, 79% of the patients maintained their same degree of potency as preoperative. Xenographic porcine jejunal submucosal grafts for the coverage of cavernosal defects after Peyronie's plaque incision allow satisfactory clinical results.

Key Words: Biomaterial grafting; Peyronie's disease; surgery.

INTRODUCTION

The fibrous inelastic scarring process involving the tunica albuginea (TA) of the corpora cavernosa caused by Peyronie's disease (PD) can result in penile curvature or deformities, leading to mechanical erectile dysfunction (ED). When PD is stable, characterized by negligible pain and stable plaque and deformity, surgical management may be offered to correct penile curvature or in those with a loss of penile rigidity. Surgical correction has included incision of the plaque and insertion of a free block of fat *(1)*, various tunical plication procedures *(2–6)*, and grafting procedures with incision or excision of the plaque with various materials (autologous, allograft, synthetic, and xenographic) *(7–18)*.

The ideal material with which to close defects in the TA after penile straightening operations has not been described. Most of the defect closure materials used in the past were not durable enough or caused recurrent fibrosis/curvature, graft contracture, or ED. Modern tissue graft materials include autologous allografts (vein, tunica vaginalis, dermis, temporalis fascia); human cadaveric graft (pericardium, dura mater); synthetic grafts (polytetrafluoroethylene); and xenografts (small intestine submucosa [SIS], dermis,

From: *Current Clinical Urology:*
Peyronie's Disease: A Guide to Clinical Management
Edited by: L. A. Levine © Humana Press Inc., Totowa, NJ

pericardium). This chapter describes the surgical technique and results of the use of an acellular xenographic porcine jejunal submucosal graft (SIS) as a closure material for the TA after plaque incision.

MATERIALS AND METHODS

From August 1998 to August 2004, there were 122 patients with PD who underwent surgical treatment with incision of the plaque and SIS (Surgisis, Cook Urological, Spencer, IN) grafting technique. The patient age ranged from 38 to 69 yr (mean 53 yr), and the mean interval between the onset of disease and surgery was 17 mo (range 12–40 mo).

The patient evaluation included a detailed medical and surgical history (i.e., the duration and progression of the symptoms, status of penile rigidity, ability to engage in sexual intercourse, and history of penile trauma or surgery). No patient had penile pain with or without an erection, and all had no progression of the penile curvature during the preceding 9 mo. All patients had full penile rigidity but were unable to obtain vaginal penetration secondary to the penile curvature. No patient who required pharmacological assistance (oral medication, intracavernosal injection [ICI], urethral insert) or a vacuum device to obtain full rigidity was included in this study. No patient had a history of penile fracture or surgery.

The physical examination focused on palpation of the penis to determine the location and extent of the plaque on the penis. Plaque sizes varied, and by ruler measurement of length and width by the same individual (L. D. K.) ranged from 1.5×4.5 cm to 3.5×6.5 cm in this group of patients.

The initial 12 patients underwent a color Doppler ultrasound examination (ATL Ultramark 9, Bothell Laboratories, Bothell, WA) after ICI of 10 μg prostaglandin E_1. Genital self-stimulation was performed manually 10 min after injection. All 12 patients had peak systolic blood flow velocities greater than 35 cm/s and end diastolic flow velocities less than 5 cm/s. The remaining 110 patients underwent an ICI with 10–20 μg of prostaglandin E_1 with genital self-stimulation. Photographic documentation of the curvature was recorded. All patients obtained a full erection with ICI. All patients had curvature greater than 60° as measured by the same examiner (L. D. K.) using a protractor. Preoperative biothesiometry was performed in all patients for documentation of baseline penile sensation.

All patients received preoperative antibiotics and general anesthesia. A circumcision incision was used, with sleeving of the skin and subcutaneous tissues to the base of the penis. The curvature was documented by creating an artificial erection, which was done by inserting a 19-gage butterfly needle into the corpus cavernosum with corpora restriction, obtained by tightening a 12-French red rubber catheter around the base of the penis (Fig. 1). Surgical loupe magnification was used to dissect the neurovascular bundle from the corpora cavernosa (Fig. 2) dorsally or the corpus spongiosum ventrally.

The center of the curvature was identified with a marking pen, and a relaxing incision was made into the plaque, extending the ends to an H shape when required (Fig. 2). With the penis stretched, using a 2-0 silk suture placed in the glans, an appropriate size porcine jejunal submucosal graft (approx 30% larger than the defect) was sutured with continuous 4-0 polyglycolic suture to cover the tunical defect (Fig. 3). The determination of graft size was accomplished by ruler measurement of the length and width of the defect with an additional 30% added to each measurement. A repeated artificial erection was performed to determine penile straightness (Fig. 4). Subcutaneous tissues and skin were closed with 4-0 chromic interrupted sutures. A 12-French Foley catheter was inserted, and a loosely

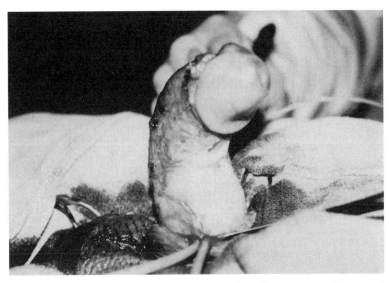

Fig. 1. Artificial erection and documentation of penile curvature. (From ref. *14*.)

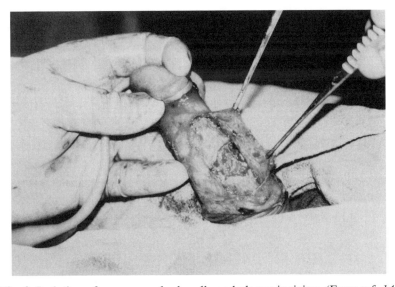

Fig. 2. Isolation of neurovascular bundle and plaque incision. (From ref. *14*.)

wrapped dressing was placed. Patients were dismissed from the hospital the following day. Sexual intercourse was permitted after 8 wk.

Home photographic documentation was obtained at 3 mo postoperatively, and all patients were examined at 3 mo postoperatively in the office. Additional assessment to determine penile length, straightness, sensation, and rigidity was performed using a special questionnaire completed by the patient at 3, 6, and 12 mo; the last two follow-ups were by telephone.

RESULTS

Dorsal curvature was the main penile deformity documented in 79 patients (65%). Twenty-two patients (18%) had lateral curvature, and 21 patients (17%) had ventral cur-

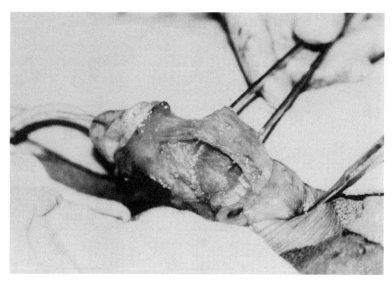

Fig. 3. Sewn-in graft. (From ref. *14.*)

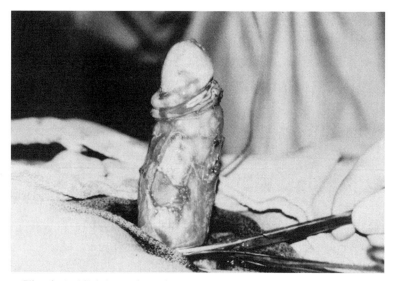

Fig. 4. Artificial erection after placement of graft. (From ref. *14.*)

vature. The degree of curvature ranged from 60 to 90°, with 18 patients having an indentation at the plaque site. All patients had plaque palpable on physical examination of the penis both preoperatively and postoperatively.

Penile curvature was straightened (<15°) in 110 patients (90%), 7 with less than 10° after follow up of 4–72 mo (mean 36 mo). Twelve patients (10%) developed recurrent curvature, of which 4 required reoperation. Four patients developed marked indentation at the graft site, and two required reoperation. The overall reoperation rate for recurrent curvature was 5% (6 of 122 patients) in the entire group.

Twenty-three patients complained about transient (2- to 12-mo duration) penile hypoesthesia (mean 3 mo). Once penile hypoesthesia resolved, postoperative biothesiometry showed no change from baseline exam in these patients. No patient complained of penile

Table 1
Postoperative Results

	No. of patients (%)
Penile straightness	
Straight (<15°)	110 (90)
Recurrent curvature	12 (10) (reoperation 4)
Penile indentation at graft site	4 (3) (reoperation 2)
Penile length change	
No change	54 (44)
Longer	68 (56)
Shorter	0 (0)
Penile sensation change	
Yes (transient)	23 (19)
No	99 (81)
Immunogenic rejection reaction	0 (0)
Postoperative erectile function	
Unaided	96 (79)
Aided	26 (21)
Oral therapy	12 (10)
ICI	8 (6)
Penile implant	6 (5)

shortening or pain. No patient developed an infection, hematoma, permanent bulging at graft site, or a local immunogenic rejection reaction (erythema, pain) to SIS (Table 1).

All patients were able to have intromission for satisfactory intercourse. Ninety-six patients (79%) were able to obtain full unaided erections; 26 patients (21%) required assistance (12 oral therapy, 8 ICI, 6 penile prosthesis) (Table 1).

DISCUSSION

Patients with PD creating penile deformity resulting in mechanical ED who have good erectile function are ideal candidates for penile straightening procedures. Despite extensive clinical experience and long-term follow-up of multiple surgical procedures for PD, no single operation is ideal for all cases of clinically significant curvature. Plaque incision rather than excision with grafting has been widely used recently; however, an ideal graft material for closure defects in the TA still eludes the urologist. The shortcomings from autologous and synthetic materials reported include graft contracture, recurrent curvature, infection, worsening ED, and morbidity associated with autologous tissue harvesting. The graft material should have good tensile strength, invoke minimal immunological response by the recipient, be easy to use, be readily available, and be inexpensive. This chapter describes the use and long-term follow up of a porcine jejunal submucosal graft for coverage of cavernosal defects after Peyronie's plaque incision.

The source of the graft is a biomaterial prepared from the porcine small intestine (jejunum). As the small intestine is processed, the graft is rendered essentially acellular, leaving the extracellular matrix material. This naturally occurring reabsorbable extracellular matrix consists of a variety of structural and functional proteins, including several types of collagen (most are type I), fibronectin, five different glycosaminoglycans, basic fibroblast growth factor, and transforming growth factor. Studies have demonstrated that the graft has shown tissue repair and remodeling characteristics and is completely reabsorbed, rather than forming a generalized fibrotic tissue when placed in vivo *(19–23)*. This regeneration of tissue remodeling after implantation has been termed *smart remodeling (24)*.

The graft averages 0.42 mm in thickness. It has a suture retention strength of 775 g/mm^2, with a burst force of 28.5 lb. These features make the graft thin but strong enough not to allow bulging at the graft site. This problem did not occur in any patient in this series. No separation of the graft was identified on palpation, and no patient developed a hematoma over the graft site.

In this series, no patient developed an infection after the procedure or demonstrated physical evidence of a local immunogenic rejection reaction (tenderness, erythema). No systemic immunological testing was performed. In preclinical studies, the submucosal graft has demonstrated greater resistance to bacterial infection compared with synthetic graft materials *(25)*. One mechanism thought responsible for this resistance is the rapid neovascularization induced by resident cytokines into the submucosal graft. The lyophilized (freeze-dried) graft is rehydrated in normal saline for a minimum of 10 min. When wet, the graft is pliable, soft, slick, and easy to handle and allows for easy suture placement.

Porcine small intestine submucosa has been used in other disciplines such as cardiovascular medicine, gastroenterology, dermatology, and orthopedics. Other human clinical trials are under way using SIS for bladder augmentation, hypospadius/epispadius repair, and sling bladder suspension procedures. Knapp et al. reported on the results of submucosal grafting and augmentation cystoplasty in animals in which the histologic results demonstrated regeneration of both epithelial and smooth muscle layers across the graft *(26)*. The lack of detection of the graft is believed to be because of the infiltration of the graft by host cells that begins the process of tissue remodeling *(19–21)*.

To date, no reports of clinical or immunological problems with human use of SIS have been reported. Weidemann and Otto reported that the use of SIS for pubourethral sling suspension procedures in humans have been studied histopathologically. The morphological findings in this study, in which the biopsy was taken from the implantation site of the SIS band under the vaginal mucosa, showed nothing more than focal residues of the SIS implant without any evidence of a specific tissue reaction. There were no changes that might point to a foreign body reaction. There was likewise no evidence of any significant immunological reaction and in particular no evidence of any chronic inflammatory reaction *(27)*.

Reoperation rate in this series was 5% (6 of 122 patients) and occurred secondarily because the graft was not made large enough. To help prevent recurrent penile curvature that occurred within the first 12 wk postoperatively, intraoperatively a suture was placed through the glans penis to stretch the penis and create the maximum size defect in the TA. It is important to make the graft size approx 30% greater than the defect. Postoperatively, it is imperative to instruct the patient to place his penis 180° opposite from his original curvature to keep the graft maximally stretched for tissue ingrowth.

To maximize surgical outcome, plaque stability and preoperative erectile function must be assessed thoroughly to minimize unrealistic expectations by patients. All 122 patients had good erectile function preoperatively; however, 26 patients (21%) developed postop ED, which occurred within the first 6 mo (range 2–6 mo). Twelve patients responded to oral phosphodiesterase 5 inhibitors. More distressing was that 8 required ICI, and 6 required placement of a three-piece inflatable penile prosthesis. The exact mechanism of the development of postoperative ED is not entirely understood, but in this series no single factor (i.e., plaque location, graft size) could be identified. Surgical placement of the penile implants (six) was not complicated by the previous grafting procedure.

CONCLUSION

Acellular porcine jejunal submucosal grafts for the coverage of cavernosal defects after Peyronie's plaque incision allow for satisfactory clinical results. The ease of surgical handling and placement, no associated comorbidities from harvesting techniques, and no adverse reactions make this material an anatomic and functional tunical substitute. It is mandatory to inform patients that surgery could possibly decrease erectile capability.

REFERENCES

1. Lowsley OS, Gentile A. An operation for the cure of certain cases of plastic induration (Peyronie's disease) of the penis. J Urol 1947; 57: 552–593.
2. Mutfi GR, Aitchison M, Bramwell SP, et al. Corporeal plication for surgical correction of Peyronie's disease. J Urol 1990; 144: 281–283.
3. Nooter RI, Bosch JL, Schroder FH. Peyronie's disease and congenital penile curvature: long-term results of operative treatment with the plication procedure. Br J Urol 1994; 74: 497–500.
4. Nesbit RM. Congenital curvature of the phallus: report of the three cases with description of corrective operation. J Urol 1965; 93: 230–234.
5. Coughlin PWF, Carson CC III, Paulson DF. Surgical correction of Peyronie's disease: the Nesbit procedure. J Urol 1984; 131: 282–285.
6. Gholami S, Lue T. Correction of penile curvature using the 16-dot plication technique: a review of 132 patients. J Urol 2002; 167: 2066–2069.
7. Devine CJ, Horton CE. Surgical treatment of Peyronie's disease with dermal graft. J Urol 1974; 111: 44–49.
8. Das S. Peyronie's disease: excision and autografting with tunica vaginalis. J Urol 1980; 124: 818–819.
9. Fallon B. Cadaver dura mater graft for correction of penile curvature in Peyronie's disease. Urology 1990; 35: 127–129.
10. Lowe DH, Ho PC, Parsons CL. Surgical treatments of Peyronie's disease with Dacron graft. Urology 1982; 19: 609–612.
11. Gelbard MK, Hayden B. Expanding contractures of the tunica albuginea due to Peyronie's disease with temporalis fascia free grafts. J Urol 1991; 145: 772–776.
12. El-Sakka AI, Rashwan HM, Lue TF. Venous patch graft for Peyronie's disease. Part II. Outcome analysis. J Urol 1998; 160: 2050–2053.
13. Hellstrom WJG, Reddy S. Application of pericardial graft in the surgical management of Peyronie's disease. J Urol 2000; 163: 1445–1447.
14. Knoll LD. Use of porcine small intestinal submucosal graft in the surgical management of Peyronie's disease. Urology 2001; 57: 753–757.
15. Levine LA, Estrada CR. Human cadaveric pericardial graft for the surgical correction of Peyronie's disease. J Urol 2003; 170: 2359–2362.
16. Usta MFB. Valacqua TJ, Sambria J, et al. Patient and partner satisfaction and long term results after surgical treatment for Peyronie's disease. Urology 2003; 62: 105–109.
17. Chun JL, McGregor A, Krishnan R, et al. A comparison of dermal and cadaveric pericardial grafts in the modified Horton-Devine procedure for Peyronie's disease. J Urol 2001; 166: 185–188.
18. Egydio PH, Lucon AM, Arap S. Treatment of Peyronie's disease by incomplete circumferential incision of the tunica albuginea and plaque with bovine pericardium graft. Urology 2002; 59: 570–574.
19. Hodde JP, Badylak SF, Brightman AO. Glycosaminoglycan content of small intestinal submucosa: a bioscaffold for tissue replacement. Tissue Eng 1996; 2: 209–217.
20. Voytik-Harbin SL, Brightman AO, Kraine M. Identification of extractable growth factors from small intestinal submucosa. J Cell Biol 1997; 67: 478–491.

21. McPherson TB, Badylak SF. Characterization of fibronectin derived from porcine small intestinal submucosa. Tissue Eng 1998; 4: 75–83.

22. Prevel LD, Eppley BL, Summerlin DJ, et al. Utilization for repair of rodent abdominal wall defects. Ann Plast Surg 1995; 35: 374–380.

23. Lantz GC, Badylak SF, Hiles MC, et al. Small intestinal submucosa as a vascular graft: a review. J Invest Surg 1993; 6: 297–310.

24. Badylak SF. Small intestinal submucosal (SIS): a biomaterial conductive to smart tissue remodeling. In: Tissue Engineering Current Perspectives (Bell E, ed.). Burkhauser, Cambridge, UK, 1993, pp. 179–189.

25. Badylak SF, Coffey AC, Lantz GC, et al. Comparison of the resistance to infection of intestinal submucosal arterial autographs vs polytetrafluoroethylene arterial prostheses in a dog model. J Vasc Surg 1994; 19: 465–472.

26. Knapp PM, Lingerman IE, Seigel YI, et al. Biocompatibility of small intestinal submucosal in urinary tract as augmentation cystoplasty graft and injectable suspension. J Endourol 1994; 8: 125–130.

27. Weidemann A, Otto M. Small intestinal submucosa for pubourethral sling suspension for the treatment of stress incontinence: first histopathological results in humans. J Urol 2004; 172: 215–218.

20

Penile Straightening With Plaque Incision or Partial Excision and Human Pericardial Grafting Technique

Laurence A. Levine, MD, FACS

SUMMARY

Penile reconstruction for Peyronie's disease may require advanced techniques of plaque incision or partial excision when the deformity is severe. This technically challenging procedure is indicated for men with good-to-excellent preoperative erectile capacity and erect penile curvature exceeding 60° or unstable penis or hinge effect caused by severe indentation or hourglass deformity. Various grafts have been used historically, including fat, dermis, fascia, vein, and more recently, processed cadaveric tissue that can be "taken off the shelf," which can shorten operative time and avoid a second incision at the donor site. These procedures require attention to detail in defining the deformity, careful elevation of the neurovascular bundle, incision or partial excision of the plaque, and proper sizing of the graft to repair the tunical defect. A comprehensive informed consent is critical to detail possible postoperative issues, including loss of penile length, diminished sexual sensation, incomplete or recurrent curvature, and, most important, erectile dysfunction. This chapter describes the plaque incision/partial excision procedure using the modified "H" incision and pericardial grafting technique.

Key Words: Penile reconstruction; penile straightening; pericardial grafting; Peyronie's disease; plaque incision or partial excision.

Surgery remains the gold standard of treatment for Peyronie's disease (PD) and is the most reliable way to correct the deformity associated with this disorder. The indications for surgical reconstruction include a stable, painless deformity, compromised ability or inability to engage in coitus as a result of deformity, or diminished rigidity. In addition, men who have extensive plaque calcification are best considered for surgical correction as these patients tend to fail all medical therapy. Last, any man who desires the most rapid and reliable result should be offered surgery.

Because all patients with PD do not present alike, no single operation is likely to treat all patients successfully. Several factors should be evaluated that will assist the surgeon in determining the appropriate surgical approach. These include the nature of the deformity in terms of curvature, hinge effect, and hourglass deformity as well as erectile capacity.

From: *Current Clinical Urology:*
Peyronie's Disease: A Guide to Clinical Management
Edited by: L. A. Levine © Humana Press Inc., Totowa, NJ

Erectile dysfunction (ED) is commonly associated with PD, and the man who has diminished preoperative rigidity needs to be counseled carefully about the surgical approach. Men with significant preoperative ED who might be corrected surgically may still have significant ED postoperatively and therefore should be counseled to proceed to penile prosthesis. On the other hand, men who have satisfactory erections with or without pharmacotherapy may be offered surgical straightening without penile prosthesis.

Several surgical algorithms for PD have been presented; the first published algorithm in 1997 suggested that when rigidity was adequate regardless of the deformity a tunica albuginea plication procedure was the preferred approach when the curvature was without significant hourglass or hinge effect or less than or equal to 60°. For the more complex, multidimensional curves of greater than 60° with or without a destabilizing hourglass or hinge effect, then plaque incision or partial excision with grafting was recommended (1).

All patients should undergo a detailed preoperative discussion as the goals for surgical reconstruction are to enhance or preserve preoperative rigidity, to straighten the penis, and to reestablish a shaft with normal caliber. We know that not all men who have undergone these procedures have been satisfied with the outcome; therefore, a detailed preoperative discussion of outcome expectations and informed consent should be obtained with every patient. The surgeon should discuss the possible side effects of surgery, including potential reduction of rigidity; diminished penile sensation; delayed ejaculation, which may take up to 6 mo to resolve; or shortening of the penis (regardless of the surgical approach). There is also a potential risk of persistent or recurrent curvature, which is unusual if disease has been stable for at least 6 mo. I counsel my patients to understand that sexual activity may not resume immediately after surgery and may take 2–6 mo to recover fully. Those patients who are not willing to accept these possible compromises should consider evaluation by a sex therapist prior to surgery.

Prior to beginning any reconstruction, penile stretched length should be measured. This is performed by measuring the dorsal shaft length from the pubis (by pushing down on the pubic fat pad) to the corona. This length uses two fixed points; measurement should be repeated pre-, intra-, and postoperatively (2).

For the patient who is a candidate for tunica plication, a variety of corporal plication procedures have been reported since the original description by Nesbit in 1965 (3). This procedure was used initially for boys with congenital chordee. A more detailed review of tunica plication options is found in Chapter 12.

This chapter focuses on the Rush University (Chicago) modification of the plaque incision and grafting procedure. This is a more complex operation than tunica plication, which is recommended for more extensive deformities, including severe curvature greater than 60° and particularly when there is advanced narrowing causing a destabilized shaft that cannot bear axial forces without buckling or hinging.

Multiple graft materials have been recommended, including dermis, vein, and more recently, nonautologous and processed cadaveric tissues such as pericardium (Mentor Corp., Santa Barbara, CA); dermis (AlloDerm, Life Cell, Branchburg, NJ); and porcine small intestinal submucosa (Cook Biotech, West Lafayette, IN). All of these grafts appear to be satisfactory. The primary concern in this operation is the preoperative erectile status. In a review of our experience using Tutoplast® processed pericardial graft (Mentor Corp.), we attempted to determine factors that might predict postoperative ED (4). Our analysis revealed that the only factors that indicated an increased risk of diminished rigidity included those men with ventral curvature for which up to 50% of patients experienced diminished erections in spite of good erections preoperatively, when the men were over 60 yr of age regardless of their history of vascular risk factors, and most importantly, when the patient described a preoperative reduction in erectile capacity.

In those men who described no compromise to preoperative erectile capacity and were simply unable to engage in intercourse because of severe deformity, 15% of these men noted some reduction in postoperative rigidity but were still able to obtain satisfactory erections for coitus spontaneously or with phosphodiesterase 5 inhibitor therapy (i.e., sildenfafil, vardenafil, tadalafil). On the other hand, in men who noted diminished erectile capacity preoperatively and graded their erections as a 7–8 out of 10, 30% noted further reduction in rigidity postoperatively. Fortunately, all of these men who had graded their own erections preoperatively as 7 out of 10 ("stuffable rigidity") or greater were able to respond to oral pharmacotherapy for adequate sexual function. Two men, who had erections of graded as less than 7 out of 10 were advised preoperatively to undergo prosthesis placement but insisted on an attempt to straighten their penes with grafting but without a prosthesis, ultimately did require insertion of a penile prosthesis.

Therefore, with this procedure informed consent is critical, focusing on issues of potential reduction of rigidity, which may require temporary or permanent use of a pharmacological or other aid, diminished penile sensation, delayed ejaculation, or shortening of the penis, even with the grafting procedure, which is designed to lengthen the shortened/scarred aspect. There is also the potential risk of persistent or recurrent curvature, which is unusual if the disease is stable for at least 6 mo preoperatively. Patients are also counseled to expect variations in penile shape, sensation, and rigidity over the first 6–12 mo postoperatively as the graft heals and undergoes tissue reabsorption. Should there be any significant graft contraction or thickening resulting in recurrent curvature during the early postoperative period, the use of an external vacuum device is recommended. I have not routinely recommended the use of a postoperative vacuum device as this typically adds an additional $400–500 expense, which may not be covered by insurance. Last, the "off-the-shelf grafts" appear to be gaining popularity as they are readily available, do not require another incision to harvest, and shorten operating room time—all of which reduce the cost of surgery. My preferred graft is the Tutoplast processed pericardium (5).

SURGICAL PROCEDURE

The erect penile deformity is evaluated following injection of papaverine (60 mg) or alprostadil (20 µg) with saline infusion (Fig. 1). The penis is degloved with a circumcising incision performed approx 1.5–2 cm proximal to the corona. When correcting the more common dorsal or lateral curvature with the incision/partial excision and grafting technique, the neurovascular bundle (NVB) is elevated over the area of the maximum curvature. This should be performed with loupe magnification to avoid injuries to these delicate structures. I prefer to take a bilateral approach with an incision in Buck's fascia running adjacent to the urethra. This avoids the majority of the dorsal nerve fibers and allows elevation of the NVB with exposure of the lateral aspects of the tunica albuginea. This is particularly useful when there is a narrowing or hinge effect in these areas. It is best only to elevate the tissue in the area of maximum deformity to reduce the likelihood of injury to nerve fibers or perforating vessels from the dorsal artery to the deep cavernosal system. If there is extension of the fibrotic tissue into Buck's fascia, then a plane can be carefully developed to release this tethering scar so that the NVB does not result in limited complete straightening (Fig. 2). Hemostasis throughout the procedure is best accomplished with bipolar electrocautery.

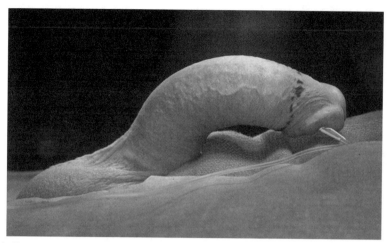

Fig. 1. Severe dorsal curve with dorsal left lateral indentation causing hinge effect.

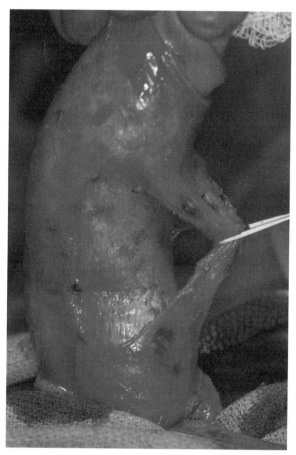

Fig. 2. Elevation of neurovascular bundle, exposing area of maximum curvature and narrowing.

If there is no significant narrowing of the shaft, then a simple transverse incision should be made centered over the area of maximum curvature and carried out to the 3 and 9 o'clock positions on the shaft bilaterally. Longitudinal extensions of the incision (modified H incision) can be made at a 30° angle to the transverse incision (Fig. 3A–D). By doing this

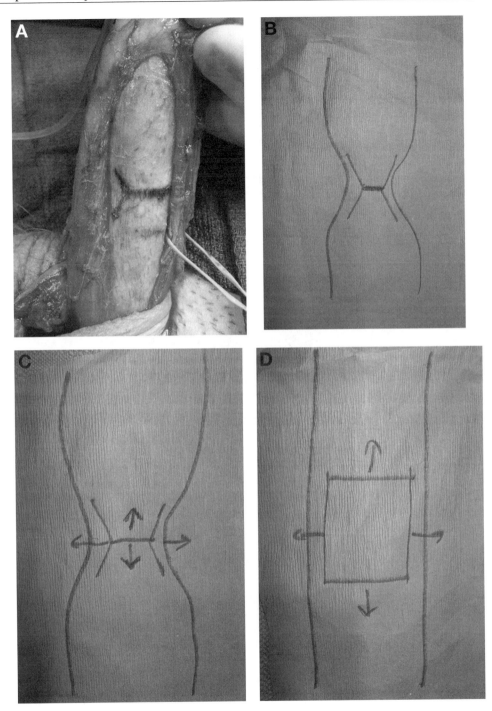

Fig. 3. Modified H incision: (**A**) lateral aspect of planned H incision with wings extending at 30° angle to longitudinal axis of shaft; (**B**) modified H incision in area of maximum curvature and narrowing with expansion of incision tunica defect develops; (**C**) expansion of incision results in lengthening and girth enhancement in this area; and (**D**) correction of deformity with tunical defect to be repaired with graft.

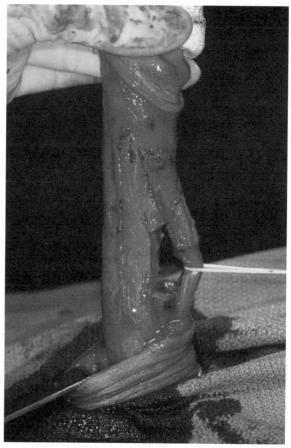

Fig. 4. Defect in tunic apparent with penis on stretch; all aspects of defect should be measured on stretch.

when the incision is expanded both longitudinally and transversely, the result will be a rectangular defect that will resume normal caliber in this area of the shaft. If there is extensive narrowing, deep indentation, or extensive calcification of the tunica, I recommend that this tissue be excised to allow reestablishment of a normal shaft caliber. Great care should be made to limit injury to the underlying cavernosal vascular tissue when releasing the scar or excising a portion of tunic.

Once the plaque is opened or excised, the penis should be placed on full stretch, and 4-0 PDS™ stay sutures (Ethicon, Somerville, NJ) are placed in the four corners of the defect. The stretched length of the penis is now remeasured (Fig. 4) and is typically 1–3 cm longer than preoperatively. All aspects of the tunical defect must be measured carefully. This may be the most critical step in this procedure to obtain the best geometric outcome.

The stay sutures stretch the defect in both the longitudinal and transverse directions to obtain the full length of the defect. Great care should be taken to measure the transverse aspect to ensure correct measurement. I place another stay suture at the midline (12 o'clock position) of the defect and then measure on stretch from the lateral aspect to the midline and then from the midline to the contralateral corner. It is remarkable how long this transverse may measure; do not be fooled to make it smaller as this may result

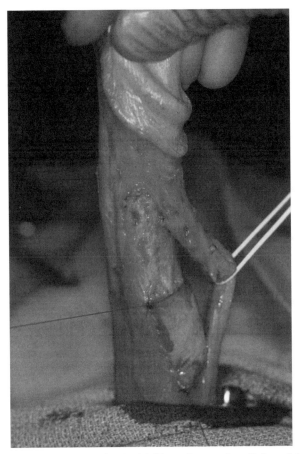

Fig. 5. Defect repaired with Tutoplast pericardial graft in place.

in recurrent narrowing. Typically, one tunical incision or partial excision is needed for straightening and reestablishing caliber. The defects to be patched range from 2 to 4 cm long by 4 to 7 cm in transverse width.

The Tutoplast processed pericardial graft can then be configured to the defect typically by adding 10%, which will allow for any minor shrinkage. Using the previously placed stay sutures, the graft is secured to all aspects to the tunica albuginea in a running fashion (Fig. 5). I prefer suturing from the tunica to the graft, which results in better contour. Once the graft is in place, erection is reestablished with the infusion pump. If there is persistent deformity that warrants further reconstruction, then another incision and grafting may be necessary, or a tunica plication can be performed contralateral to the curvature. In a recent analysis, we found that an added plication did not compromise postoperative rigidity or result in any significant shortening *(4)*.

To reduce the likelihood of subgraft hematoma formation, the midline of the graft can be secured to the septal fibers with two or three simple 4-0 PDS sutures. Subgraft hematomas occur in an unpredictable fashion. In the past, I made an effort to aspirate the accumulated blood postoperatively in the office and found that doing this provided no particular benefit unless the hematoma was causing patient discomfort. Therefore, on most occasions I leave the hematoma to reabsorb spontaneously with time.

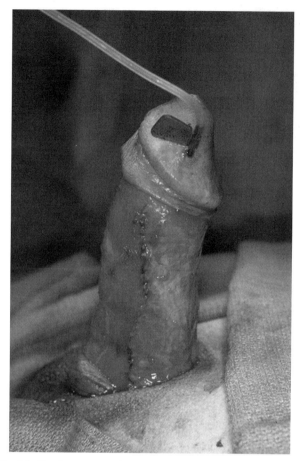

Fig. 6. Buck's fascia reapproximated with running 4=0 chromic suture.

The grafting procedure may also be performed for severe (>90°) ventral curvature, but as noted, there is a heightened risk of postoperative ED (~50%).

Buck's fascia is reapproximated bilaterally with a running 4-0 chromic suture (Ethicon, Somerville, NJ); this should use just the very edge of the fascia so it does not compromise the neurovascular tissue within it. This reapproximation will provide support for the graft as well as tamponade bleeding under the fascia (Fig. 6). The shaft skin is reapproximated with horizontal mattress sutures of 4-0 chromic. Men who are uncircumcised should undergo a circumcision as paraphimosis has occurred in patients who are left uncircumcised.

A combination dressing is applied in the following fashion: A first layer of Xeroform® (Tyco Health Care, Mansfield, MA) is placed circumferentially over the circumcising incision covered by a single dry sterile dressing, and then a lightly applied Coban® dressing (3M, St. Paul, MN) is applied from distal to the proximal base, which is molded to the shaft of the penis (Fig. 7). The Coban dressing is removed on postoperative day 3, and on postoperative day 14, the patient is seen in the office and instructed on penile massage and stretch therapy to help encourage recovery. This is done twice per day for 5–10 min for 1 mo.

Over the past 3 yr, in those patients who have undergone the incision and grafting with Tutoplast (Mentor Corp., Santa Barbara, CA) processed pericardium, we have instituted

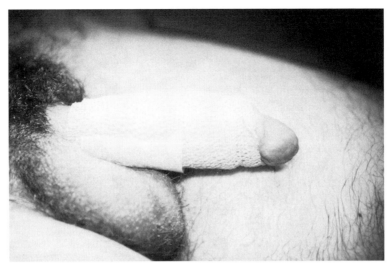

Fig. 7. Coban dressing in place, lightly applied from distal to proximal allowing exposure of glans.

a sexual rehabilitation protocol using sildenafil citrate (Viagra, Pfizer, New York) by which 25–50 mg are taken at bedtime beginning on postoperative night 10 and continuing through night 50. A noncontrolled study of patients who followed this rehabilitation protocol vs those who did not showed a trend of less postoperative dysfunction and more rapid recovery to satisfactory erections ($p > 0.05$) *(4)*. Overall sexual activity may resume 6 wk following surgery. If erections are suboptimal, then a phosphodiesterase type V inhibitor (e.g., sildenafil, vardenafil, tadalafil) is recommended to enhance erectile response. For those patients who need further assistance with their postoperative rigidity, vacuum devices may be used either alone or in concert with the phosphodiesterase 5 inhibitor medication.

In a published review of our initial experience with the Tutoplast pericardial graft repair for advanced Peyronie's deformity, we found that in 40 consecutive men with a mean age of 50 yr who had a mean curvature of 69° (range 40–140°) and in whom 65% had significant indentation, 98% were satisfactorily surgically straightened (defined as curvature less than 20°) at a mean follow-up of 18 mo (range 2–40 mo) *(5)*. Of these individuals, all were sexually active, 70% required no pharmacological assistance, and as noted, 15% of men had reduction of their erections when they had a grade 9–10 out of 10 erection preoperatively, but 30% had reduction of rigidity when their rigidity was graded as 7–8 out of 10. Objective evaluation of length change measured dorsally both pre- and postoperatively revealed that 58% of patients had a mean increased penile length of 1.4 cm, 33% had mean shortening of 1.7 cm, and 10% were unchanged.

It is therefore my opinion that the incision or partial excision and grafting procedure remains an effective procedure for the properly selected patient. The most critical selection features for this operation are a deformity that makes intercourse severely compromised or impossible in the man who has minimal or no associated ED preoperatively.

REFERENCES

1. Levine LA, Lenting EL. Experience with a surgical algorithm for Peyronie's disease. J Urol 1997; 158: 2149–2152.
2. Levine LA, Greenfield JM. Establishing a standardized evaluation of the man with Peyronie's disease. Int J Impot Res 2003; 15(suppl 5): S103–S112.

3. Nesbit RM. Congenital curvature of the phallus: report of three cases with description of corrective operation. J Urol 1965; 93: 230.

4. Greenfield JM, Estrada CR, Levine LA. Erectile dysfunction following surgical correction of Peyronie's disease and a pilot study of the use of sildenafil citrate rehabilitation for postoperative erectile dysfunction. J Sexual Med 2005; 2: 241–247.

5. Levine LA, Estrada C. Human cadaveric pericardial graft for the surgical reconstruction of Peyronie's disease. J Urol 2003; 170: 2359–2362.

21

Surgical Straightening With Tunica Incision and Grafting Technique

Single Relaxing Incision Based on Geometrical Principles

Paulo H. Egydio, MD, PhD

SUMMARY

This single geometrically determined incision is a standardized procedure that may be used for the correction of any penile curvature whether or not associated with tunical constriction regardless of plaque characteristics, resulting in maximum penile length gain.

Key Words: Graft; induratio penis plastica; penile induration; Peyronie's disease; surgery; surgical technique; tissue engineering; tunica albuginea.

INTRODUCTION

Peyronie's disease (PD) is characterized by the development of scar tissue in the tunica albuginea, making it less elastic and consequently causing penile bending *(1)*. The principle goal for surgery is not removal of the plaque but of the penile deformity. When the penis bends, it becomes shorter, and the functional penile length is reduced.

This can hinder sexual intercourse as it reduces the ability to penetrate—or facilitates the penis escaping from—the vagina during intercourse. A bent penis has a short and a long side. If an attempt is made to straighten it by shortening the longer *(2–6)* side, this may leave the patient dissatisfied with the final penile length. This reduction in length is proportional to the degree of curvature.

The focus of surgical treatment should therefore be the restoration of the functional penile length. The alternative that offers the maximum gain in penile length is the elongation of the short side *(7–12)*.

Fibrous plaque excision gives rise to uncertain results because the plaque is not palpable in 30% of the cases *(13)* and may be multifocal *(14)*, and changes in the tunica are diffuse and not restricted to the plaque itself *(15,16)*. On the other hand, relaxing incisions can correct all types of curvature and may be applied whether or not the cases are associated with fibrous plaque.

From: *Current Clinical Urology:*
Peyronie's Disease: A Guide to Clinical Management
Edited by: L. A. Levine © Humana Press Inc., Totowa, NJ

A relaxing incision alone can correct all types of curvature, whether or not associated with a plaque or shaft constriction, by expansion. Besides, it produces a simpler tunical defect and consequently an easier grafting procedure. There are different types of relaxing incision that have been suggested for each specific type of penile curvature whether or not associated with constriction (8,9), but there is no established standard procedure (17–19). Some surgeons even define the size of the tunical incision to be made based on the size of the available graft material that has already been chosen. In these cases, the surgery has not been based on the degree of penile curvature but on the size of the graft material available.

The technique described here uses a single incomplete circumferential relaxing incision forked at the ends by the precise application of geometrical principles (11,12) to determine the exact site for the incision in the tunica or plaque so that the shorter side shall be made as long as the longer side and to create a simpler defect in the tunica albuginea to make the grafting placement easier. In cases of erectile dysfunction (ED) that require penile prosthesis (20,21), the prosthesis can be implanted at the time of the geometrically determined straightening procedure. The size of the prosthesis will be compatible with the longer side as it is the shorter side that is to be lengthened (12).

PATIENT SELECTION

The role of surgery in the management of PD is determined by the severity of curvature and the degree of the patient's disability to have sexual intercourse, and it is the treatment of choice for patients with moderate-to-severe penile curvature and stable disease. Stable disease is characterized by duration of the symptoms for at least 12 mo, without progression or regression of the plaque or deformity and without pain during erection or physical examination for at least 6 mo (22).

The surgical treatment aims at correcting penile curvature that either precludes or makes intercourse difficult despite adequate erection, that is, full rigidity maintained up to ejaculation. Difficult intercourse is characterized by difficulty in penetration or the penis escaping from the vagina because of either penile shortening or instability. Penile instability makes penile bending easier at the point of curvature because of changes in the penile axis or penile constriction associated with reduced rigidity at this point.

PREOPERATIVE ASSESSMENT

Medical and sexual history, physical examination, pharmacologically induced erection, combined with color duplex Doppler ultrasound are used to evaluate penile deformity and preoperative erectile status.

The best candidate for penile grafting reconstruction is the one with normal spontaneous erection sustained up to ejaculation and no relevant comorbid risk factors; corroboration by normal erectile response to pharmacologically induced erection, preferably together with normal duplex Doppler ultrasound, should be made. Normal pharmacotesting in the physician's office means good erectile rigidity sustained for at least 10–15 min, which means there is normal veno-occlusion but not necessarily normal arterial function in up to 10% of patients (23). Color duplex Doppler ultrasound is the most informative and least invasive means of evaluating vasculogenic ED. PD associated with ED should be evaluated for either veno-occlusive dysfunction or arteriogenic ED.

Patients with mild ED but good hemodynamic penile workups (pharmacologically induced erection and Doppler ultrasound) with good response to oral medication are can-

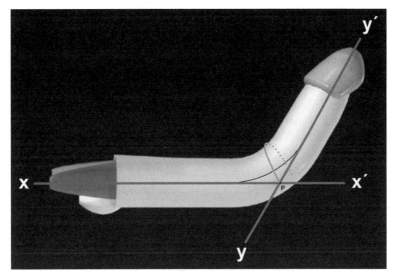

Fig. 1. The intersection of the tangential lines to the penile axis x-x' and y-y' determines the point of maximum curvature P. A circumferential line is drawn from point P in the bisectrix of the angle formed by the lines x-x' and y-y'.

didates for penile grafting reconstruction. On the other hand, those with intractable ED that requires penile prosthesis may have the latter implanted in combination with the straightening grafting procedure, with the size of the prosthesis compatible with the longer side of the penis.

The penile deformity is recorded by dorsal and lateral photographs of full erection from which the angle of curvature is measured.

SURGICAL TECHNIQUE: GEOMETRICAL PRINCIPLES

The penis is degloved after a circumcision incision. One of the cavernous bodies is punctured using a 21-gage scalp needle. Full erection is achieved by saline injection. When necessary, both cavernous bodies may be punctured. Magnifying loupes (2.5×) are used for better visualization. In cases of dorsal curvature, two lines tangential to the penile axis are drawn on the proximal and distal straight segments (x-x' and y-y', respectively) toward the area of curvature of the erect penis (Fig. 1). From the point of maximum curvature P situated at the intersection of the lines x-x' and y-y', a circumferential line is drawn to bisect the angle formed by these lines (Fig. 1).

The point at which this circumferential line crosses the neurovascular bundle (NVB) in the dorsal region and the urethra in the ventral region determines the place at which these structures must be separated from the tunica albuginea. The transverse incision in the tunica will be later made along this circumferential line. Then, the erection is reversed. Two paraurethral incisions (u-u') at the point where the circumferential line crosses the urethra are made to dissect Buck's fascia and its NVB from the tunica around the complete circumference of the penis in all types of curvature, except at the level of the urethra (Fig. 2A,B). A new erection is induced, and the circumferential line is drawn again, this time on the tunica where the circular incision will be made (Fig. 2C). This incision is forked at the ends so that the defect created has a rectangular shape, which makes the grafting procedure easier (Fig. 3A).

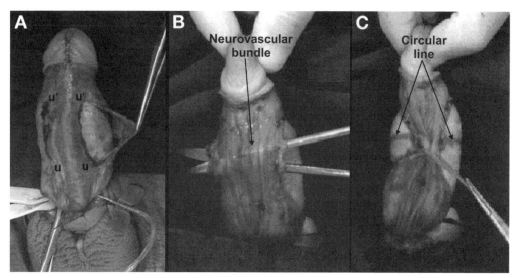

Fig. 2. (**A**) Paraurethral incisions (u-u') in Buck's fascia. (**B**) Dissection of Buck's fascia and the neurovascular bundle from the tunica albuginea. (**C**) Drawing of the circumferential line at the point of maximum curvature.

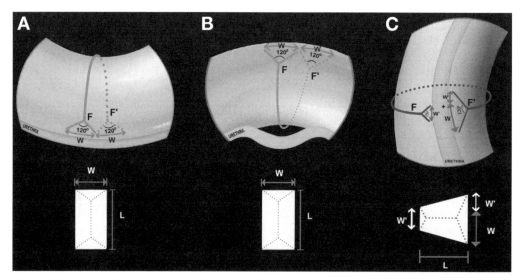

Fig. 3. Bifurcation of the transverse incision and the correspondent defects in the tunica albuginea in cases of dorsal and dorsolateral (**A**), ventral or ventrolateral (**B**), and lateral (**C**) curvatures. W, width of the defect; L, length of the defect; F and F' are the points from which the transversal incision is forked.

The width W of the tunical defect should be the same as the difference between the long and the short sides of the penis. This measurement is calculated by the distance between any two complete circumferential lines perpendicular to the penile axis drawn on the straight penile segments (i.e., outside the area of curvature; before d-d' and after e-e') (Fig. 4). The difference W between d-e and d'-e' will be the size of the defect on each side of the urethra in cases of dorsal curvature (Fig. 3A). The length L of the defect is the distance between the ends of the forks round the circumference of the fully erect penis (Fig. 3A).

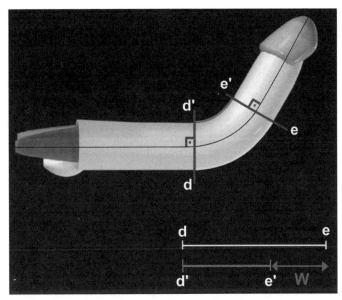

Fig. 4. W is equal to the difference between the distance of the two points of the long side (d-e) of the penis minus the equivalent distance (d'-e') in the short side measured outside the curvature area (□ = 90°).

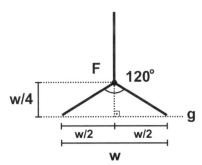

Fig. 5. Geometrical explanation to produce a tripod-shaped bifurcation for a more stable structure and to produce simpler tunical defect. g, line that determines the position of the extremities of the intended forked incision on each side of the penis; W, width of the tunical defect; F, the point at which the bifurcation will begin to produce an angle of 120°. This is defined by measuring a quarter of W back from g along the circular line around the penis.

First, it is necessary to establish a line on each side of the penis to determine the position of the extremities of the intended forked incision. This line must be positioned close and parallel to the urethra for cases of dorsal, dorsolateral, and lateral curvature and about 0.5 cm from the dorsal groove on each side and parallel to it for cases of ventral or ventrolateral curvature. Now, a distance equivalent to a quarter of W is measured back from this line along the circumference. This gives the position of points F and F' at which the bifurcation on each side will begin (Fig. 5). Thus, a simple defect is produced as stable as a tripod (Fig. 3A–C).

Once the position of the circumferential line forked at the ends is determined, the incision is made in the tunica albuginea, producing a rectangular defect of an already known size. The complete penile straightening is achieved by a 5-mm incision in the intercaver-

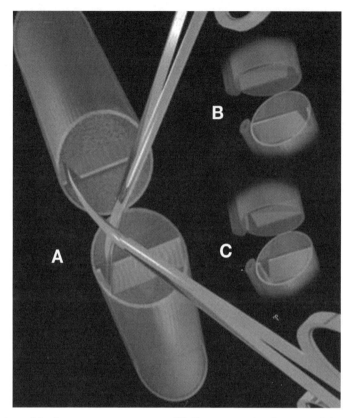

Fig. 6. (A) Cutting of the intercavernous septum. **(B)** Septum cutting in cases of dorsal, dorsolateral, or lateral curvature. **(C)** Septum cutting in cases of ventral or ventrolateral curvature.

nous septum on each side of its intersection with the transverse incision (Fig. 6). To facilitate the graft suturing, a 5-mm dissection is made between the four edges of the defect and the respective adjacent cavernous bodies. The graft is sutured, and a new induced erection demonstrates the complete penile straightening (Fig. 7).

In cases of ventral curvature, the technique is similar, with the following differences: the forking of the transverse incision is made in the dorsal region near the intercavernous septum and is maintained and not separated in this region (Figs. 3B and 8B). The urethra is dissected from its bed, and the graft is placed between the urethra and the cavernous body (Fig. 8C). A new erection is induced to demonstrate complete penile straightening (Fig. 8A,D).

Dorsolateral curvatures with a larger dorsal component and ventrolateral curvatures with a greater ventral component are corrected using the same technique, respectively, as for dorsal or ventral curvatures.

In cases of lateral curvature (Fig. 9A), the technique is similar with the following differences: to avoid a triangular defect that would make the grafting procedure more difficult, a trapezoidal defect is created by adding an additional 0.5–1 cm (W') to the width W and on the opposite side. The length of the tunical defect L is measured in the same way as described for the other types of curvature (Fig. 3C). Thus, a defect of triangular shape is avoided, which would make the graft procedure more difficult (Fig. 9).

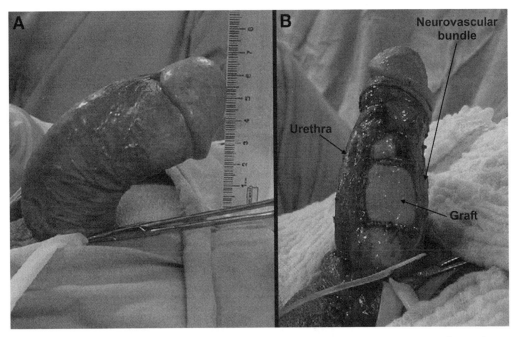

Fig. 7. (A) Preoperative dorsal curvature. **(B)** Final result after straightening and graft suturing.

All the defects are covered with bovine pericardium trimmed to sizes 1–2 mm wider and longer than the respective defects because this extra margin is taken up by the poliglecaprone 4.0 continuous suture. During this suturing, it is important to maintain the tunica on stretch. A new erection is induced to certify the penile straightening. The mean (SD, range) sizes of graft used were 2.6 (0.5, 1.7–4.1) cm for width by 7.6 (0.7, 5–10) cm for length. The increase in functional penile size was 3.1 ± 1.4 cm (varying from 1 to 7). Buck's fascia is not sutured again. An aspirative drain is placed if necessary. The penile degloving is reversed, and the incision is closed. If necessary, the foreskin is removed. A light compressive dressing is recommended.

For cases that present with floppy glans, the disassembly technique *(24)* may be applied for distal reconstruction (Fig. 10).

CAVEATS TO THE SINGLE GEOMETRICAL INCISION

- The achievement of full erection is an important step for the accurate application of geometrical principles and determination of the appropriate site for the tunica incision. Vasoactive drugs with saline solution may be injected to facilitate full erection.
- The difference between the long and short sides that will define the width of the defect may be measured between any two points on the straight portions of the penis because it will always be the same.
- To prevent ED, it is very important to ensure larger collaterals between dorsal arteries and cavernous arteries and to preserve at least one septal insertion.
- During tunica-grafting suturing, it is important to maintain the tunica stretched as when erect for better fit of the graft.

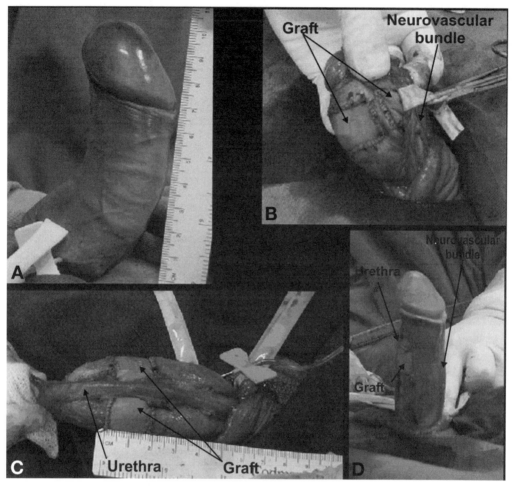

Fig. 8. (A) Preoperative ventral curvature. (B) Graft sutured beside the intercavernous septum and in front of the neurovascular bundle. (C) Graft passing behind the urethra. (D) Final result of the penile straightening.

- Septum incision on both edges of the transversal incision on the short side of the penis is fundamental for adequate lengthening of the short side and complete penile straightening; there is no association with higher incidence of ED.
- The traction of the penis after the final tunical and septal incision and tunical dissection from the spongy tissue of the cavernous body allows for complete penile straightening checking. If the NVB is restricting penile straightening, then its dissection may be extended.
- The bifurcations in the dorsal region for ventral curvatures should not cross the intercavernous septum to preserve it at this point.
- The graft is cut according to the measurements already made of the width W and length L but should be 1–2 mm wider and longer than the defect because the extra will be taken up by the suture. However, the graft should only be of this size where there is no likelihood of the material used shrinking, in which case a percentage allowance for shrinkage should be added to the dimensions of the graft.
- The length of the defect should be measured with the penis erect and outside any constricted area.

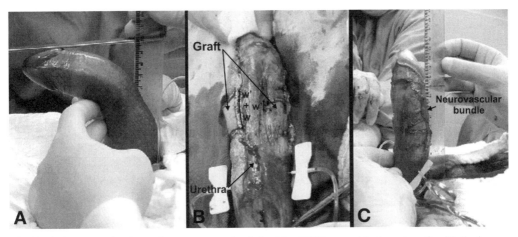

Fig. 9. (A) Preoperative lateral curvature to the right side. **(B)** Trapezoid-shaped graft with the longer side at the right and the shorter side at the left. **(C)** Final result of penile straightening.

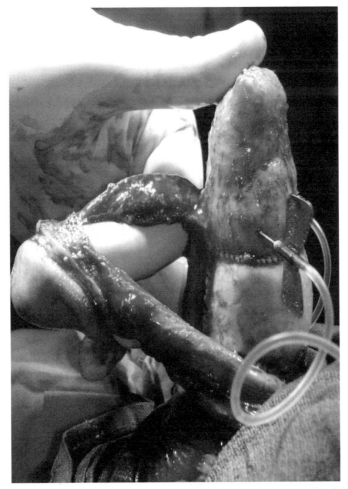

Fig. 10. Floppy glans treated by applying a disassembly technique to expose distal shaft of the penis for distal reconstruction. In the middle shaft of the penis, a graft placement was done to treat dorsal curvature.

POSTOPERATIVE CARE AND PATIENT FOLLOW-UP

When the surgery is performed with sedation and local anesthesia and no drain or Foley catheter is used, the patient can be discharged on the same day. A light compressive dressing is recommended and should be maintained for 3 to 5 d. When spinal anesthesia is used, the Foley catheter and drain when used are withdrawn, and the patient is discharged on postoperative day 1.

It is recommended that the penis be kept in an upright position for 2–3 wk to help reduce swelling. Although the patient may have spontaneous erections, a 6-wk period of sexual abstinence is recommended. If the patient is not experiencing spontaneous erection within 7–10 d after surgery, then a phosphodiesterase inhibitor is recommended to stimulate nocturnal or early morning erections. This is preferable to the application of a vacuum device.

It is recommended that in certain cases a phosphodiesterase inhibitor be used as an aid to sexual intercourse after 6 wk to achieve a better erection and avoid erectile problems caused by anxiety. Psychogenic dysfunction is common on the return to sexual activity but should be treated. Once the patient has regained confidence, the medication should be discontinued.

It is very important to avoid penile trauma to prevent a new manifestation of PD at some other site in the tunica. It is recommended that the partner be checked regarding vaginal stenosis and problems with lubrication; partners should be treated accordingly and instructed on the avoidance of trauma. Rapid ejaculation should be treated. After a 6-mo follow-up, alprostadil-induced erections are used to check penile straightening.

OUTCOME

Between April 1999 and July 2004, 192 patients with the following characteristics underwent surgery: preoperative normal erection sustained up to ejaculation; no relevant comorbid risk factors (such as diabetes mellitus, hypertension, coronary artery disease, peripheral vascular disease, alcoholism, smoking, and neurological or endocrine disorders); normal response to pharmacologically induced erection; and color duplex Doppler ultrasound with peak systolic velocity above 40 cm/s and end diastolic velocity under 3 cm/s in both cavernous arteries during the 10–20 min of evaluation after an induced erection. The mean age for this group was 52 (22–72) yr. Penile deformities were distributed among dorsal (47%), dorsolateral (30%), lateral (12%), ventral (6%), and ventrolateral (5%). No infection, retraction, or rejection of the graft occurred. In 15.6% (30/192) of the patients with PD associated with penile shaft constriction at the site of the curvature, the technique corrected both deformities. The cases with greatest curvature showed the biggest gain in penile length.

Prostaglandin-induced erection in the follow-up revealed penile straightening in 88% of patients (169 of 192) and residual curvature of up to 15° in 11% (21 of 192) and of up to 30° (which does not hinder penile functioning for sexual intercourse) in 1% (2 of 192). The gain in functional penile size was maintained in patients whose penile straightening was maintained and reduced by up to 0.5 cm in those who developed curvature postoperatively.

The preoperative erection status was maintained in this selected group of patients who during the follow-up period of 28.5 ± 11.3 mo (6–63 mo) had resumed continuous satisfactory sexual activity.

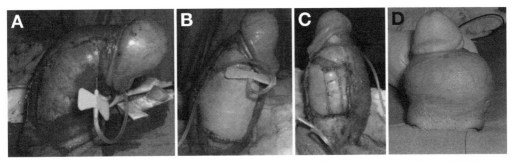

Fig. 11. (**A**) Preoperative dorsal curvature. (**B**) and (**C**) Immediate postoperative: left and right graft view. (**C**) Graft-grafting suturing with 4.0 poliglecaprone continuous suture. (**D**) Bulge at 5-mo follow-up.

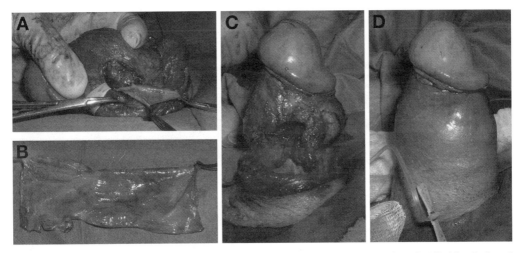

Fig. 12. (**A–D**) Further surgery. (**A**) Opened graft to graft suture. (**B**) Removed graft. (**C**) After induced erection, left without graft. (**D**) After penile regloving.

COMPLICATIONS

In one case at 2-mo follow-up, the patient had developed a small bulge, which increased in size over the follow-up period, on the site of the graft (Fig. 11).

This patient had further surgery after 5 mo, and a graft-to-graft suture was found to have opened with a consequent hematoma. The original graft was removed, and erection was induced to test for leakage. As no leakage was seen, the patient was maintained without the graft (Fig. 12). There are two lessons to be learned from this complication. First, the graft-to-graft suturing must be done with nonabsorbable suture. Second, for the purpose of research the graft should allow delayed reabsorption.

SUMMARY OF THE BENEFITS WITH COMMENTS

The technique presented here is based on a long circumferential incision forked at the ends in the tunica albuginea or plaque, irrespective of the characteristics and location of the plaque *(11,12,25,26)*. It may be used to correct all types of curvature, whether or not associated with constriction.

The dissection of Buck's fascia and the NVB was standardized for all cases by means of two paraurethral incisions. Usually, at this level the circumflex veins may be cauterized because of their small caliber, which results in a reduced number of ligatures. The dorsal dissection may be limited to the area of curvature or extended in cases in which it is restricting complete penile straightening.

The extended circumferential incision makes it possible to break all the lines of force, allowing curvature correction on more than one plane (dorsolateral or ventrolateral) at the same time.

For lateral curvatures, the correction based on a rectangular tunical defect would require the cutting of the intercavernous septum in both dorsal and ventral regions. As the risk of ED produced by the incisions is unknown (27), a trapezoid-shaped defect is preferred so one of the intercavernous septum insertion points is preserved.

Tripod-shaped forkings of 120° produce a simpler configuration of the tunical defect, resulting in geometrically shaped grafts that can be easily sutured. These forkings also permit the relaxation of constricted areas of the tunica and the correction of associated constrictive lesions.

When geometrical principles and induced erection are used, the size of the defect in the tunica albuginea can be calculated before the incision is made, and this makes the preoperative preparation of the graft possible. In the future, with the development of tissue engineering, this measurement may be made in the office after intracavernous injection creating of a full erection, and it will be possible to calculate the size of the graft needed.

As the majority of patients have penile curvature at only one site, only one incision and graft are necessary. If there are two significant curvatures at different points of the penis, then two grafts should be prepared as described. Complementary plication that not only damages the healthy side but also leads to penile shortening should be avoided.

The present technique opens the way for the standardization of a single tunical incision procedure, reproducible in multicenter studies, and may lead to a more objective understanding of the advantages and disadvantages of the different types of graft material (28–30).

CONCLUSIONS

This single geometrically determined incision is a standardized procedure that may be used for correction of any penile curvature whether or not associated with tunical constriction at the same site regardless of plaque characteristics, resulting in maximum penile length gain.

REFERENCES

1. Carson CC, Lue T, Levine L, et al. Symposium on Peyronie's disease, April 12, 1997. Int J Impot Res 1998; 10: 121–122.
2. Nesbit RM. Congenital curvature of the phallus: report of three cases with description of corrective operation. J Urol 1965; 93: 230–232.
3. Pryor JP. Correction of penile curvature and Peyronie's disease: why I prefer the Nesbit technique. Int J Impot Res 1998; 10: 129–131.
4. Yachia D. Modified corporoplasty for the treatment of penile curvature. J Urol 1990; 143: 80–82.
5. Daitch JA, Angermeier KW, Montague DK. Modified corporoplasty for penile curvature: long-term results and patient satisfaction. J Urol 1999; 162: 2006–2009.
6. Gholami SS, Lue TF. Correction of penile curvature using the 16-dot plication technique: a review of 132 patients. J Urol 2002; 167: 2066–2069.
7. Devine CJ Jr, Horton CE. Surgical treatment of Peyronie's disease with a dermal graft. J Urol 1974; 111: 44–49.

8. Gelbard MK. Relaxing incisions in the correction of penile deformity due to Peyronie's disease. J Urol 1995; 154: 1457–1460.

9. Lue TF, El-Sakka AI. Venous patch graft for Peyronie's disease. Part I: technique. J Urol 1998; 160: 2047–2049.

10. Hellstrom WJ, Reddy S. Application of pericardial graft in the surgical management of Peyronie's disease. J Urol 2000; 163: 1445–1447.

11. Egydio PH, Lucon AM, Arap S. Treatment of Peyronie's disease by incomplete circumferential incision of the tunica albuginea and plaque with bovine pericardium graft. Urology 2002; 59: 570–574.

12. Egydio PH, Lucon AM, Arap S. A single relaxing incision to correct different types of penile curvature: surgical technique based on geometrical principles. BJU Int 2004; 94: 1147–1157.

13. El-Sakka AI, Rashwan HM, Lue TF. Venous patch graft for Peyronie's disease. Part II: outcome analysis. J Urol 1998; 160: 2050–2053.

14. Rollandi GA, Tentarelli T, Vespier M. Computed tomographic findings in Peyronie's disease. Urol Radiol 1985; 7: 153–156.

15. Somers KD, Sismour EN, Wright GL Jr, et al. Isolation and characterization of collagen in Peyronie's disease. J Urol 1989; 141: 629–631.

16. Anafarta K, Beduk Y, Uluoglu O, et al. The significance of histopathological changes of the normal tunica albuginea in Peyronie's disease. Int Urol Nephrol 1994; 26: 71–77.

17. Ralph DJ, Minhas S. The management of Peyronie's disease. BJU Int 2004; 93: 208–215.

18. Hellstrom WJ, Bivalacqua TJ. Peyronie's disease: etiology, medical, and surgical therapy. J Androl 2000; 21: 347–354.

19. Gholami SS, Gonzalez-Cadavid NF, Lin CS, et al. Peyronie's disease: a review. J Urol 2003; 169: 1234–1241.

20. Montague DK, Angermeier KW, Lakin MM, et al. AMS three-piece inflatable penile prosthesis implantation in men with Peyronie's disease: comparison of CX and Ultrex cylinders. J Urol 1996; 156: 1633–1635.

21. Levine LA, Dimitriou RJ. A surgical algorithm for penile prosthesis placement in men with erectile failure and Peyronie's disease. Int J Impot Res 2000; 12: 147–151.

22. Carson CC, Gelbard MK, Jordan GH. Peyronie's disease: how to choose a surgical procedure. Contemp Urol 1999, 11: 12–43.

23. Pescatori ES, Hatzichristou DG, Namburi S, Goldstein I. A positive intracavernous injection test implies normal veno-occlusive but not necessarily normal arterial function: a hemodynamic study. J Urol 1994; 151: 1209–1216.

24. Perovic SV, Djordjevic ML. The penile disassembly technique in the surgical treatment of Peyronie's disease. BJU Int 2001; 88: 731–738.

25. Egydio PH, Lucon AM, Arap S. A single relaxing incision to correct different types of penile deformity in Peyronie's disease: geometrical principles. J Urol 2003; 169(suppl): 275.

26. Seftel AD. Treatment of Peyronie's disease by incomplete circumferential incision of the tunica albuginea and plaque with bovine pericardium graft [editorial comment]. J Urol 2002; 168: 869.

27. Lue TF, El-Sakka AI. Lengthening shortened penis caused by Peyronie's disease using circular venous grafting and daily stretching with a vacuum erection device. J Urol 1999; 161: 1141–1144.

28. Chun JL, McGregor A, Krishnan R, et al. A comparison of dermal and cadaveric pericardial grafts in the modified Horton-Devine procedure for Peyronie's disease. J Urol 2001; 166: 185–188.

29. Carson CC, Chun JL. Peyronie's disease: surgical management: autologous materials. Int J Impot Res 2002; 14: 329–235.

30. Leungwattanakij S, Bivalacqua TJ, Yang DY, et al. Comparison of cadaveric pericardial, dermal, vein, and synthetic grafts for tunica albuginea substitution using a rat model. BJU Int 2003; 92: 119–124.

22

Minimally Invasive Intracorporal Incision of Peyronie's Plaque

Anthony J. Bella, MD, FRCSC
and Gerald B. Brock, MD, FRCSC

SUMMARY

Surgical management of Peyronie's disease remains an area of evolving technique. Although few surgeons agree on the optimal procedure, most are comfortable with the concept that the chosen procedure should be as minimally invasive as possible and restore shape and function with the lowest risk to the individual. Currently, there exists no best procedure able to accomplish all of these ideal end points. Most surgeons experienced in management of Peyronie's disease utilize a wide range of procedures, from plications to incisions and excisional techniques with grafts obtained from either autologous or exogenous sources. In this chapter, we report on our experience with an intracorporal incisional technique directed at men with small, discrete, dorsally located penile plaques. The ability for us to incise the scar from the interior of the corpora reduces pain and limits the need for us to widely mobilize the neurovascular bundle in these men.

Key Words: Intracorporal repair; minimally invasive incisional Peyronie's repair; Peyronie's disease.

INTRODUCTION

Over the past decade, greater understanding of the pathogenesis of Peyronie's disease (PD) has occurred. Innovative studies attempting to link the development of this condition with certain human lymphocyte antigen (HLA) subtypes and other states of altered wound healing hold the promise of novel therapeutic approaches in the future. Currently, however, no effective medical therapy exists that reliably "cures" the penile deformity of PD. In the context of this reality, failure of conservative or nonsurgical treatment of PD often necessitates surgical intervention when intercourse is made difficult by the penile deformity and the disease has been present for at least 12 mo. Acceptable surgical candidates should have stable curvature and plaque size for at least 6 mo, a preoperative assessment of erectile function, and clear understanding of treatment options and objectives *(1)*.

The ideal surgical approach for a patient with PD would correct penile curvature, maintain erectile function, and cause minimal morbidity with rapid postoperative patient recovery (Table 1). Unfortunately, contemporary surgical approaches, including penile

From: *Current Clinical Urology:*
Peyronie's Disease: A Guide to Clinical Management
Edited by: L. A. Levine © Humana Press Inc., Totowa, NJ

Table 1
Characteristics of the Ideal
Surgical Repair of Peyronie's Disease

Correction of curvature
Preservation of rigidity, length, and width
Minimally invasive with few complications
Rapid recovery

Table 2
Limitations of Current Surgical Approaches

Tunical plication	Plaque incision and grafting
Plaque progression	Penile pain with tumescence
Penile shortening	Induration at base of penis
Palpable nodules	Penile shaft numbness
Recurrence (absorbable suture material)	Impaired veno-occlusive mechanism
Ruptured suture material	Diminished rigidity during erection

Table 3
Goals of Minimally Invasive Peyronie's Repair

Preserve dorsal neural and vascular structures
Minimize risk of sensory loss postcorrection
Preserve rigidity by preserving tunica
Eliminate use of graft
Shorten operative time
Minimize complications
Shorten recovery period

Table 4
Advantages of Minimally
Invasive Intracorporal Plaque Incision

Small tunical incision
Limited neurovascular dissection
Preservation of tunical integrity
Correction under visual monitoring possible
Minimal risk of sensory loss
Eliminate use of graft
Shorter recovery period

shortening (Nesbit and plication), incision or excision of the plaque with grafting, and penile prosthesis implantation supplemented with remodeling, carry an inherent risk of side effects, including postoperative erectile dysfunction, penile length and girth loss, and sensory deficits (Table 2) *(2,3)*.

Until better understanding of the molecular biology of PD allows for the development of novel nonsurgical therapies, surgical techniques that minimize corporal disruption may offer the patient effective, better tolerated treatment options (Table 3). In this chapter, a novel minimally invasive intracorporal plaque incision technique is described. This surgical option is suitable for patients with discrete plaques less than 2 cm in size and has resulted in good correction of curvature, minimal difficulties with erectile function, and high patient-reported satisfaction at a median follow-up of 25 mo (Table 4) *(4)*.

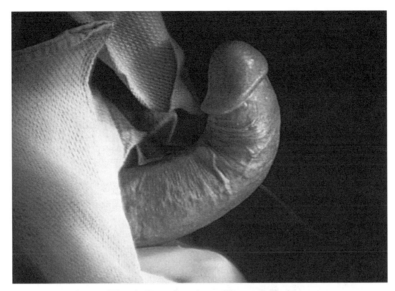

Fig. 1. Preoperative saline erection.

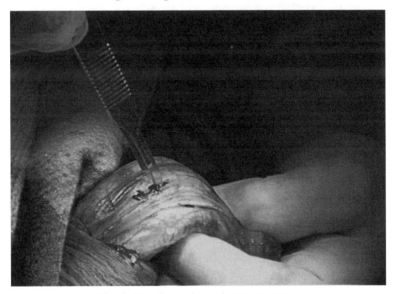

Fig. 2. The 5-mm lateral corporotomy.

OPERATIVE TECHNIQUE

Preoperative surgical planning for this dorsally located plaque is confirmed using an initial saline erection (Fig. 1). A standard, subcoronal circumferential skin incision is made, and the skin is mobilized to the base of the penis. A limited mobilization of the neurovascular bundle is performed, freeing a small 1- to 2-cm span overlying the palpable Peyronie's plaque. Minimizing dissection decreases the possibility of incurring neurovascular injury. A 5-mm corporotomy is made laterally at the level of the plaque, allowing access for the triangular blade (Fig. 2). Prior to doing so, blunt scissors are used for blunt subtunical dissection medially toward the plaque (Fig. 3). This allows for atraumatic introduction of the 5-mm triangular blade along the wall of the tunica to the level of the plaque (Fig. 4). The plaque is then incised from within the corpora as the elevated

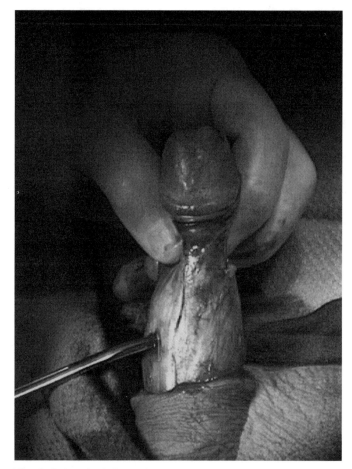

Fig. 3. Subtunical dissection medially toward palpable plaque.

neurovascular bundle allows placement of an index finger on the plaque at the exterior of the corpora (Fig. 5).

In this manner, controlled incisions are made at multiple levels of the plaque while palpating from the exterior. These incisions are not made through the full thickness of the tunica, leaving the outer layer intact. Saline erection is performed to confirm correction and determine if further plaque incision is needed (Fig. 6). A limited, single pair of ventrally placed tunical incisions may be required in select cases to maintain the plaque in an open position (Fig. 7). Disruption of the plaque minimizes or eliminates the need for placement of plication sutures, thereby minimizing penile shortening. If required, the small lateral corporotomies are closed with 2-0 absorbable monofilament sutures. Buck's fascia is reapproximated, and the skin incision is closed with chromic gut suture. A sterile dressing and compressive wrap are applied. Patients are discharged either the same day or the following morning and are instructed to return for dressing removal after 5–7 d.

RESULTS

The initial results of this technique with 23 patients and a median follow-up of 25 mo have been promising. The median curvature treated was 60° (range 30–90°), with 21

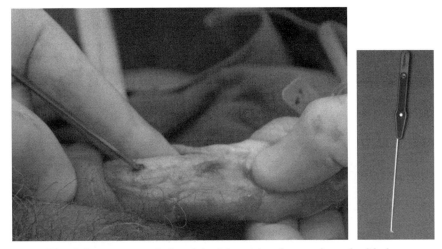

Fig. 4. Intracorporeal plaque incision using 5-mm triangular blade.

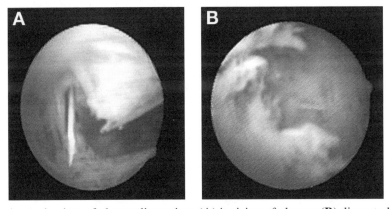

Fig. 5. Endoscopic view of plaque disruption: (**A**) incision of plaque; (**B**) disrupted plaque.

patients having dorsally located plaques. Curvature correction, considered to be residual penile curvature less than 10° degrees, was successful in 21 of 23 patients. Results from a standardized telephone survey (91% response rate) showed rigidity of erections sufficient for intercourse in 80% of men, with additional erectogenic therapy (sildenafil) required by 5 patients. Eighty-five percent of patients were either satisfied or very satisfied with their surgical outcome at 2-yr follow-up (4). Limitations of the minimally invasive Peyronie's repair are given in Table 5.

COMPLICATIONS

Penile shortening was reported by the majority of patients (85%) but did not adversely affect overall erectile function. At clinical follow-up, all but two patients reported correction of curvature. One patient achieved only 50% correction but had regained functional ability to resume sexual intercourse. After initial correction of a 60° dorsal curvature, a second patient had a recurrence after 3 mo with a left-sided curvature. A single patient has also reported partial glans hypoesthesia (4).

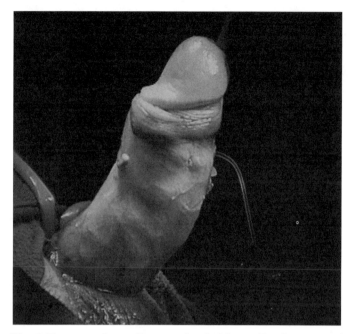

Fig. 6. Postprocedure saline erection (without plication sutures).

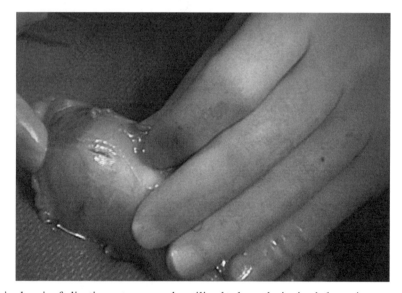

Fig. 7. A single pair of plication sutures may be utilized to keep the incised plaque in an open position.

Table 5
Limitations of Minimally Invasive Peyronie's Repair

Limited single-center experience with 2-yr follow-up
Select patients: inappropriate for extensive or complex curvatures
May require opposite-side plication
Risk of neurovascular injury

CONCLUSIONS

Minimally invasive approaches to Peyronie's repair such as the intracorporal incision technique represent new alternatives for men considering surgical correction of their disease. Correction of curvature, maintenance of erectile function, and high patient-reported satisfaction coupled with a low incidence of complications and shortened operative and recovery times support intracorporal incision as a primary treatment option. As this technique is limited to discrete plaques measuring less than 2 cm, we continue to utilize grafting techniques when there is an extensive plaque, an hourglass deformity, or a complex curvature.

REFERENCES

1. Dean RC, Lue TF. Peyronie's disease: advancements in recent surgical techniques. Curr Opin Urol 2004; 14: 339–343.
2. Tornehl CK, Carson CC. Surgical alternatives for treating Peyronie's disease. BJU Int 2004; 94: 774–783.
3. Kendirci M, Hellstrom WJ. Critical analysis of surgery for Peyronie's disease. Curr Opin Urol 2004; 14: 381–388.
4. Bella AJ, Beasley KA, Obied A, Brock GB. Minimally invasive Peyronie's repair: initial experiences with a new technique. J Sex Med 2004; 1(1S): 88.

23 Surgical Straightening With Penile Prosthesis

Steven K. Wilson, MD and Culley C. Carson, III, MD

SUMMARY

Peyronie's disease (PD) is an incurable, chronic condition producing scarring fibrosis of the tunica albuginea and is associated with penile deformity and erectile dysfunction. Although men afflicted with PD usually have a number of treatment options, those who also present with erectile dysfunction (ED) arising from it are not easily treated. Surgical straightening procedures that have been used to treat PD may not restore erectile function, and failure to straighten the penis with corrective surgery may be the result of erectile inadequacy during the postoperative period. For those men with PD and associated ED, penile prosthesis implantation will provide penile rigidity and straightening. This chapter discusses penile prosthesis implantation as a surgical option for patients with PD, placing emphasis on the choice of devices and surgical techniques. Implant choices are critical in the success of these procedures, and modeling to attain maximum straightening is the preferred method for correcting penile deformity after prosthesis implantation. Newer techniques hold the promise of high success rates and low morbidity.

Key Words: Erectile dysfunction; penile implant; penile modeling; penile prosthesis; Peyronie's disease.

Peyronie's disease (PD) is an incurable, benign condition characterized by the formation of fibrotic plaques in the tunica albuginea of the corpora cavernosa. The French physician François Gigot de la Peyronie described a series of five patients with "plastic penile deformity" in 1743 (1). De la Peyronie suggested the etiology might be chronic irritation from sexual activity or inflammatory sexually transmitted disease and that treatment was bathing in the waters of Barège in southern France.

Although the etiology of this condition has yet to be elucidated, as men age, the elasticity of the tunica albuginea is decreased, and repeated trauma may cause traumatic separation of the tunical layers and stimulate a healing cascade, resulting in a scar tissue plaque. As scar replaces or is deposited in the elastic tunica, penile compliance is impaired, and a shortened, curved, or tethered erection is noted. The scar tissue may become so prominent that it has been proposed to inhibit blood flow distal to the area of fibrosis, resulting in the complaint of proximal rigidity with distal flaccidity. This rigidity of the tunica albuginea may also impair the veno-occlusive mechanism, resulting in veno-occlusive dysfunction

From: *Current Clinical Urology:*
Peyronie's Disease: A Guide to Clinical Management
Edited by: L. A. Levine © Humana Press Inc., Totowa, NJ

or venous leak erectile dysfunction (ED). Thus, the association of ED and PD is a common condition *(2)*.

Over the ensuing 262 yr since description of the condition, hundreds of treatments, including oral medications, injections, external treatments, and various surgical procedures, have been suggested. As can be appreciated from other chapters in this book, there is no specific nonsurgical therapy that has been unequivocally successful for this condition. Indeed, medical treatment of PD has been disappointing *(3)*. Since the introduction of sildenafil citrate in 1998, the treatment of PD has been revolutionized. Prior to sildenafil's release, soft curved erections could only be treated with penile prosthesis implantation. With the facilitation of erection with phosphodiesterase 5 inhibitors, many patients and partners are able to tolerate the curvature and resume coital function. In addition, surgical straightening complicated by the development of ED required treatment with injection or vacuum constriction therapy. Patients now with ED as a result of a penile straightening procedure can be successfully treated by supplementing their erections with oral therapy *(4)*.

The initial article describing penile modeling over an inflatable penile prosthesis as a treatment for Peyronie's deformities in patients with associated ED was published in 1994 *(5)*. Since that publication, penile modeling has achieved widespread acceptance as a first-line therapy for patients with PD and ED.

CANDIDATES FOR SURGICAL CORRECTION
OF PEYRONIE'S DISEASE

PD has two phases: The early inflammatory phase is characterized by penile pain on erection, progressive curvature or hourglass deformity of the erect penis, and palpable plaque formation. After 12–18 mo, a chronic phase begins. The patient has a stable, painless plaque that may occasionally be calcified. This fibrotic thickening of the tunica albuginea prohibits expansion and is manifest as shortening of the affected side on tumescence as the noncompliant tunica fails to stretch with erection.

Clinical expression results in various appearances. The penis may be curved to one side, dorsal or ventral. The penis may appear to have undergone torsion. The penis may have areas of restricted girth or an hourglass deformity when erect. Many complain of flail penis or hinging—tumescence at the base but distal flaccidity that make penetration difficult. Of the plaques, 70% are dorsal, making upward deflection the most common presentation *(3)*. The less-frequent downward deflections and lateral bending are more likely to interfere with sexual intercourse and are more likely to precipitate physician consultation. Some men exhibit all the manifestations and present with a shortened, corkscrew, flail penis or even profound ED.

Surgery must be directed at correction of the stable deformity after the acute inflammation has resolved. Several criteria have been established as guidelines for considering surgical intervention *(6)*. The disease should be past the acute inflammatory stage as indicated by lack of pain on erection and stability of the degree of impaired erection. The progression of penile curvature and associated ED should have been stable for at least 3 mo. Because nonsurgical therapy has such a poor track record of effectiveness, trial of conservative therapy may only allow plaque maturation before surgical intervention. Trials of oral or injectable medications while resolution of the inflammatory phase continues often give the patient an opportunity to pursue resolution actively and increase motivation for a surgical solution. Difficulty with intercourse must be well documented in the clinical record. Some urologists believe surgery for PD for a palpable induration or curvature without functional sexual limitation is meddlesome *(2)*.

Once the disease is fully stable, the surgical management consists of either correction of the penile deformity or insertion of a penile prosthesis in those patients who have concomitant ED. The method of correction of the penile deformity in sexually functioning patients is controversial. Surgical correction without prosthesis implantation can be broken into two categories with numerous technical variations contained within each group *(6,7)*. The first category includes operations that shorten the long side by plicating or removing tunical tissue—variations of the Nesbit procedure originally described for congenital curvature of the penis. The second type of corrective surgery lengthens the short side and includes variations of the Horton-Devine operation. These procedures are accomplished by incision/excision of the plaque with grafting.

Patients undergoing corrective surgery without prosthesis placement must be aware of the risk to their erectile function with any of these procedures *(6,8)*. Some patients will have the deformity corrected but then need pharmacological therapy to maintain an erection. If the resulting ED is severe enough, then they may require a secondary placement of a penile implant. Because 70% of Peyronie's plaques are dorsal, many corrective surgeries require elevation of the dorsal neurovascular bundle and can result in glanular hypoesthesia or anesthesia *(6)*. Although loss of glanular sensation is rare, ED and penile shortening are fairly common with these operations and may be caused by the surgery or by the shortening inherent in PD *(8)*.

It is difficult to assess the medical literature and quantify the association of ED and PD. The distinction between whether the ED is caused by lack of tumescence (proximal or distal flaccidity) or whether the dysfunction is purely a functional inability to perform because of the curvature is not clearly elucidated. ED in PD may be linked with associated, independent vascular risk factors because the average age of patients with this condition is over 50 yr. Others have suggested that the noncompliant fibrotic tunica albuginea predisposes to veno-occlusive disease by reduced venous occlusion *(2)*. Thus, the older the patient afflicted with this condition, the more likely he is to report significant erectile problems *(9)*.

In patients with PD with associated ED, the curvature is corrected by prosthesis implantation with or without modeling. In a distinct minority of these patients, additional corporoplasty with plaque incision/excision and possible grafting may be necessary if the implanted cylinders and modeling are not sufficient *(10)*. Other chapters in this book outline surgical therapy without prosthesis implantation; the remainder of this chapter focuses on the appropriate use of penile implant surgery in the treatment of PD.

PROSTHESIS PLACEMENT IN PEYRONIE'S DISEASE

Men with both ED and PD should be considered candidates for prosthesis placement. Curvature with penile flaccidity distal to the plaque resulting in flail penis and erection with decreased duration from veno-occlusive dysfunction are frequent presenting complaints *(11)*. Because surgical intervention without prosthesis placement can result in penile shortening and subsequent ED, the pool of candidates for prosthesis implantation can be expanded to include men with a short penis and partial erections. All patients with PD who are older than 50 yr, especially those with vascular comorbidities, are counseled to consider penile prosthesis. Many of these older men demonstrate poor axial rigidity distal to the plaque after a penile injection of vasoactive agents.

In addition, penile duplex Doppler studies may demonstrate nonsymptomatic impairment of penile blood flow (arterial or venous) in these older subjects *(11)*. Doppler studies should include adequate vasoactive agent injection and photographic documentation of penile deformity to assist in planning of surgical correction. Patient photographs may also be helpful in preoperative patient counseling. Although these studies are most helpful for nonprosthetic correction, they can be useful when placing a penile implant with modeling or plaque incision.

SEMIRIGID, MALLEABLE, AND MECHANICAL IMPLANTS

Physicians have long recognized that the simple placement of a pair of intracorporal rods is usually enough to straighten the curvature of most patients with PD without the need for adjunctive straightening maneuvers. Many different styles of semirigid or malleable prosthetic devices have been successfully used for men with PD, including soft silicone rods without embedded wires *(12,13)*. The surgery is not difficult because the Peyronie's plaques are subtunical and usually do not compromise the corporal space.

Prosthetic girth is an important factor in correction of the curvature. It is important to dilate large enough to insert a 13-mm (for malleable) or 12-mm (for mechanical Dura II) prosthesis (American Medical Systems, Minnetonka, MN). The additional girth when compared with smaller diameter models helps overcome the deformity because girth (i.e., axial rigidity), not length, is believed to be the most important contributing factor to penile rigidity and successful intromission *(13)*. Proper sizing of the length of rods is imperative in a patient with PD. Despite the apparent shortening of one side of the penis because of the disease process, the operating surgeon should always endeavor to place rods of the same length. If there is any question of length, slightly shorter rods should be used. Indeed, downsizing rod implants 0.5–1 cm in patients without PD improves comfort and concealment without compromising glans support *(14)*.

After implantation of intracorporal rods, it is necessary to judge the straightening and assess possible glansular deviation and support. Ghanem et al. reported that 35% of patients were not satisfied with the degree of straightening after simple rod implantation with a variety of different models (Duraphase, Mentor Accuform, Mentor Corp., Santa Barbara, CA; AMS 650, American Medical Systems, Minnetonka, MN) *(15)*. Montorsi et al. reported poor patient and partner satisfaction with PD and semirigid rod implants *(16)*. More than 60 mo after surgery, 48 men and 29 partners were interviewed. Only 48% of patients and 40% of partners were satisfied with the results. Of these, 52% of patients and 60% of partners complained of poor length or girth.

Review of the medical literature indicated that 19–42% of patients with PD will require adjunctive straightening procedures after simple rod implantation *(12,14–16)*. If the deformity persists after insertion of the rod cylinders, it is easy to overcome by making transverse relaxing incisions in the tunica albuginea on the short side of the penis with electrocautery *(17)*. This results in lengthening of the concave portion and resultant straightening. It is not necessary to close the tunical defects when inserting a semirigid device; in fact, the open tunica albuginea adds the required length to the short side to accomplish the desired straightening.

Use of the subcoronal incision for placement of malleable or mechanical prostheses in PD has an advantage over the traditional penoscrotal approach *(18)*. This incision will facilitate degloving of the penis if additional straightening by relaxing incision of the short side is needed. The subcoronal incision is only useful in circumcised men or uncircumcised men who consent to concomitant circumcision in conjunction with the implantation. Preputial edema and eventually phimosis or paraphimosis frequently results from use of the subcoronal approach and failure to circumcise. If circumcision is not desired, then a longitudinal ventral penile incision is an effective substitute and does not require removal of the foreskin (14).

TWO-PIECE INFLATABLE PROSTHESIS

There are two published reports on the use of two-piece penile prostheses in Peyronie's patients. In the first, Levine and Dimitriou described a surgical algorithm for prosthesis placement in 46 men with PD for whom several different devices were used. The Ambicor was employed in 17 men; successful straightening was noted in all men with curvature less than or equal to 60°. There were no mechanical failures or infections during a mean follow-up of 39 mo (range 1–74 mo) (10). In a second series, the mechanical reliability and safety of the Ambicor device was examined in 131 men with ED, of whom 20 also had PD. In this series, successful straightening was noted in the entire group. There were no mechanical failures at a mean follow-up of 43 mo (19). We have only anecdotal experience with the Ambicor prosthesis in correction of curvature in patients with PD and ED.

The Hydroflex and Dynaflex implants are historical prostheses no longer marketed that are earlier models of the Ambicor cylinders. These implants performed similar to rods and provided good axial rigidity with proper girth sizing. The cylinders, even if sized properly in girth, do not have the same intrinsic rigidity as semirigid rods and were not as reliable in straightening an erection without additional corporoplasty as rods or the three-piece inflatable implants. If adjunctive relaxing incisions are needed to finish straightening, it is not necessary to cover the gaps because the implant has a girth restriction and should not aneurysm through the opened tunica (20). One problem with the predecessor cylinders of the Ambicor is that the devices acted as tissue expanders with consequent erection deterioration. This required the subsequent substitution of longer cylinders of a three-piece device in 2–3 yr irrespective of the preoperative presence of PD (20,21). Levine and associates have not reported this complication despite the similarity of the cylinder construction (19).

INFLATABLE PENILE PROSTHESIS
AND THE MODELING PROCEDURE

One of the original inventors of the AMS inflatable penile prosthesis conceived the modeling procedure early in the development of inflatable implants (22). Dr. Brantley Scott had noted orthopedic surgeons modeling broken bones over metal rods and postulated that the concept might be useful in correction of PD deformities. Unfortunately, during Dr. Scott's active clinical years, the available cylinders had no fabric insert and were only one layer of pure silicone. The limitless distensibility of the single-layer cylinder construction did not provide enough rigidity against deformation to act as a fulcrum to disrupt the plaque. Carson et al. in 1983 reported the use of these devices for PD and like Knoll's report in 1985, over half the patients required relaxing incisions often with reinforcement using Gore-Tex or other synthetic grafting (23).

In the late 1980s, the partially nondistensible and controlled expansion (CX) cylinders replaced the original Scott (AMS 742a) cylinder. The new cylinders consisted of a three-layer construction with a woven polyurethane fabric (similar to Dacron or Lycra) sandwiched between two silicone layers. This minimally elastic fabric prevented aneurysmal dilatation when the cylinder was bent or encountered weakened tunica. In addition, Mentor introduced a competitive three-piece implant with cylinders constructed of a tough plastic similar to polyurethane called Bioflex. While Scott conceptualized the modeling procedure, Wilson and Delk began developing the technique in 1987 and reported the first large series in 1993 using both AMS and Mentor cylinders *(5)*.

Ten years after the first report, the modeling procedure for treatment of PD has achieved worldwide acceptance. Modeling has been successfully reported with AMS 700 CX, but the AMS 700 Ultrex has had limited success because of the enhanced distensibility of its cylinders *(5,17,24)*. In a textbook chapter, Ralph and Pryor wrote, "Operative modeling of the penis over prosthesis may look and sound horrible, but gives a good result in any deformity" *(2)*.

THREE-PIECE IMPLANTS

AMS CX, CXR, or CXM cylinders of equal length are placed, and the corporotomy is closed with interrupted sutures. Alternately, Mentor Alpha I or Mentor Titan cylinders can be placed in a similar fashion. All these cylinders do not expand in length. Mentor Alpha NB, Mentor Titan NB, and AMS Ultrex are not recommended. The downsized Mentor cylinder tends to aneurysm through the suddenly open corporotomy if the corporotomy closure ruptures during modeling. The AMS Ultrex, because it is a lengthening cylinder, tends to exaggerate the curvature and does not generate enough axial rigidity if modeling is needed to overcome the curve without additional tunical incisions. Montague et al. reported additional corporoplasty was necessary in 26% of patients with PD undergoing the modeling procedure if Ultrex cylinders were implanted compared with none of the patients implanted with CX cylinders *(24)*. Along with Fishman, we have had similar poor experiences using Ultrex cylinders for modeling patients with PD *(25,26)*.

Cylinder size is determined from intracorporal measurement. Rear tip extenders are usually used. Because PD tends to shorten the penis, the corporal measurements may differ by 1–2 cm. When there is confusion about the measurements, it is best to use a shorter rather than a longer measurement. It is important, if possible, to place cylinders and rear tip extenders of equal length on both sides to optimize the postoperative appearance. It is not necessary to exit the input tubing from the corpora deep in the scrotum. In fact, the smaller the corporotomy, the less chance it will rupture during modeling. Thus, the tubing is routinely routed along the cylinder for a short distance before exiting from the corporotomy. It is important to use interrupted closure of the corporotomy because a running closure is more likely to rupture during modeling, and the rupture of a running closure results in frayed tunical edges that are difficult to reclose adequately.

The pump is connected to the filled reservoir or a syringe and maximum inflation of the cylinders is achieved. Maximally inflating correct size three-piece cylinders as a tissue expander will straighten the Peyronie's deformity in more than 50% of cases (Fig. 1). The intrinsic rigidity of these nondistally expanding cylinders will frequently straighten the curve without modeling or any adjunctive procedures. If the curvature is less than 20 or 30°, the surgeon can count on the implant straightening further over the next year of use, and the patient will achieve a straight penis. Similarly, hourglass deformities become symmetrical with use as the cylinders stretch the fibrotic tissue. If significant curvature persists, then the technique of modeling may be employed.

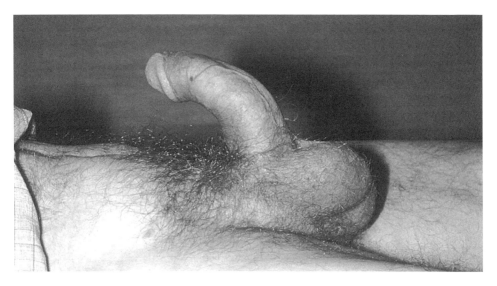

Fig. 1. Patient with Peyronie's curvature after penile prosthesis implantation.

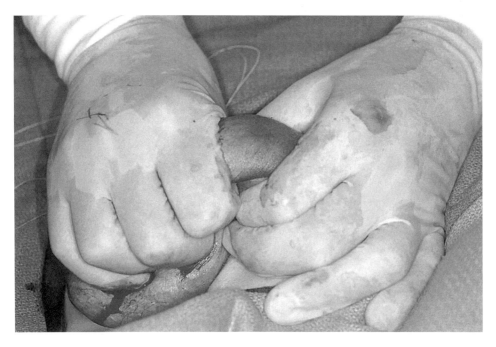

Fig. 2. Modeling technique for penile curvature correction.

THE MODELING PROCEDURE: STEP BY STEP

After closure of the corporotomy incision, the cylinder input tubing is cross-clamped with rubber-shod clamps to protect the pump from high pressures during modeling. Another safety maneuver is to protect the sutured corporotomies by placing the thumb on one corporotomy and the first two fingers on the other. This maneuver supports the closure and minimizes suture breakage during forcible inflation and vigorous modeling.

The penis is bent in a direction opposite the curvature in a maneuver similar to breaking a twig in both hands (Fig. 2). Forcible bending pressure is held for 90 s. After 90 s, the clamps are removed, and additional fluid can be added to the cylinders. This is possible because the restricted corporal space has been expanded. The clamps are then reapplied, corporotomies protected, and the modeling procedure repeated for another 90 s. The intervals of 90 s are arbitrary but have been successful in the majority of cases. Using a fixed amount of time reinforces the principal that persistent bending rather than a quick fracture of the plaque is necessary to achieve straightening. Modeling probably results in splitting and rupturing of the fibrotic plaques. The operating surgeon can often hear snapping or feel movement of the cylinders as previous nonpliant tunica is expanded.

Two modeling sessions are all that are usually necessary. The cylinders are deflated completely after the second session and reinflate to only about 75%. Maximum inflation is needed for correcting the curvature, but patients rarely pump to the maximum during intercourse. Straightening of the penis should be judged at 75%, not maximal, inflation. If the resultant erection has less than a 20–30° curvature or wasp waisting, then these deformities will usually correct themselves with regular prosthesis usage over the next year (27). Patients may be counseled to inflate and model at home if they complain of residual deformity. After prosthesis implantation, it is important to inform the patient prior to discharge that the penis may be curved when flaccid but will be straighter when erect. The reason is that the cylinders seem to act as a stent in flaccidity, curving the penis to the short side.

During early modeling experience, modeling was occasionally not sufficient to achieve satisfactory results. The original publication reported 8% of patients required additional corporoplasties (5). In these patients, the penis was degloved, and multiple small relaxing incisions were made on the concave side of the erect penis. Opening of the transverse incision resulted in lengthening along the short side of the curvature and additional straightening.

Tunical incisions after prosthesis insertion are best accomplished with electrocautery because sharp incision may result in damage to the cylinders. The current should be set less than 35 W because Mentor cylinders can be damaged with higher settings (28).

Tunical defects greater than 2 cm in axial length are recommended to be closed with a graft (10). It was once recommended that the incisions could be left open, the prosthesis left partially inflated for 2 mo, and the gaps would granulate in (23). Most of these gaps encouraged aneurysmal bulging of the cylinder, particularly with the Mentor models. The CX should be less likely to require a graft because its fabric wrap controls its girth expansion and prevents bulging out the defect, but we have seen this cylinder protrude out the defect, particularly if the defect is greater than 2 cm in any dimension. Many patients will complain of the feeling of the defect if a graft is not employed (29). Graft materials can include Gore-Tex, Dacron, or autologous grafts such as dermis, small intestine submucosa, or cadaveric pericardium (30).

Excessive compliance, as with tunica vaginalis grafts, may not adequately support the inflatable cylinders. Hakim and associates have reported less than full-thickness relaxing incisions facilitated by the diathermy with resultant straightening in PD without necessity of grafting (28).

COMPLICATIONS OF THE MODELING PROCEDURE

After 10 yr of use of the modeling procedure on hundreds of patients, the rate of urethral laceration attributable to modeling remains at 4%. The laceration always occurs near the meatus and is heralded by blood at the meatus. Visual confirmation of the laceration is obtained by spreading the meatus after noting blood on the Foley catheter or glans penis. If blood is seen at the meatus and no erosion is visualized externally, then flexible cystoscopy may assist in the diagnosis. On several occasions, urethral laceration has occurred by modeling on the first postoperative visit. If urethral laceration occurs, then it is possible to remove only the offending cylinder. The remainder of the prosthesis remains in situ, and the tubing leading to the removed cylinder is plugged. A Foley catheter is left in place for 48 h. It is not necessary to close the fossa navicularis defect. At 8 wk, the cylinder may be replaced. Some patients may be satisfied with a one-cylinder erection, particularly when the Mentor cylinder was employed.

In the initial report, 8% of the patients required additional corporoplasties (5). A study published in 2001, however, showed no subsequent patients needing adjunctive maneuvers for straightening except modeling (27). Reviewing the early cases showed several reasons for the additional corporoplasties. When the Ultrex cylinders were used, there was a high likelihood of failure of adequate straightening with modeling, and this cylinder is no longer recommended for patients with PD. The other cases were believed caused by failure to fully complete the modeling technique. Persistent and aggressive modeling almost always obviates the need for additional corporoplasty.

In the latter publication (27), there was a small, but statistically significant, difference in the 5-yr survival from revision for mechanical cause for the AMS cylinders when compared with the Mentor cylinders, both with and without modeling (27). Cylinder failure was the usual cause of failure of the AMS device. Occasionally during modeling, we noted abrasion of the outer layer of silicone that caused staining of the inner fabric with blood. Thus, the modeling may abrade the outer layer of silicone, predisposing the cylinder to early failure. AMS addressed this problem in late 2000 with the addition of a Paralene coating to non-tissue-contacting surfaces of the cylinders (31). This coating increases the lubricity of the silicone surface, thereby reducing friction and wear. Paralene has been demonstrated in bench testing to add millions of stress cycles before detectable wear is measured (31). Since the addition of the Paralene coating, we have not noted early cylinder failure in the AMS device during modeling.

The current experience of both of our centers for the last 5 yr gives support to the conclusion that modeling the penis over an inflated penile prosthesis causes no increased risk of mechanical malfunction or reoperation when compared with patients who have prosthesis insertion without the modeling maneuver.

PATIENT OUTCOMES AND SATISFACTION

Although there are few series that adequately evaluated patient or partner satisfaction and long-term outcomes, there are several studies that suggested good patient and partner acceptance. Montorsi et al. showed poor patient and partner satisfaction with the semirigid rod implants but far improved satisfaction in their center for patients implanted with AMS 700 CX penile prostheses for Peyronie's disease (16,32). In reviewing the results of a multicenter study of the AMS 700 CX implants and comparing outcomes from patients with and without PD, Carson et al. showed equal success in both groups in mechanical function but somewhat poorer satisfaction with the patients with PD because of penile size *(33)*. Interestingly, no patient in the Peyronie's group had penile glans hypoesthesia. The satisfaction therefore appears to be reduced by the penile size restriction caused by the loss of penile compliance caused by PD itself.

REFERENCES

1. Carson CC. François Gigot de la Peyronie (1678–1747). Invest Urol 1981; 19: 62–63.
2. Ralph D, Pryor JP. Peyronie's disease. In: Textbook of Erectile Dysfunction (Carson CC, Kirby R, Goldstein I, eds.). Isis Medical Media, Oxford, UK, 1999, pp. 515–527.
3. Mulcahy JJ, Wilson SK. Management of Peyronie's disease with penile prosthesis. Int J Imp Res 2002; 14: 1–5.
4. Carson CC. Therapeutic strategies for managing erectile dysfunction: a step-care approach. Am Osteopath Assoc 2002; 102(12 suppl 4): S12–S18.
5. Wilson SK, Delk JR. A new treatment for Peyronie's disease: modeling the penis over an inflatable penile prosthesis. J Urol 1994; 152: 1121–1123.
6. Tornehl CK, Carson CC. Surgical alternatives for treating Peyronie's disease. BJU Int 2004; 94: 774–783.
7. Levine LA, Lenting EL. Experience with a surgical algorithm for Peyronie's disease. J Urol 1997; 158: 2149–2152.
8. Melman A, Holland TF. Evaluation of the dermal graft inlay technique for the surgical treatment of Peyronie's disease. J Urol 1979; 120: 421–422.
9. Stecker JF, Devine CJ. Evaluation of erectile dysfunction in patients with Peyronie's disease. J Urol 1985; 133: 680–681.
10. Levine LA, Dimitriou RJ. A surgical algorithm for penile prosthesis placement in men with erectile failure and Peyronie's disease. Int J Impot Res 2000; 12: 147–151.
11. Carson CC. Penile prosthesis implantation in the treatment of Peyronie's disease and erectile dysfunction. Int J Impot Res 2000;12(suppl 4): S122–S126.
12. Carson CC, Hodge GB, Anderson EE. Penile prosthesis in Peyronie's disease. Br J Urol 1983; 55: 417–421.
13. Subrini L. Surgical treatment of Peyronie's disease using penile implant: survey of 69 patients. J Urol 1984; 132: 47–49.
14. Mulcahy JJ. Unitary, inflatable, mechanical and malleable penile implants. In: Textbook of Erectile Dysfunction (Carson CC, Kirby R, Goldstein I, eds.). Issis Medical Media, Oxford, UK, pp. 413–421.
15. Ghanem HM, Fahmy I, El Meliegy A. Malleable penile implants without plaque surgery in the treatment of Peyronie's disease. Int J Imp Res 1998; 10: 171–173.
16. Montorsi F, Guazzoni G, Bergamaschi F, Rigatti P. Patient-partner satisfaction with semirigid penile prostheses for Peyronie's disease: a 5-yr follow-up study. J Urol 1993; 150: 1819–1821.
17. Carson CC. Penile prosthesis implantation in the treatment of Peyronie's disease. Int J Impot Res 1998; 10: 125–128.
18. Eigner EB Kabalin JN, Kessler R. Penile implants in the treatment of Peyronie's disease. J Urol 1991; 145: 69–71.
19. Levine LA, Estrada CR, Morgentaler A. Mechanical reliability and safety of and patient satisfaction with the Ambicor inflatable penile prosthesis: results of a two center study. J Urol 2001; 166: 932–937.
20. Wilson S. Penile prosthesis implantation: pearls, pitfalls and perils. In: Male Infertility and Sexual Dysfunction (Helstrom WJG, ed.). Springer, New York, 1997, pp. 529–549.
21. Wilson SK, Cleves MA, Delk JR. Long-term results with Hydroflex and Dynaflex penile prostheses: device survival comparisons to multi-component inflatables. J Urol 1996; 155: 1621–1624.
22. Wilson SK. Management of penile implant complications. In: Topics in Clinical Urology, Diagnosis and Management of Male Sexual Dysfunction (Mulcahy JJ, ed.). Igaku-Shoin, New York, 1997, pp. 231–235.

23. Knoll LD, Furlow WL, Benson RC. Management of Peyronie's disease by implantation of inflatable penile prosthesis. Urology 1990; 36: 406–408.

24. Montague DK, Angermeier KW, Lakin MM, Ingleright BJ. AMS 3-piece inflatable penile prosthesis implantation in men with Peyronie's disease: comparison of CX and Ultrex cylinders. J Urol 1996; 156: 1633–1635.

25. Fishman IJ. Editorial comment. J Urol 1996; 156: 1635.

26. Kowalczyk JJ, Mulcahy JJ. Penile curvatures and aneurismal defects with the Ultrex penile prosthesis corrected with insertion of the AMS 700 CX. J Urol 1996; 156: 398–401.

27. Wilson SK, Cleves MA, Delk JR. Long-term follow-up of treatment for Peyronie's disease: modeling the penis over an inflatable penile prosthesis. J Urol 2001; 165: 825–829.

28. Hakim LS, Kulaksizoglu H, Hamill BK, et al. Guide to safe corporotomy incisions in presence of underlying inflatable penile cylinders: results of in vitro and in vivo studies. J Urol 1995; 155: 366–368.

29. Carson CC. Reconstructive surgery using urological prostheses. Curr Opin Urol 1999; 9: 233–239.

30. Carson CC, Chun JL. Peyronie's disease: surgical management: autologous materials. Int J Impot Res 2002; 14: 329–335.

31. Data on file. American Medical Systems, Minnetonka, MN.

32. Montorsi F, Guazzoni G, Barbieri L, et al. AMS 700 CX inflatable penile implants for Peyronie's disease: functional results, morbidity and patient-partner satisfaction. Int J Impot Res 1996; 8: 81–85.

33. Carson CC, Mulcahy JJ, Govier FE. Efficacy, safety and patient satisfaction outcomes of the AMS 700 CX inflatable penile prosthesis: results of a long term multicenter study. J Urol 2000; 164: 376–380.

Index